WO 300
RAT
(ORD)

Regional Anesthesia

THE REQUISITES IN ANESTHESIOLOGY

SERIES EDITOR **Roberta L. Hines,** M.D.
Chair and Professor
Department of Anesthesiology
Yale University School of Medicine
New Haven, Connecticut

OTHER VOLUMES IN THE REQUISITES™   Adult Perioperative Anesthesia
IN ANESTHESIOLOGY SERIES

Cardiac and Vascular Anesthesia

Pediatric Anesthesia

Critical Care

Obstetric and Gynecologic Anesthesia

Pain Medicine

Ambulatory Anesthesia

Regional Anesthesia

THE REQUISITES IN ANESTHESIOLOGY

James P. Rathmell, M.D.

Professor
Department of Anesthesiology
University of Vermont College of Medicine
Burlington, Vermont

Joseph M. Neal, M.D.

Staff Anesthesiologist
Department of Anesthesiology
Virginia Mason Medical Center
Seattle, Washington

Christopher M. Viscomi, M.D.

Associate Professor
Department of Anesthesiology
University of Vermont College of Medicine
Burlington, Vermont

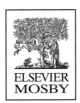

ELSEVIER
MOSBY

ELSEVIER
MOSBY

The Curtis Center
170 S Independence Mall W 300E
Philadelphia, Pennsylvania 19106

REGIONAL ANESTHESIA: THE REQUISITES IN ANESTHESIOLOGY   ISBN: 0-323-02042-9

NOTICE

Anesthesiology is an ever-changing field. Standard safety precautions must be followed, but as new research and clinical experience broaden our knowledge, changes in treatment and drug therapy may become necessary or appropriate. Readers are advised to check the most current product information provided by the manufacturer of each drug to be administered to verify the recommended dose, the method and duration of administration, and contraindications. It is the responsibility of the treating physician, relying on experience and knowledge of the patient, to determine dosages and the best treatment for each individual patient. Neither the Publisher nor the editor assumes any liability for any injury and/or damage to persons or property arising from this publication.

Library of Congress Cataloging-in-Publication Data

Rathmell, James P.
 Regional anesthesia: the requisites in anesthesiology / James P. Rathmell, Joseph M. Neal,
   Christopher M. Viscomi. — 1st ed.
    p.   ; cm.
 ISBN 0-323-02042-9
 1. Conduction anesthesia. 2. Anesthesiology I. Neal, Joseph M.   II. Viscomi, Christopher M.
 III. Title.
 [DNLM: 1. Anesthesia, Conduction—methods.   2. Anesthetics, Local—administration & dosage.
   WO 300 R234r 2004]
 RD84.R38 2004
 617.9'6—dc22

                                                     2004042567

International Standard Book Number 0-323-02042-9

Acquisitions Editor: Natasha Andjelkovic
Developmental Editor: Anne Snyder
Project Manager: Daniel Clipner

Printed in the United States of America

Last digit is the print number: 9   8   7   6   5   4   3   2   1

"To our families who have been supportive throughout. The Rathmells: Bobbi, Lauren, James and Cara; the Neals: Kay, Erin and Pete; the Viscomis: Denise, Alta, and Jack."

Preface

The *Requisites in Anesthesiology* series is designed for the trainee in anesthesiology who is preparing for the board-certification examination or for the seasoned practitioner who is in search of a concise review of subject matter in preparation for re-certification. While this volume on *Regional Anesthesia* is aimed toward those preparing for examinations, we have made every effort to make the text a stand-alone reference that can serve as a rapid and practical review of material used in the daily practice of anesthesiology.

This volume is constructed in five major sections: Anatomy and Physiology; Pharmacology; Regional Anesthetic Techniques; Safety, Complications, and Outcomes; and Specialty Considerations. The first two sections cover relevant structure and function of the nervous system and the pharmacology of drugs commonly used in performing regional anesthesia. Discussions of various agents include the mechanisms of action and toxicity, dosing guidelines, and comparisons of the advantages and disadvantages of agents within each class. When data are available to support the advantage of one agent over another, detailed explanations are included. The pharmacology section also includes a chapter covering the pharmacology of various local anesthetic additives, including vasoconstrictors and the preservatives found in currently available preparations.

The third and largest section details specific regional anesthetic techniques. For each technique, we have presented a concise review of the anatomy, indications and contraindications for the specific block, and a description of how the technique is performed. Original drawings aid the reader in understanding many techniques. Safety, complications and outcomes associated with regional anesthesia are covered in the fourth section. We

have discussed common complications like postdural puncture headache and the use of epidural blood patch for treatment as well as uncommon complications like epidural abscess and hematoma formation. Current guidelines regarding neuraxial blockade and anticoagulation are reviewed, as are the data regarding perioperative outcomes associated with use of regional anesthesia. Several common, but specialized regional techniques did not easily fit within our general descriptions of each technique. Thus, we created a fifth and final section of the text dedicated to a discussion of specific regional anesthetic techniques that are commonly limited to the subspecialty areas of obstetrics, pediatrics, and perioperative pain management.

Throughout this volume, we have extracted material from the text and assembled highlighted boxes with brief lists of details that we feel are the key concepts within each chapter. This should prove particularly useful for those who want to skip from section to section, reading in depth only when they reach areas of particular interest. We have made every attempt to be thorough yet concise. Inevitably, some topics will be covered in greater depth than others. Our hope is that the core material regarding regional anesthesia that every practicing anesthesiologist should be familiar with has been covered in sufficient detail. Where choice among agents or techniques is based largely on the preference of each clinician rather than advantages in safety of efficacy, we have tried to make this clear. We hope that you find this new book useful in your review of regional anesthesia.

James P. Rathmell, M.D.
Joseph M. Neal, M.D.
Christopher M. Viscomi, M.D.

Color Plates

Plate 1   Interscalene anatomy. Note the brachial plexus exiting through the interscalene groove, and how the phrenic nerve lies on top of the anterior scalene muscle (inset). (Redrawn from Brown DL: *Atlas of Regional Anesthesia*, Second Edition, WB Saunders, Philadelphia, 1999, p. 26, Fig. 3-2.)

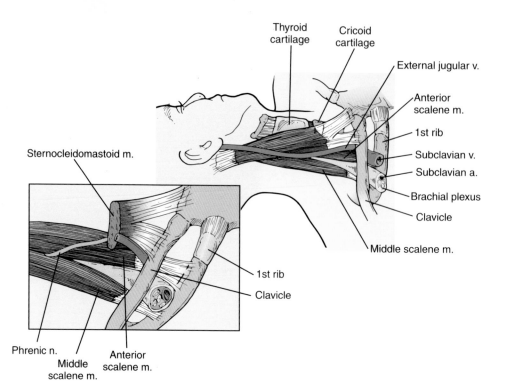

Thyroid cartilage
Cricoid cartilage
External jugular v.
Anterior scalene m.
1st rib
Subclavian v.
Subclavian a.
Brachial plexus
Clavicle
Middle scalene m.

Sternocleidomastoid m.

1st rib
Clavicle

Phrenic n.
Middle scalene m.
Anterior scalene m.

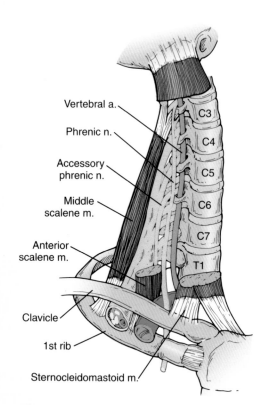

Vertebral a.
Phrenic n.
Accessory phrenic n.
Middle scalene m.
Anterior scalene m.
Clavicle
1st rib
Sternocleidomastoid m.

C3
C4
C5
C6
C7
T1

Plate 2   Relationship of the brachial plexus to the interscalene groove, clavicle, first rib, and subclavian artery. Note the compactness of the plexus at this level. (Redrawn from Brown DL: *Atlas of Regional Anesthesia*, Second Edition, WB Saunders, Philadelphia, 1999, p. 20, Fig. 2-9.)

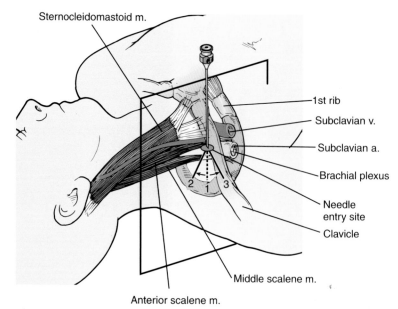

Sternocleidomastoid m.

1st rib
Subclavian v.
Subclavian a.
Brachial plexus
Needle entry site
Clavicle
Middle scalene m.

Anterior scalene m.

Plate 3   Plumb-bob approach. Note how the limited 20° cephalad and caudad needle traverse is made strictly within the parasagittal plane. (Redrawn from Brown DL: *Atlas of Regional Anesthesia*, Second Edition, WB Saunders, Philadelphia, 1999, p. 39, Fig. 34-7.)

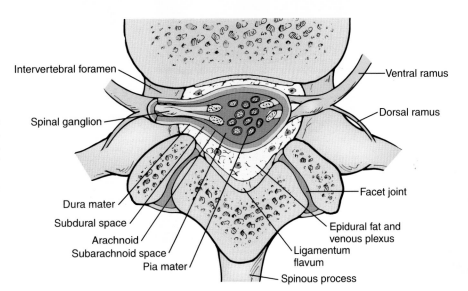

Plate 4   Epidural space anatomy. Fat and veins fill the epidural space. Spinal nerve roots, within dural cuffs, exit through the intervertebral foramina. (Redrawn from Miller RD: Atlas of regional anesthesia procedures. In: *Anesthesia*, Fifth Edition, Churchill Livingstone, Philadelphia, 2000, Plate 6.)

Intervertebral foramen

Spinal ganglion

Ventral ramus

Dorsal ramus

Facet joint

Dura mater

Subdural space

Arachnoid

Subarachnoid space

Pia mater

Epidural fat and venous plexus

Ligamentum flavum

Spinous process

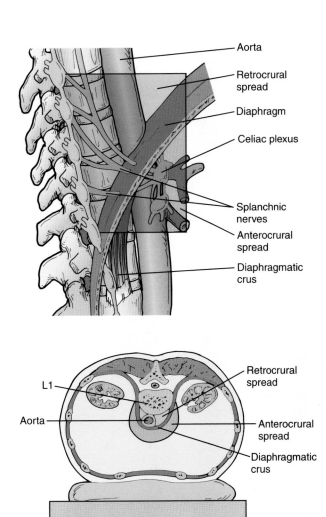

Aorta

Retrocrural spread

Diaphragm

Celiac plexus

Splanchnic nerves

Anterocrural spread

Diaphragmatic crus

Retrocrural spread

L1

Aorta

Anterocrural spread

Diaphragmatic crus

Plate 5   Celiac plexus block – retrocrural and anterocrural relationships. (Redrawn from Brown DL: *Atlas of Regional Anesthesia*, Second Edition, WB Saunders, Philadelphia, 1999, p. 288.)

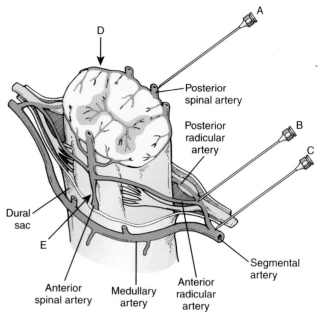

Plate 6 Arterial blood supply to the spinal cord, cross-sectional view. Note how the segmental (**A**), radicular (**B**), and possibly the posterior spinal (**C**) arteries are potentially vulnerable to needle injury (as illustrated by needles). Also note on the left side of the figure how vascular anomalies may present: (**D**) fused posterior spinal and posterolateral spinal arteries or (**E**) narrowing of the anterior spinal artery. (Redrawn from Bridenbaugh PO, Greene NM, Brull SJ: Spinal (subarachnoid) neural blockade. In: Cousins MJ, Bridenbaugh PO (eds), *Neural Blockade in Clinical Anesthesia and Pain Management*, Third Edition, Lippincott-Raven, Philadelphia, 1998, p. 211, Fig. 7-10.)

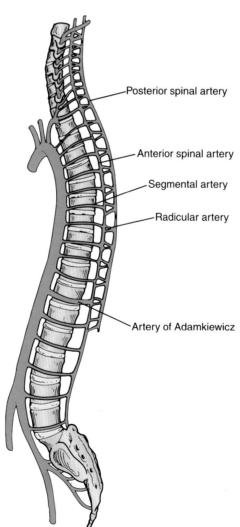

Plate 7 Arterial blood supply to the spinal cord, longitudinal view. Note the pathway from segmental → radicular → anterior and posterior spinal arteries. (Redrawn from Covino BG, Scott DB: *Handbook of Epidural Anaesthesia and Analgesia*, Grune & Stratton, Orlando, 1985, p. 21, Fig. 1-19.)

Contents

ANATOMY AND PHYSIOLOGY

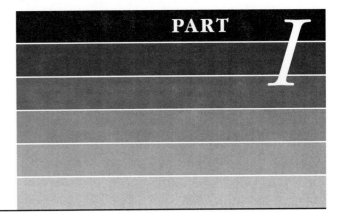

PART

I

An Introduction to Neuroanatomy and Neurophysiology Relevant to Pain and Regional Anesthesia

JAMES P. RATHMELL

BASIC ANATOMY AND PHYSIOLOGY OF THE NEURON

Overview of the Sensory Neuron

A typical neuron is made up of a cell body, multiple small branches close to the cell body called dendrites, and a single, long projection called an axon. The cell bodies of sensory neurons are located in the dorsal root ganglia, adjacent to the spinal cord. Each sensory neuron has a single axon with a short branch projecting centrally to the spinal cord and a long branch extending to the periphery (Fig. 1-1 on p. 4). Sensory axons terminate in skin, joints, muscle, viscera, or connective tissue. There are a number of specialized nerve endings (see further discussion below) that convert various sensory stimuli (mechanical, thermal, chemical) into trains of electrical impulses within the axon. The frequency and intensity of the electrical impulses, in part, encode the intensity of the sensory input. The electrical impulses travel from the axon's peripheral branch to the central projection, where the signals are relayed to a second-order neuron within the spinal cord.

Axon and Peripheral Nerve Structure

Axons are cylindrical projections of cell membrane that extend from the neuron's cell body. The cytoplasm within the axon is continuous with the cytoplasm of the entire neuron. All axons are encased within myelin sheaths. Several unmyelinated axons are contained within the myelin of a single Schwann cell, while myelinated axons are encased within several layers of myelin from a single Schwann cell (Fig. 1-2 on p. 4). The myelin sheath surrounding the axon is interrupted periodically; these points of interruption in the myelin sheath are called nodes of Ranvier.

Peripheral nerves contain axons that conduct toward the central nervous system (afferent axons, largely sensory neurons) as well as away from the central nervous system (efferent axons, largely motor neurons) (Fig. 1-3 on p. 5). Each nerve is encased within a thin connective tissue layer called the endoneurium. Bundles of axons are enclosed in a squamous epithelium that is several cell layers in thickness called the perineurium. One or more perineural bundles are enclosed in an outermost connective tissue layer, the epineurium, which contains the blood vessels supplying the nerve cells themselves. Diffusion of local anesthetic to the target axons is affected by many factors, including the thickness of the perineurium (the only tissue layer that presents a significant barrier to diffusion), the presence or absence of myelin, the size of the axons, and the position of the axons within the nerve bundle (superficial or deep).

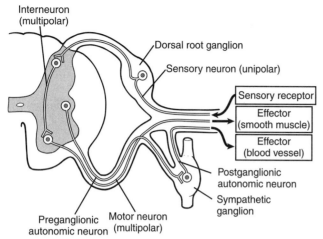

Figure 1-1   The neuron. The unipolar sensory neuron with the cell body located within the dorsal root ganglion and projections to the periphery and the dorsal horn of the spinal cord. Multipolar interneuron with its numerous dendrites. Multipolar motor neuron with a long peripheral axon. Preganglionic and postganglionic autonomic neurons are also illustrated. (Redrawn from Strichartz GR: Neural physiology and local anesthetic action. In: Cousins MJ, Bridenbaugh PO (eds), *Neural Blockade*, Third Edition, Lippincott-Raven, Philadelphia, PA, 1998, p. 36.)

Nerve Membranes and Impulses

Nerve impulses, or action potentials, travel along unmyelinated axons as a continuous wave. However, only the periodic unmyelinated regions, or the nodes of Ranvier, are depolarized along myelinated axons. Thus, nerve impulses skip from node to node along myelinated axons, a process called saltatory conduction. Because only small areas must depolarize, the speed of conduction along myelinated axons is far greater than the rate in unmyelinated axons.

Nerve cells generate electrical impulses through ionic concentration gradients and selective ionic permeability of the neuronal cell membrane. The concentration of potassium (K^+) is about ten times greater inside the cell than outside and the concentration of sodium (Na^+) is about ten times higher outside the cell than within. A protein pump within the cell membrane (Na^+/K^+ pump) uses cellular energy in the form of ATP to maintain the ionic gradients across the resting cell membrane. The resting membrane potential is typically -70 mV to -80 mV. Upon activation, specific sodium channels open leading to a rapid inward movement of sodium ions (depolarization phase). As the membrane potential rises, this leads to a smaller gradient driving inward movement of sodium and activation of voltage-dependent potassium channels that, in turn, permit a large outward movement of potassium (repolarization

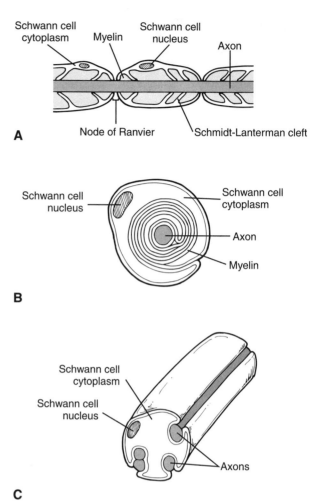

Figure 1-2   Diagram of the axon. A, Longitudinal cross-section showing the axon surrounded by the myelin (Schwann cell). The periodic regions without myelination between Schwann cells are called nodes of Ranvier. **B,** Short-axis cross-section of a myelinated axon demonstrating the multiple layers of myelin from a single Schwann cell enveloping a single axon. **C,** A Schwann cell and its group of non-myelinated axons. (Redrawn from Strichartz GR: Neural physiology and local anesthetic action. In: Cousins MJ, Bridenbaugh PO (eds), *Neural Blockade*, Third Edition, Lippincott-Raven, Philadelphia, PA, 1998, p. 37.)

phase). Thus, inward currents carried by sodium ions lead to depolarization and outward currents of potassium ions lead to repolarization (Fig. 1-4 on p. 5). Impulses are propagated along the axon as currents are conducted within the cytoplasm to adjacent areas. Local anesthetics act by interfering with the function of sodium channels. In the presence of local anesthetics, sodium channels are less likely to open in response to a depolarizing stimulus. When the local anesthetic concentration is high enough, the function of a sufficient number of sodium channels is impaired to completely block the generation of nerve impulses.

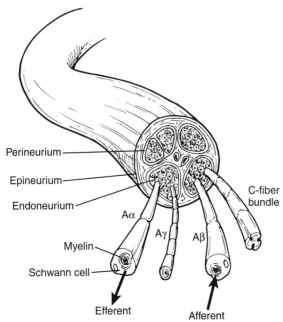

Figure 1-3   The peripheral nerve. The thin connective tissue layer of the epineurium surrounds the entire nerve bundle. The perineurium is comprised of several layers of squamous epithelium and envelopes groups of axons to form nerve bundles. The endoneurium is a thin connective tissue layer surrounding each individual axon. (Redrawn from Strichartz GR: Neural physiology and local anesthetic action. In: Cousins MJ, Bridenbaugh PO (eds), *Neural Blockade,* Third Edition, Lippincott-Raven, Philadelphia, PA, 1998, p. 38.)

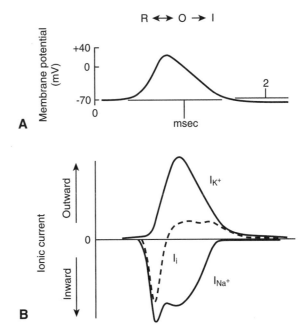

Figure 1-4   Components of the action potential. A, Changes in membrane potential during cell depolarization. **B,** Individual ionic currents during the action potential. Note the initial inward sodium current (depolarization) followed by an outward potassium current (repolarization). (Redrawn from Strichartz GR: Neural physiology and local anesthetic action. In: Cousins MJ, Bridenbaugh PO (eds), *Neural Blockade,* Third Edition, Lippincott-Raven, Philadelphia, PA, 1998, p. 38.)

Mechanism of Action: Local Anesthetics

Local anesthetics act by interfering with the function of sodium channels

In the presence of local anesthetics, sodium channels are less likely to open in response to a depolarizing stimulus

When the local anesthetic concentration is high enough, the function of a sufficient number of sodium channels is impaired to completely block the generation of nerve impulses

NOCICEPTION

Pain is induced by physical, thermal, or chemical stimuli that can potentially induce tissue injury. Between the site of the stimulus and pain perception, a complex sequence of electrochemical events takes place, which are collectively called *nociception* (Fig. 1-5) (Box 1-1).

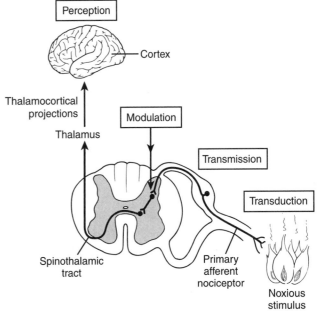

Figure 1-5   Overview of nociceptive pathways. (Redrawn from Katz NL, Ferrante FM: Nociception. In: Ferrante FM, VadeBoncouer TR (eds), *Postoperative Pain Management,* Churchill Livingstone, New York, 1993.)

Box 1-1   Components of Nociception
Transduction
Transmission
Modulation
Perception

Box 1-2   Stimuli Leading to Increased Firing in Nociceptive Free Nerve Endings
Mechanical distortion
Heat
Acidic pH
Elevated K$^+$
Lipidic acids
Specific peptides (e.g. substance P)

Transduction

A number of different stimuli can lead to the perception of pain. These stimuli can be broadly grouped into mechanical, thermal, and chemical stimuli. Mechanical forces, heat, and chemical changes result in increased firing in nerve terminals within tissue – this process is referred to as *transduction*.

Mechanical distortion of tissue can lead to the perception of pain. Two groups of specialized nerve endings, Pacinian corpuscles and tendon tension organs (muscle spindles), are typically activated by low-threshold mechanical distortion in tissue (Fig. 1-6). Free nerve endings begin firing at significantly higher levels of mechanical distortion and are referred to as high-threshold receptors. Thermal and chemical stimuli lead to increased firing in free nerve terminals. Thermal activation begins at temperatures exceeding 40–42° C. Changes in the chemical milieu at the peripheral sensory terminal, such as acidic pH, elevated potassium levels, lipidic acids, and a variety of peptides, can also lead to increased firing in afferent axons. There is little or no spontaneous activity in the afferent axons that carry pain signals. The rate of firing in these afferent axons generally increases in proportion to the magnitude of the stimulus over the range of typical stimulus intensities (Box 1-2).

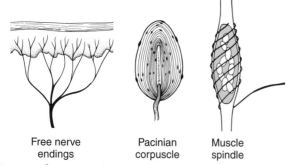

| Free nerve endings | Pacinian corpuscle | Muscle spindle |

Figure 1-6   Specialized nerve endings involved in nociception. (Redrawn from Sensory receptors and their basic mechanisms of action. In: Guyton AG (ed), *Textbook of Medical Physiology*, WB Saunders, Philadelphia, PA, 1981.)

Transmission

Afferent Axons

Various stimuli cause increased firing in afferent axons which carry signals from the site of peripheral stimulation toward the spinal cord where the signals are relayed to higher centers within the central nervous system. This process is called *transmission*. Afferent axons can be classified in a number of ways: according to size, degree of myelination, conduction velocity, or by modality of stimulation which results in activity. Large myelinated axons are called Aβ fibers, small myelinated axons are called Aδ fibers, and unmyelinated axons are called C fibers (Box 1-3). The conduction velocity is proportional to the degree of myelination, (Aβ > Aδ > C). The majority of axons which carry nociceptive information are Aδ and C fibers (Box 1-3).

Fibers that conduct at Aδ velocities (poorly myelinated) generally carry low- and high-threshold mechanical stimuli and often have specialized transduction organs at their peripheral terminus (Pacinian corpuscle, tendon stretch organ). Other groups of Aδ fibers begin to fire at temperatures which are mildly noxious and increase their firing rates up to very high temperatures (52–55° C).

Fibers that conduct at C velocities (unmyelinated) comprise the bulk of nociceptive afferent axons. Most of these afferents are activated by high-threshold mechanical stimuli, thermal stimuli, and chemical stimuli. They typically have no specialization at the distal terminus and are said to have free nerve endings. These neurons respond to a variety of different stimuli and are called C-polymodal nociceptors.

Anatomy of the Dorsal Horn

Within the peripheral nerve, large and small afferent axons are anatomically intermingled. As the nerve root approaches the spinal cord, there is a tendency for the large myelinated afferents to move medially and the smaller unmyelinated afferents laterally. Thus, large fibers tend to enter the dorsal root entry zone of the spinal

Box 1-3 Afferent Axons

TYPE OF AXON	DEGREE OF MYELINATION	CONDUCTION VELOCITY	FUNCTION
Aβ fibers	Well myelinated	Fast	Not involved in nociception; responsible for tactile sensation and proprioception
Aδ fibers	Poorly myelinated	Intermediate	Low- and high-threshold mechanical stimuli; heat
C fibers	Unmyelinated	Slow	High-threshold mechanical, thermal, and chemical stimuli (most nociceptive afferent axons fall into this class)

cord more medially and small fibers laterally. A significant population of unmyelinated afferents also exists within the ventral roots and this is likely to account for the pain reported during ventral root stimulation.

Based on microscopic appearance, the gray matter of the spinal cord can be divided into anatomical regions or laminae, called Rexed's laminae after the neuroanatomist who first described their microscopic appearance (Fig. 1-7). Four principal classes of neurons are involved in nociception (Box 1-4).

Lamina I (marginal zone) contains large neurons oriented across the cap of the dorsal gray matter. Some of these neurons project to the thalamus via the contralateral spinothalamic tract while others project intra- and inter-segmentally within the spinal cord. These neurons respond to intense muscle and cutaneous stimulation.

Lamina II (substantia gelatinosa) neurons receive a large portion of their input from Aδ and C fibers. They respond to thermal, chemical, and mechanical stimuli. These neurons exhibit complex and prolonged response to nociceptive input.

Laminae IV and V (nucleus proprius) cells fall into two broad categories: those that respond to innocuous Aβ

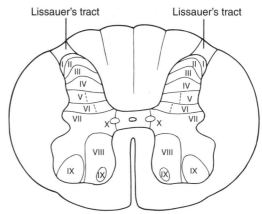

Figure 1-7 Rexed's laminae. (Redrawn from Katz NL, Ferrante FM: Nociception. In: Ferrante FM, VadeBoncouer TR (eds), *Postoperative Pain Management*, Churchill Livingstone, New York, 1993.)

input (low-threshold mechanical and thermal stimuli) and those that respond to a broad range of stimuli carried through Aβ, Aδ, and C fibers. This latter group of neurons responds to stimuli ranging from intensities that are

Box 1-4 Spinal Cord Dorsal Horn Neurons Involved in Nociception

DORSAL HORN LAMINA	NAME	FUNCTION
Rexed lamina I	Marginal layer	Projections to the thalamus; respond to intense muscle and cutaneous stimuli
Rexed lamina II	Substantia gelatinosa	Large proportion of input from Aδ and C fibers; respond to mechanical, thermal, and chemical stimuli; prolonged response to nociceptive input
Rexed laminae IV and V	Nucleus proprius	Two general groups of neurons: those that respond to Aβ input (low-threshold mechanical and thermal stimuli) and those that respond to a broad range of stimuli carried through Aβ, Aδ, and C fibers (wide-dynamic-range neurons)

non-noxious to those that are very noxious and thus they are termed wide-dynamic-range (WDR) neurons. Response of WDR neurons can account for many of the characteristics of neuropathic pain.

Functional Characteristics of Dorsal Horn Neurons

Several physiologic properties of dorsal horn neurons can account for characteristics of pain reported clinically (Box 1-5). Dorsal horn neurons gradually increase their rate of firing following repetitive stimulation of C nociceptive afferents; this phenomenon is called "windup." The increase in firing rate is also accompanied by an increase in the size of the peripheral receptive field. Spinal cord windup accounts for the clinical observation that following tissue trauma, the area of injury and the surrounding tissue become painful even to light touch (allodynia).

A second characteristic of dorsal horn neurons called convergence accounts for referred pain. Depending on the spinal level, dorsal horn neurons respond to stimuli that converge from anatomically distinct organs. Thus, stimulation of sympathetic afferents by coronary artery occlusion converges to activate the same group of spinal cord neurons that receive nociceptive input from cutaneous and deep receptors in the left upper extremity.

Ascending Spinal Tracts

Activity evoked in the spinal cord by painful stimuli reaches supraspinal sites within the central nervous system via long inter-segmental tracts within the ventrolateral quadrant of the spinal cord, the spinothalamic, spinoreticular, and spinomesencephalic tracts (Fig. 1-8). The importance of the spinothalamic tracts is shown when surgical lesions are placed through the ventrolateral aspect of the spinal cord (e.g. percutaneous cordotomy). Following such a lesion, the threshold for visceral and somatic pain rises dramatically below and on the side contralateral to the lesion. The sensory level following cordotomy also indicates that ascending tracts travel several segments rostrally before crossing midline to join the contralateral spinothalamic tract. The spinoreticular and spinomesencephalic projections are likely involved in arousal and other behaviors associated with pain (e.g. arousal, affective components of pain perception) (Box 1-6).

Supraspinal Systems

Medulla

Spinoreticular projections carry fibers to the medullary reticular formation. Medullary cell bodies (particularly neurons within the nucleus gigantocellularis) are activated by nociceptive input, and in turn send projections to the thalamus. The medullary reticular formation likely acts as a relay for rostral transmission of nociceptive information.

> ### Box 1-5 Functional Characteristics of Dorsal Horn Neurons Leading to Clinically Observed Characteristics of Pain Following Nerve Stimulation or Injury
>
> *Spinal cord windup* – Dorsal horn neurons gradually increase their rate of firing following repetitive stimulation of C nociceptive afferents; this phenomenon is called "windup." Spinal cord windup accounts for the clinical observation that following tissue trauma, the area of injury and the surrounding tissue become painful even to light touch (allodynia).
>
> *Allodynia* – Pain following a normally non-painful stimulus (e.g. light touch causes pain). Allodynia is pathognomonic for neuropathic pain.
>
> *Convergence* – Depending on the spinal level, dorsal horn neurons respond to stimuli that converge from anatomically distinct organs. Thus, stimulation of sympathetic afferents by coronary artery occlusion converges to activate the same group of spinal cord neurons that receive nociceptive input from cutaneous and deep receptors in the left upper extremity.

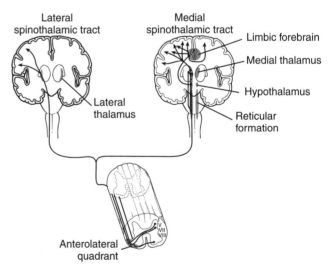

Figure 1-8   Ascending pain pathways. (Redrawn from Katz NL, Ferrante FM: Nociception. In: Ferrante FM, VadeBoncouer TR (eds), *Postoperative Pain Management*, Churchill Livingstone, New York, 1993.)

Box 1-6   Ascending Spinal Pathways Involved in Nociception

The ascending pain pathways lie in the anterolateral portion of the spinal cord.

Spinothalamic tract (pain localization and intensity)

Spinoreticular tract (arousal and behavior associated with pain)

Spinomesencephalic tract (arousal and behavior associated with pain)

Box 1-7   Role of Supraspinal Structures in Nociception

ANATOMIC STRUCTURE	ROLE IN NOCICEPTION
Medulla oblongata	Relay to higher centers; descending inhibitory modulation of nociceptive impulses entering the dorsal horn of the spinal cord
Thalamus	Somatotopic organization of pain stimuli and integration of somatosensory and limbic activity
Parietal lobe (primary somatosensory cortex)	Sensory/discriminative aspects of pain perception
Frontal lobe	Affective/motivational aspects of pain perception through frontal-limbic connections
Limbic system	Affective and motivational aspects of pain behavior through frontal-limbic connections

Thalamus

Spinothalamic axons project to specific regions within the thalamus (ventrobasal complex; medial thalamic nuclei; intralaminar nuclei). The role of the thalamus in nociception is complex. The ventrobasal complex receives nociceptive projections that are highly somatotopically organized and likely subserves discriminative pain. The medial thalamic nuclei are associated with visceral sensory activity and subserve integration of somatosensory and limbic activity. The intralaminar nuclei receive projections from the spinothalamic tract and send projections to wide areas of the cerebral cortex. Lesions in this region raise sensory thresholds and electrical stimulation produces reports of contralateral burning pain. Clinical reports in patients with lesions within the thalamus indicate the complexity of thalamic function in nociception. One recent report chronicles the evolution of changes in thermal and pain perception in a patient with a slowly expanding arteriovenous malformation within the thalamus (Greenspan et al. 1997).

Cortex

Discrete areas within the somatosensory cortex receive nociceptive input, primarily from the thalamus. However, the role of the cortex in pain perception is confusing. Removal of large areas of the cortex leaves pain perception intact. However, epileptic activity and direct electrical stimulation of the cortex can produce pain. The primary somatosensory cortex (parietal lobe) is thought to subserve the sensory/discriminative aspects of pain perception. The frontal lobe receives diffuse projections from medial thalamic nuclei and is thought to subserve the affective/motivational aspects of pain perception through frontal-limbic connections.

Limbic System

Pain has an overriding affective/motivational component that goes beyond the initiating stimulus. Frontal lobotomies were once used for intractable pain. However, such patients continued to report pain if questioned, but seldom asked for medications and no longer seemed to care about their pain. Complex interconnections between the limbic system and other supraspinal regions receiving nociceptive input are responsible for the affective and motivational aspects of pain behavior (Box 1-7).

Modulation of Nociceptive Input

Electrical stimulation of the periaqueductal gray region within the midbrain and the periventricular gray matter lateral to the hypothalamus produces profound analgesia in humans. Such regions have been found to contain high concentrations of endogenous opioid neurotransmitters. The periventricular gray matter and the periaqueductal gray matter are interconnected and also connect anatomically with the rostroventral medulla. The rostroventral medulla sends descending projections via the dorsolateral funiculus to laminae I, II, and V of the dorsal horn (Fig. 1-9 on p. 10). Norepinephrine, serotonin, and systemically administered opioids all likely produce their nociceptive effects through activation of these descending inhibitory pathways. The dorsal horn also contains high concentrations of α-adrenergic receptors as well as μ-opioid receptors. This accounts for the observation that clonidine (α_2-agonist) inhibits discharge of nociceptive neurons when applied locally to

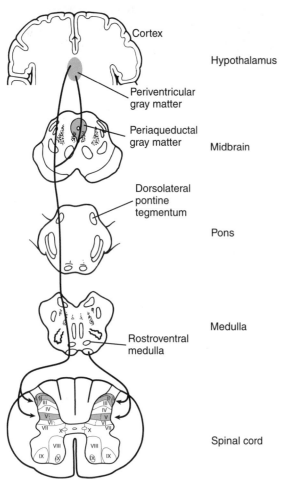

Cortex

Hypothalamus

Periventricular
gray matter

Periaqueductal
gray matter

Midbrain

Dorsolateral
pontine
tegmentum

Pons

Medulla

Rostroventral
medulla

Spinal cord

Figure 1-9   Descending modulatory pathways. (Redrawn from Katz NL, Ferrante FM: Nociception. In: Ferrante FM, VadeBoncouer TR (eds), *Postoperative Pain Management*, Churchill Livingstone, New York, 1993.)

the spinal cord. Neuraxial injection of opioids also produces intense analgesia via local binding to μ-opioid receptors in the dorsal horn and resultant inhibition of nociceptive transmission (Box 1-8).

Box 1-8   Anatomic Localization of Opioid Receptors

Opioid receptors are found in high density at specific anatomic locations within the spinal cord and higher centers within the medulla, midbrain, and hypothalamus. Opioid binding leads to inhibitory modulation of nociceptive input. Systemic administration of opioids leads primarily to binding within higher brain centers resulting in an increase in descending inhibition. Opioid administration directly at the spinal level leads to direct inhibitory modulation at the spinal cord level through opioid receptors located on dorsal horn neurons. High densities of opioid receptors are found in the following locations within the central nervous system:

> Periventricular gray matter (hypothalamus)
> Periaqueductal gray matter (midbrain)
> Substantia gelatinosa (Rexed lamina II, spinal cord dorsal horn)

SUGGESTED READING

Greenspan JD, Joy SE, McGillis SLB, Checkosky CM, Balanowski SJ: A longitudinal study of somesthetic perceptual disorders in an individual with a unilateral thalamic lesion, *Pain* 72:13–25, 1997.

Katz NL, Ferrante FM: Nociception. In: Ferrante FM, VadeBoncouer TR (eds), *Postoperative Pain Management*, Churchill Livingstone, New York, 1993.

Strichartz GR: Neural physiology and local anesthetic action. In: Cousins MJ, Bridenbaugh PO (eds), *Neural Blockade*, Third Edition, Lippincott-Raven, Philadelphia, PA, 1998, pp. 35–54.

Yaksh TL: Organizational anatomy of pain pathways. In: Bailin M (ed), *The Harvard Electronic Anesthesia Library*, Lippincott, Williams & Wilkins, Philadelphia, PA, 2001.

Sensory receptors and their basic mechanisms of action. In: Guyton AG (ed), *Textbook of Medical Physiology*, WB Saunders, Philadelphia, PA, 1981, pp. 588–596.

PHARMACOLOGY

PART

II

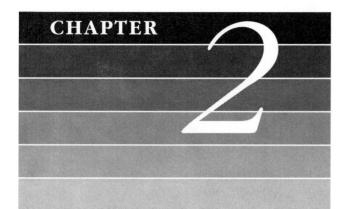

CHAPTER 2

Pharmacology of Local Anesthetics

CHRISTOPHER M.VISCOMI

INTRODUCTION

Before the reader launches into a description of specific regional anesthetic techniques, it is essential to understand the local anesthetics used to perform neural blockade. Each regional block is a unique pairing of anatomic localization and optimal anesthetic agent: a properly located needle serving as a conduit to deliver appropriately selected pharmaceutical agents.

Local anesthetics are the pharmacologic cornerstone of regional anesthesia. They produce temporary and complete blockade of neuronal transmission when they are applied near axons. This may result in complete interruption of nerve impulse conduction, allowing abolition of all sensation from the area innervated by the nerves that are blocked. Alternatively, dilute concentrations of local anesthetics applied to the neuraxis can selectively block pain without substantial interference with motor function.

This chapter explains the basic chemical structure of local anesthetics, describes receptor pharmacology, and discusses pharmacologic properties of individual agents. The clinical utility of different classes of local anesthetics is compared. The chapter concludes with an in-depth discussion of local anesthetic toxicity.

LOCAL ANESTHETICS

Chemical Structure

Local anesthetic molecules are comprised of three basic building blocks: a lipophilic aromatic moiety (benzene ring), a hydrophilic tertiary amine, and an intermediate chain connecting the two. The chemical connection between the intermediate chain and the aromatic ring allows classification of local anesthetics as either "esters" or "amides." Fig. 2-1 on p. 14 illustrates the basic chemical structure of a local anesthetic molecule. This chemical differentiation of local anesthetics into amides and esters is clinically relevant, because the amides are more stable and have less risk of allergic reaction than the esters (Table 2-1).

In addition to their basic molecular structure, certain amide local anesthetics (mepivacaine, bupivacaine, and

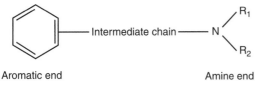

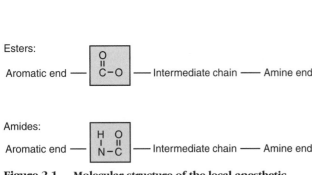

Figure 2-1 **Molecular structure of the local anesthetic molecule.**

ropivacaine) exist as stereoisomers that have differing pharmacodynamic effects. Stereoisomerism refers to subsets of identical compounds, which vary only in the arrangement of atoms around the chiral carbon (four different atoms or moieties attaching to the same carbon atom). The same group of atoms can be arranged in two different patterns around any axis of rotation. While the resulting compounds share an identical chemical formula, they form pairs of molecules that are mirror images to one another called enantiomers. Enantiomers cannot be superimposed and are referred to as chiral molecules. Chiral molecules can be described by two independent nomenclatures: (+) and (−), and R and S. The first designation, (+) and (−), refers to whether the molecule rotates polarized light to the right (+, clockwise, or dextrorotatory) or the left (−, anticlockwise, or

levorotatory). The second designation, R and S, refers to rectus and sinister, which describe the configuration of ligands around the stereogenic carbon atom. These naming systems are independent, meaning that combinations of the two systems can describe molecules. As an example, bupivacaine exists in S(−) and R(+) forms. Most local anesthetics are manufactured and used clinically as equal mixtures of the two enantiomers (racemic mixtures). In recent years, economical means of preparing the enantiomers of local anesthetics have been devised and distinct pharmacologic properties have been identified. For example, *l*-bupivacaine, the levorotatory enantiomer of racemic bupivacaine, appears to exhibit significantly less cardiac toxicity while maintaining the same anesthetic potency as the racemate. Table 2-2 summarizes the chemical structure and properties of local anesthetic agents.

Site of Action

To gain an understanding of the mechanism of local anesthetic-induced neural blockade, it is important to review the electrophysiology of neuronal conduction. Neurons maintain a negative (−70 mV) intracellular resting potential compared to the extracellular fluid. An active sodium–potassium exchange pump maintains this electrical gradient. This pump actively moves sodium out of the neuron and potassium into the neuron, creating a concentration gradient of both sodium and potassium (higher concentration of potassium intracellular compared to extracellular, higher concentration of sodium extracellular compared to intracellular). Despite this active pumping mechanism, the cell membrane is considerably more permeable to passive movement of potassium compared to sodium. This greater passive extracellular movement of potassium (compared to intracellular movement of sodium) results in a net negative intracellular charge.

With electrical excitation of the neuron, a depolarizing stimulus is conducted down an axon. A stimulus of significant magnitude changes the negative resting potential from −70 mV toward the −55 mV threshold required for complete depolarization; sodium channels in the cell membrane are activated and a sudden influx of extracellular sodium ions moves into the intracellular fluid. This influx of cations rapidly changes the membrane potential to +35 mV. The resultant propagation of voltage change down the axon is defined as the action potential (see Chapter 1, Fig. 1-4 on p. 5). Local anesthetic molecules traverse the cell membrane and then block the sodium channel from within the cell (Fig. 2-2 on p. 17). Thus, propagation of the action potential is prevented and neural signal transmission along the nerve is blocked.

	Esters	Amides
Metabolism	Plasma cholinesterase (pseudocholinesterase)	Hepatic
Serum half-life	Shorter	Longer
Allergic potential	Low	Very low
Clinical drugs	Procaine, chloroprocaine, cocaine, tetracaine	Lidocaine, mepivacaine, bupivacaine, ropivacaine, etidocaine, prilocaine

Table 2-1 **Properties of Amide and Ester Local Anesthetic Agents**

Clinical Caveat: The Dibucaine Number

Dibucaine is an amide local anesthetic occasionally used for topical anesthesia. An interesting aspect of the pharmacology of dibucaine is that it strongly binds normal plasma (pseudo)cholinesterase. This binding of plasma cholinesterase inhibits the enzyme. Atypical pseudocholinesterases are not bound nearly as strongly and thus produce less inhibition of enzymatic activity. The type of plasma cholinesterase an individual has is genetically determined. The simplest classification is "homozygous" (normal), "heterozygous" (mixture of normal and atypical plasma cholinesterases), and "homozygous atypical" (all atypical enzyme).

When individuals are suspected of having atypical plasma cholinesterase (typically on the basis of prolonged duration of paralysis after receiving succinylcholine or mivacurium), a "Dibucaine Number" can be ordered as a laboratory blood test. The following table describes possible results:

GENETIC TYPE	DURATION OF SUCCINYLCHOLINE EFFECT	DIBUCAINE NUMBER (% INHIBITION OF PLASMA CHOLINESTERASE ACTIVITY)	APPROXIMATE INCIDENCE
Homozygous (normal)	6 minutes	80	998/1000
Heterozygous	15–25 minutes	50	1/475
Homozygous atypical	1–6 hours	20	1/3300

Metabolism

Ester local anesthetics are primarily metabolized by ubiquitous plasma cholinesterases (pseudocholinesterase). These enzymes are made by the liver, and are found throughout the vascular system and in the cerebrospinal fluid (CSF). They degrade numerous drugs of relevance to the anesthesiologist, including ester local anesthestics, succinylcholine, and mivacurium. Because of the widespread distribution of these enzymes, plasma degradation of ester local anesthetics is typically rapid. In contrast, amide local anesthetics undergo degradation by hepatic enzymes and typically have a longer serum half-life.

Allergic Potential

The majority of local anesthetic allergic reactions reported by patients represent misinterpretation of the associated clinical event. Allergic reactions may occur from preservatives added to some local anesthetics (sulfites, methylparaben). Actual allergic reactions to local anesthetics are quite rare, but are more common with ester local anesthetics as compared to amides. This is likely due to the breakdown products of ester local anesthetics, such as *para*-aminobenzoic acid (PABA), which has been implicated in many allergic reactions, including those to sunscreen products. There are only a few convincing reports of allergic reactions to preservative-free amide local anesthetics.

It is therefore important to assess accurately a patient's report of "local anesthetic allergy." A frequent scenario reported by the patient as "an allergy to local anesthetic" occurs when the patient receives a local anesthetic injection in a dental office. On close questioning, the symptoms are usually attributable to intravascular injection of local anesthetic solution (often with epinephrine). Rarely are actual allergic manifestations (urticaria, bronchospasm, or anaphylaxis) part of the history (see Chapter 5). If there is a history suggestive of true allergy, it may be worthwhile to perform allergy testing to preservative-free local anesthetics.

Pharmacokinetics: Protein Binding and Lipid Solubility

Physical and chemical properties of local anesthetics exert a major influence on their potency, toxicity, and clinical effects. One of the most important clinical characteristics of a local anesthetic is its duration of action – essential knowledge for optimally matching local anesthetics to specific surgical requirements. Duration correlates with the degree of local anesthetic protein binding (typically to alpha-1 acid glycoprotein). Long-duration local anesthetics, such as bupivacaine and ropivacaine, are highly protein bound. High protein affinity local anesthetics bind to nerve sodium channel proteins for long periods of time, and therefore have a long duration of action. In the serum, local anesthetics bind to albumin and alpha acid glycoprotein, which also promotes long serum half-life.

Fig. 2-3 on p. 17 describes a continuum for local anesthetic duration and speed of onset. In general, short-acting local anesthetics have a fast onset of clinical effect,

Table 2-2   Physicochemical Properties of Local Anesthetics

Drug (Brand Name)	Type (Year Introduced)	Chemical Structure	Relative Potency Frog Sciatic Nerve	Rat Sciatic Nerve	pK$_a$	Lipid Solubility	Rat Sciatic Binding
Cocaine	Ester	CH$_2$—CH—CHCOOCH$_3$ / NCH$_3$—CHOOC$_6$H$_5$ / CH$_2$—CH—CH$_2$	—	—	—	—	—
Procaine (Novocaine)	Ester (1905)	H$_2$N—⟨⟩—COOCH$_2$CH$_2$N(C$_2$H$_5$)$_2$	1	1	8.9	0.6	5.8
Benzocaine	Ester (1900)	H$_2$N—⟨⟩—COOC$_2$H$_5$	—	—	3.5	—	—
Tetracaine (Pontocaine)	Ester (1930)	H$_9$C$_4$·N(—⟨⟩—COOCH$_2$N(CH$_3$)$_2$)	16	8	8.5	80	75.6
2-Chloroprocaine (Nesacaine)	Ester (1952)	H$_2$N—⟨Cl⟩—COOCH$_2$N(C$_2$H$_5$)$_2$	4	1	8.7	—	—
Lidocaine (Xylocaine)	Amide (1944)	(CH$_3$)$_2$⟨⟩—NHCOCH$_2$N(C$_2$H$_5$)$_2$	4	2	7.72	2.9	64.3
Mepivacaine (Carbocaine)	Amide (1957)	(CH$_3$)$_2$⟨⟩—NHCO—N(CH$_3$) piperidine	2	2	7.6	0.8	77.5
Prilocaine (Citanest)	Amide (1960)	CH$_3$⟨⟩—NHCOCH—NH—C$_3$H$_7$	3	2	7.7	0.8	55
Ropivacaine (Naropin)	Amide (1996)	(CH$_3$)$_2$⟨⟩—NHCO—N(C$_3$H$_7$) piperidine	6	6	8.1	14	94
Bupivacaine (Marcaine, Sensorcaine)	Amide (1963)	(CH$_3$)$_2$⟨⟩—NHCO—N(C$_4$H$_9$) piperidine	—	8	8.1	27.5	95.6
Etidocaine (Duranest)	Amide (1972)	(CH$_3$)$_2$⟨⟩—NHCOCHN(C$_2$H$_5$)(C$_2$H$_5$ C$_3$H$_7$)	16	8	7.74	141	94

Adapted with permission from Covino BG and Vassallo HG, *Local Anesthetic: Mechanisms of Action and Clinical Use*, New York: Grune & Stratton, 1976, and deJong RH, *Local Anesthetics*, Springfield, IL: Charles C Thomas, 1977.

while long-duration anesthetics have a slower onset of clinical effects.

Serum protein binding also protects against drug toxicity, because only free drug (those molecules not bound to serum proteins) can induce toxicity. However, once serum proteins are saturated with local anesthetic molecules, any additional administration or absorption of local anesthetic rapidly causes toxicity. Indeed, patients can very rapidly progress from having no signs of local anesthetic toxicity to manifestations of severe cardiac toxicity when highly protein-bound local anesthetics are used.

Clinical Caveat: Influence of Hypoproteinemia on Protein Binding and Local Anesthetic Toxicity

Patients with low circulating protein levels are at particular risk for local anesthetic toxicity:

Neonates and infants (particularly those <56–60 weeks of post-conceptual age)

Malnourished patients or those with advanced cancer

Patients with advanced liver disease

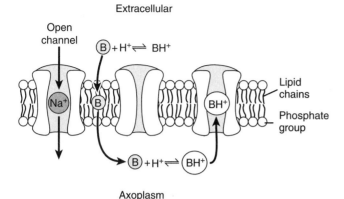

Figure 2-2   Mechanism of action of local anesthetics. Penetration of the base (non-ionized) local anesthetic molecule and reversible block of sodium channel. (Redrawn from DiFazio CA, Rowlingson JL: Additives to local anesthetic solutions. In Brown DL (ed), *Regional Anesthesia and Analgesia*, WB Saunders, Philadelphia, 1996, p. 233, Fig. 14-2.)

Lipid solubility correlates with potency: the more lipid soluble the drug, the more potent. Lipid solubility facilitates penetration of the neuronal cell membrane, which accelerates local anesthetic binding to the intracellular portion of the sodium channel. Lipid solubility is highly influenced by the side chains of the benzene ring.

Ionization and pK$_a$

Local anesthetics are weak bases (pK$_a$ = 7.6–9.0) that are commercially prepared as an acidic solution, typically at pH 4–5. The pK$_a$ defines the pH where half of the drug is ionized and half non-ionized. The ionized and non-ionized forms have different, but important, clinical effects. The non-ionized form penetrates the nerve membrane, while the ionized form binds to proteins on the intracellular side of the sodium channel (Fig. 2-4 on p. 18). Because the pH of local anesthetic formulations is significantly less than the pK$_a$ of the local anesthetics themselves, the ratio of non-ionized to ionized molecules is 1:1,000–1:10,000. Sodium bicarbonate can be added to local anesthetic solutions to raise the pH of the solution, thereby increasing the non-ionized form. Other factors being equal, local anesthetics with more basic pK$_a$ (e.g. bupivacaine) have a slower onset of local anesthetic effect due to the lesser amount of non-ionized local anesthetic molecules at physiologic pH. This relative lack of

the non-ionized form impairs local anesthetic movement across the cell membrane, and thus delays block onset (Fig. 2-4 on p. 18).

Individual Local Anesthetic Agents

Local anesthetics vary widely in structure, tissue penetration, duration, and toxicity. Practitioners must be able to choose appropriate local anesthetics for a given clinical application. Common local anesthetics used in clinical practice and their applications are shown in Table 2-3.

Ester Local Anesthetics

Cocaine

Cocaine, which is extracted from the dried leaves of the coca plant, was the first clinically used local anesthetic. August Bier used cocaine in the first spinal anesthetic in 1897. In contemporary practice, cocaine is used almost exclusively for topical airway anesthesia. Even in this limited role, cocaine's use is diminishing because suitable alternatives exist that have less potential for abuse.

Topical mucous membrane application of cocaine results in very rapid anesthesia and vasoconstriction. At excessive doses, cocaine's vasoconstrictive properties are linked to hypertension, coronary ischemia, and arrhythmias (Box 2-1). Mixtures of lidocaine with phenylephrine or oxymetazoline are safer alternatives to cocaine for anesthetizing and vasoconstricting mucous membranes.

Procaine

Procaine was synthesized in 1904 in an attempt to develop a safer alternative to cocaine. Unfortunately, procaine combines a short duration and limited tissue penetration. Procaine is still occasionally used for skin infiltration and short-duration (30–45 minutes) spinal anesthesia, although discharge readiness may be slightly longer than that seen with equipotent doses of spinal lidocaine.

2-Chloroprocaine

This ester local anesthetic is synthesized by adding a chloride to the benzene ring of procaine. In comparison to procaine, it has a more rapid onset and a slightly longer duration of action. The principal uses of chloroprocaine are in obstetric and ambulatory anesthesia, because of its rapid onset when used in epidural anesthesia. Chloroprocaine is frequently chosen for urgent forceps or cesarean deliveries

Figure 2-3   Onset and duration of local anesthetics.

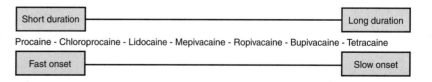

Short duration ——————————————— Long duration

Procaine - Chloroprocaine - Lidocaine - Mepivacaine - Ropivacaine - Bupivacaine - Tetracaine

Fast onset ——————————————— Slow onset

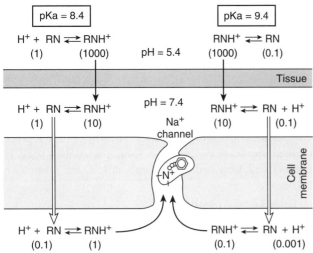

Figure 2-4   Effect of ionization on activity. The proportion of local anesthetic in the base (non-ionized) form will depend on its own pK_a and the pH of the solution. A drug with a pK_a of 8.4 is 3 pH units (10^3) away from its 50% equilibrium point when prepared in a commercial solution at pH 5.4, producing roughly the ratio shown. When injected into body tissue, the pH rises and the ratio approaches equality, but is still a factor of 10 away. For a solution with a pK_a that is higher, the ratio is even further from equality. Since only the non-ionized form will penetrate lipid membranes, the higher pK_a solutions will usually have slower onset because of less effective drug at the site of action. (Redrawn from Mulroy MF: *Regional Anesthesia: An Illustrated Procedural Guide*, Little, Brown, 1989, p. 8.)

in parturients with indwelling epidural catheters. Like other ester local anesthetics, chloroprocaine is rapidly metabolized by plasma cholinesterases. Since serum half-life is approximately 40 seconds, fetal accumulation is extremely unlikely.

Chloroprocaine was the subject of intense scrutiny in the early 1980s after reports were published of cauda equina syndrome. These reports had in common the unintentional subarachnoid injection of large doses of chloroprocaine during attempted epidural anesthesia, with resulting total spinal anesthesia. After resolution of subarachnoid block, patients were left with lower extremity paralysis and bowel/bladder dysfunction (cauda equina syndrome). The combination of the preservative sodium bisulfite and low pH have been implicated as the primary etiologic factors.

Clinical Controversy: Local Anesthetic Preservatives and Toxicity

Sodium metabisulfite – neurotoxic under conditions of acidosis and tissue hypoxia
Methylparaben – increased allergic potential
Benzyl alcohol – a common preservative in multi-dose vials, unknown toxic potential
Ethylenediaminetetraacetate (EDTA) – chelates calcium, may cause localized hypocalcemia with muscle tetany, which can manifest as back pain after epidural analgesia

---

A second preservative that is used in some chloroprocaine formulations is ethylenediaminetetraacetate (EDTA). EDTA chelates calcium. A side effect associated with epidural chloroprocaine containing EDTA as a preservative is a 2–5% incidence of severe lower back muscle spasms that present as the block is resolving and last for several hours. This is speculated to be the result of EDTA exiting the epidural space via the intervertebral foramina, which, by chelating calcium, causes localized hypocalcemia with resultant muscle tetany. There may be other causes of severe short-lived back pain after epidural chloroprocaine, as back pain has been reported even after use of preservative-free chloroprocaine.

Tetracaine

Tetracaine is used in spinal and ophthalmic anesthesia, and is occasionally used for topical airway anesthesia. The latter application has declined with the recognition that

---

Table 2-3   Common Clinical Applications of Individual Local Anesthetic Agents*

	Spinal Anesthesia	Epidural	Peripheral Nerve Blocks	Field Blocks	Usual Concentration
Procaine	X			X	10%
Chloroprocaine		X	X		2–3%
Lidocaine	X	X	X	X	1–5%
Mepivacaine		X	X		1–2%
Tetracaine	X				1%
Ropivacaine		X	X		0.1–0.75%
Bupivacaine	X	X	X	X	0.1–0.75%

* X denotes common clinical applications of particular local anesthetics. Chloroprocaine is used only occasionally in gynecologic nerve blocks (paracervical, pudendal).

tetracaine has a narrow margin between therapeutic and toxic doses that may lead to serious systemic toxicity after mucosal application. Lidocaine is a far safer alternative for mucous membrane anesthesia. Commonly used in spinal anesthesia, tetracaine is uniquely dependent upon the co-administration of epinephrine to yield acceptable surgical anesthesia. Indeed, plain tetracaine has an initial failure rate of >30%. Tetracaine with epinephrine has the longest duration of action of the available spinal anesthetic agents, with lower extremity anesthesia lasting approximately 4 hours.

Tetracaine is less chemically stable compared to lidocaine and bupivacaine. This instability may result in an occasional failed spinal anesthetic due to degradation of the local anesthetic during storage. For this reason, the drug is frequently lyophilized to prolong shelf life. However, poor clinical technique is far more likely to cause failed spinal anesthesia than unstable tetracaine.

Amide Local Anesthetics

Lidocaine

Lidocaine was synthesized by Neils Lofgren in 1948, and remains the most widely used local anesthetic. It combines significant potency, fast onset, intermediate duration, good tissue penetration, and minimal cardiac toxicity. Lidocaine is widely used for infiltration, intravenous regional, major nerve block, topical airway, and neuraxial anesthesia.

In animal models, lidocaine neurotoxicity is concentration and time dependent. Clinically, excessive concentrations of lidocaine can occur within localized areas surrounding the cauda equina or an exiting nerve root during continuous spinal anesthesia. This appears to be the mechanism that resulted in several cases of cauda equina syndrome reported in association with use of small-diameter microcatheters for continuous spinal anesthesia. These microcatheters were available in the USA during the early 1990s and were as small as 32 gauge in diameter. The extremely small lumen and long length of these catheters produced significant resistance to injection and flow of solution through the catheter. This resistance resulted in a small degree of turbulence as the local anesthetic exited the catheter into the intrathecal space. Without turbulence, the local anesthetic mixed poorly with the CSF, and high concentrations of the local

anesthetic could be produced locally around neural structures, resulting in direct neurotoxicity. Spinal microcatheters have since been withdrawn from the US market. Single-shot spinal anesthesia can be associated with transient neurologic symptoms (TNS), the etiology of which is uncertain. Because of its considerably higher frequency with lidocaine, some speculation has focused on TNS as a minor neurotoxic reaction.

Mepivacaine

Mepivacaine has a similar pharmacokinetic profile to lidocaine, with slightly longer duration and better tissue penetration. It is used primarily for intermediate-duration peripheral nerve blocks, and as a spinal agent in Europe. Mepivacaine was used in obstetric epidural anesthesia until the mid-1980s, when one study suggested neonates whose mothers had received the agent for epidural analgesia during labor had lower neurobehavioral scores in the first day of life. This study and neonatal neurobehavioral scoring have both been criticized, but mepivacaine has never regained popularity in obstetric epidural anesthesia.

Prilocaine

Prilocaine is widely used for intravenous regional anesthesia outside of the USA. Within the USA, prilocaine was withdrawn from use for this application following several cases of methemoglobinemia. Prilocaine is metabolized to nitro- and *ortho*-toluidene, which can oxidize hemoglobin to methemoglobin. In the USA, prilocaine is used commercially in topical eutectic mixture of local anesthetics (EMLA) cream, as well as in proprietary mixtures of local anesthetics specifically marketed for airway anesthesia. Significant methemoglobinemia has been reported in both of these applications.

Clinical Caveat: Methemoglobinemia

Methemoglobinemia occurs with agents that oxidize hemoglobin to the Fe^{3+} form. It is most commonly seen with nitrates, such as nitroglycerin

Prilocaine and benzocaine (present in local anesthetic sprays used for oropharyngeal anesthesia in endoscopy and bronchoscopy) are metabolized to o-toluidene, which can oxidize hemoglobin and cause clinical methemoglobinemia

Pulse oximetry is not capable of evaluating methemoglobinemia because the peak infrared absorption of MetHb is not interrogated by conventional pulse oximetry. Very high levels of methemoglobin are often interpreted by pulse oximetry as a SpO_2 of 85%

The diagnosis can be made by arterial blood gas analysis using a co-oximeter. In addition, the blood sample will appear brown. Metabolic acidosis is usually pronounced

Treatment is IV methylene blue 1 mg/kg, and oral ascorbic acid 300–600 mg

Etidocaine

This drug is rarely used in contemporary practice. Its high protein binding is similar to bupivacaine, as is its onset, duration of action, and cardiac toxicity profile. Because it produces more motor block than sensory block, it is most useful when muscle relaxation is beneficial, such as during hip arthroplasty. Reports of patients receiving etidocaine and then experiencing pain and concurrent motor weakness are largely exaggerated. This scenario is easily avoided by giving a final epidural dose of bupivacaine to prolong sensory block.

Bupivacaine

Bupivacaine is the prototypical long-acting amide local anesthetic. Bupivacaine is highly protein bound, which is consistent with long duration and potential for cardiotoxicity. Indeed, the cardiotoxicity of bupivacaine prompted the development of ropivacaine and l-bupivacaine. Bupivacaine is popular for use in a wide array of applications, including infiltration, peripheral nerve block, and neuraxial anesthesia. Because of systemic toxicity, it is not used for IV regional anesthesia.

In the obstetric and acute postoperative pain settings, continuous epidural infusions of dilute concentrations of bupivacaine (typically combined with a lipophilic opioid) provide excellent analgesia without significant motor block. Bupivacaine's relative separation of sensory and motor blockade is highly desirable in these two settings.

Clinically used concentrations of bupivacaine vary from 0.05% (epidural continuous infusions for labor analgesia and acute pain management) to 0.75% (spinal anesthesia and peripheral nerve blocks). The 0.75% concentration is specifically contraindicated for obstetric epidural anesthesia due to concerns about cardiotoxicity. It is worth noting that the practice patterns in use when bupivacaine cardiotoxicity was seen during obstetric epidural anesthesia are no longer prevalent. Contemporary epidural anesthesia incorporates use of multiorifice catheters (which allow a more accurate aspiration test), test dosing regimens, incremental dosing, and low concentrations of local anesthetic via continuous infusion.

l-Bupivacaine

Levo-bupivacaine is the levorotatory enantiomer of bupivacaine. Cardiac toxicity studies in animals indicate that l-bupivacaine is approximately 35% less cardiotoxic compared to racemic bupivacaine. Central nervous system toxicity is probably very similar to racemic bupivacaine. l-Bupivacaine is used in the same concentrations, doses, and applications as racemic bupivacaine.

Ropivacaine

Ropivacaine is a long-acting amide local anesthetic. This drug was specifically designed and formulated to minimize cardiotoxicity. Ropivacaine is primarily used in epidural anesthesia/analgesia and peripheral nerve block applications. Ropivacaine appears to be approximately

---

Box 2-2   Comparing the Clinical Characteristics of Bupivacaine, l-Bupivacaine, and Ropivacaine

Bupivacaine (racemic mixture) is the prototypical long-acting amide local anesthetic that possesses less motor block compared to sensory block. This separation of motor and sensory blockade is particularly advantageous with epidural analgesia in obstetrics and postoperative pain management. Unfortunately, bupivacaine is highly cardiotoxic.

Ropivacaine also possesses a relative separation of sensory and motor blockade. When the same mass of ropivacaine and bupivacaine are administered epidurally, ropivacaine achieves similar sensory block and less motor block. With extremely dilute (0.03–0.05%) epidural infusions, ropivacaine appears to be 20–35% less potent compared to bupivacaine. This potency differential is not clinically apparent at concentrations typically used for epidural infusion. Ropivacaine is also about 40% less cardiotoxic and 30% less neurotoxic compared to racemic bupivacaine.

l-Bupivacaine is the levorotatory chiral isolate of unfractionated bupivacaine. l-Bupivacaine is about 35% less cardiotoxic compared to racemic bupivacaine, and approximately equipotent in terms of neurotoxicity. There are some reports suggesting slightly less motor block with l-bupivacaine compared to racemic bupivacaine.

  In summary:
Potency: Bupivacaine = l-Bupivacaine > Ropivacaine
Motor block: Bupivacaine ≥ l-Bupivacaine >
    Ropivacaine
Cardiotoxicity: Bupivacaine > l-Bupivacaine >
    Ropivacaine
Neurotoxicity: Bupivacaine = l-Bupivacaine >
    Ropivacaine

40% less cardiotoxic as compared to racemic bupivacaine in animal models. In dilute epidural infusions, ropivacaine is somewhat less potent (~20%) compared to bupivacaine. This potency differential may diminish the reduced toxicity advantages of ropivacaine if practitioners increase its dose in an effort to offset lower potency (Box 2-2).

LOCAL ANESTHETIC TOXICITY

Local anesthetics have a long history of safe clinical application, but toxicity may nevertheless occur. Local anesthetic toxicity is categorized as localized neurotoxicity and systemic toxicity (central nervous system or cardiac) from high serum levels of local anesthetics. Adjuvants mixed with local anesthetics can also have independent toxicity (e.g. cardiac arrhythmias from epinephrine) (see Chapter 3 for further details).

Neurotoxicity

Direct nerve injury from local anesthetics is receiving increased scrutiny, particularly with regards to spinal anesthesia. Toxicity can result from either local anesthetics themselves or from additives, preservatives, antiseptics, or the pH of the formulation. Schwann cell injury and axonal degeneration are the hallmarks of neurotoxicity. The mechanism of local anesthetic-induced neurotoxicity is multifactorial. Direct nerve injury is evident when isolated nerves are exposed to high concentrations of local anesthetics, particularly lidocaine and tetracaine. Local anesthetics also change the biologic milieu surrounding neurons, including localized alteration of prostaglandin production, altered ionic permeability, and changes in neural blood flow.

In the 1970s, chloroprocaine with sodium bisulfite preservative was occasionally unintentionally administered intrathecally during attempted epidural anesthesia. This injection typically caused total spinal anesthesia, but also caused permanent cauda equina syndrome after resolution of the total spinal anesthetic. Laboratory investigation implicated the sodium bisulfite preservative as the primary neurotoxin.

Individual local anesthetics are associated with specific neurotoxic manifestations. As previously mentioned, 2-chloroprocaine was linked to cauda equina syndrome following unintentional subarachnoid injection, and post-block resolution back pain of uncertain etiology.

As compared with bupivacaine, lidocaine has a significantly greater potential for direct neurotoxicity, particularly when isolated nerves are exposed to high concentrations of lidocaine over long periods of time. Hyperbaric 5% lidocaine and tetracaine have been associated with cauda equina syndrome after continuous (and very rarely, single-shot) spinal anesthesia. In these cases, spinal microcatheters were used to administer supernormal (up to 300 mg) doses of hyperbaric 5% lidocaine. Because spinal microcatheters (25–32 gauge) greatly limit the speed of drug administration, maldistributed local anesthetics presumably pooled near the catheter tip. As a result of the lordotic lumbar spine curvature, neurotoxic concentrations of lidocaine remained in the lumbosacral cistern. Spinal microcatheters were withdrawn from the US market in the mid-1990s, but are undergoing testing for possible reintroduction.

Single-shot spinal anesthesia can cause transient pain ("transient neurologic symptoms" or TNS), manifest as back and posterior leg discomfort with radicular symptoms lasting 1–3 days after spinal anesthesia. The etiology of TNS is unclear, but some have speculated that this syndrome represents a form of neurotoxicity. Transient neurologic symptoms occur more frequently with lidocaine than bupivacaine, which may relate to lidocaine's greater neurotoxicity in isolated nerve preparations. This difference in neurotoxicity may also be partially explained by high bupivacaine concentrations being difficult to prepare: high concentrations of bupivacaine will cause precipitation in solution.

Clinical Caveat: Transient Neurologic Symptoms (TNS)

TNS typically presents 4 to 12 hours after resolution of spinal anesthesia and lasts for 12 to 72 hours

TNS describes unilateral or bilateral back and buttock discomfort that radiates into the posterior thighs. There are no associated neurologic signs or weakness. TNS is treated conservatively with non-steroidal anti-inflammatory drugs, heat, rest, and reassurance

The incidence of TNS is increased with the use of lidocaine, lithotomy or knee arthroscopy position, and ambulatory surgery

The incidence is highest with lidocaine, lowest with bupivacaine, and intermediate with other local anesthetics. TNS is not affected by local anesthetic concentration, baricity, or lidocaine doses >40 mg. Low-dose lidocaine (25–40 mg) is associated with a highly reduced, but not zero, incidence of TNS

It is important to differentiate neurotoxicity from other causes of nerve injury. Direct trauma to a nerve from the regional anesthetic needle can occur. Intraneural injection may cause nerve injury from the combination of mechanical disruption of nerve fascicles plus neurotoxicity from the injected local anesthetic. Nerve fibers or the spinal cord are also subject to pressure injury from expanding hematoma or abscess. For example, epidural hematoma can cause paraplegia following neuraxial anesthesia in patients concomitantly anticoagulated with low molecular weight heparin. Other causes of neural injury include positioning injuries, surgical trauma, and injuries related to the use of a limb tourniquet.

Systemic CNS Toxicity

Systemic local anesthetic toxicity can present as central nervous system effects (seizures) or cardiac toxicity. Seizures result from high plasma concentrations of local anesthetics. Depending on the site of injection, signs of systemic toxicity may present immediately or up to several hours later. With intra-arterial injection, seizures immediately follow injection of very small amounts of local anesthetic (<15 mg lidocaine or <2.5 mg bupivacaine) if the local anesthetic is injected into an artery directly supplying the brain. An example of this would be direct injection of local anesthetic into a vertebral or carotid artery during stellate ganglion, cervical plexus, or interscalene block. Much more commonly, seizures occur from systemic absorption of large doses of local anesthetics used in neural blockade, or from unrecognized intravascular injection of local anesthetic solution during a regional anesthetic injection. An example of this latter clinical situation would be unrecognized placement of an epidural catheter into an epidural vein.

It is important to appreciate systemic toxicity as it relates to serum levels of local anesthetics. First, the site of injection of the local anesthetic has a significant bearing on the resulting serum level. Highly vascular areas, such as with intercostal nerve blocks typically result in much higher local anesthetic serum levels as compared to the same dose of local anesthetic injected near the femoral artery during a femoral nerve block. Figure 2-5 illustrates differences in serum levels of local anesthetics after various nerve blocks. Clinical application of this information includes strict adherence to safe doses of local anesthetics when performing blocks that cause high serum levels of local anesthetics. Table 2-4 lists the

Table 2-4	Recommended Maximal Local Anesthetic Doses*	
	Local Anesthesia without Epinephrine	**Local Anesthesia with Epinephrine**
Lidocaine	4–5 mg/kg	7 mg/kg
Mepivacaine	5–6 mg/kg	8–9 mg/kg
Bupivacaine, ropivacaine, *l*-bupivacaine	2.5–3.0 mg/kg	2.5–3.0 mg/kg

* Note of caution: These data are based on toxicity in animals and how well the information translates to humans receiving nerve blocks under usual clinical circumstances is uncertain. Indeed, peak plasma levels of local anesthetic in actual clinical practice correlate poorly with patient weight or body mass index. Combinations of local anesthetics produce additive toxicity.

recommended maximal dose of local anesthetic for major regional blocks.

A second key concept is that with some local anesthetics (such as lidocaine or mepivacaine), systemic toxicity progresses in a stepwise fashion from CNS to cardiovascular manifestations. Conversely, potent local anesthetics (racemic bupivacaine) can nearly simultaneously progress from CNS signs to cardiovascular collapse.

Figure 2-6 illustrates the typical progression of symptoms with lidocaine. Patients must be closely observed and actively questioned about the occurrence of these symptoms during and following a regional anesthetic injection. Depending on the site of injection, systemic toxicity signs may present immediately (after intravascular injection) or up to several hours later (after subcutaneous injection as occurs with plastic surgery tumescence techniques). Recognition of symptoms that

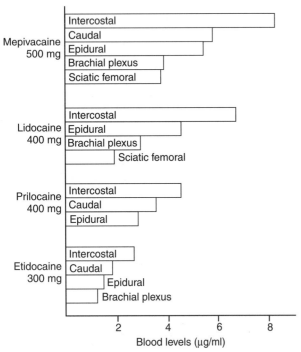

Figure 2-5   Local anesthetic peak plasma concentrations as a function of regional technique. (Redrawn from Stoelting RK, Miller RD: *Basics of Anesthesia*, Fourth Edition, Churchill-Livingstone, Philadelphia, 2000, p. 85, Fig. 7-6.)

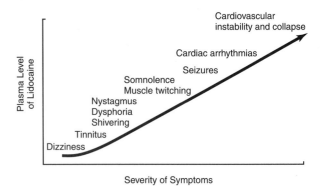

Figure 2-6   Patient symptoms with progressive rise in lidocaine plasma levels. (Note: This progression of symptoms may not apply to drugs like bupivacaine where cardiovascular instability and collapse may present without the appearance of any other signs or symptoms of intravascular injection.)

occur at lower serum levels of local anesthetic (tinnitus, circumoral numbness, subjective feeling of doom) should cause the anesthesiologist to cease the local anesthetic injection immediately. Patients who are heavily sedated will not be able to provide this valuable information, and indeed even mild sedation can interfere with the appreciation of a local anesthetic test dose, with or without epinephrine.

Management of Seizures

Prevention strategies center on limiting the total local anesthetic dose, avoiding intravascular injection by attempting to aspirate blood from the block needle prior to injection and again several times during the block, and fractionated administration of local anesthetic while closely observing and questioning the patient for any symptoms of local anesthetic toxicity.

Should a seizure occur, treatment priorities include maintenance of oxygenation and ventilation, and termination of the seizure. Usually a small dose of thiopental (50 mg) will terminate the seizure, while 100% O_2-bag-mask ventilation will maintain respiratory support. Intubation is rarely necessary because most local anesthetic-induced seizures are self-limited.

Systemic Cardiovascular Toxicity

Although most local anesthetics exhibit antiarrhythmic effects, bupivacaine, ropivacaine, and etidocaine have proarrhythmic potential. Numerous electrophysiologic effects have been noted, manifesting as prolonged PR and QT intervals, prolonged QRS complex, AV block, ventricular tachycardia, and ventricular fibrillation (Fig. 2-7). The exact mechanism of these effects is not clear, but probably involves local anesthetic binding to cardiac conduction system sodium channels. Bupivacaine avidly binds to sodium channels in the cardiac conduction system, but dissociates from these channels slowly ("fast-in, slow-out"). This is in contrast to lidocaine, which rapidly binds to cardiac conduction system proteins, but then dissociates quickly ("fast-in, fast-out"). Because sodium channels remain blocked by bupivacaine, it is difficult to escape aberrant rhythms and reestablish normal electrophysiologic conditions within the cardiac conduction system. Quantitatively, the binding of bupivacaine to cardiac conduction system sodium channels is approximately 1000% longer than lidocaine, which explains in part why bupivacaine is 9 times more cardiotoxic than lidocaine. Ropivacaine and *l*-bupivacaine appear to have substantially less cardiotoxicity compared to bupivacaine, but are still 4 to 5 times more cardiotoxic than lidocaine.

In general, there is a clear stepwise progression in symptoms of local anesthetic toxicity as free (not protein bound) local anesthetic serum levels rise (see Fig. 2-6 on p. 22). However, sudden bupivacaine cardiotoxicity is reported to occur without prior symptoms, probably related to the high serum protein and pulmonary glycoprotein binding of bupivacaine. As bupivacaine initially enters the systemic circulation, these proteins are protective against the cardiac toxicity of "free" (unbound) bupivacaine, but once these protein-binding sites are saturated, additional bupivacaine rapidly results in toxicity. Indeed, bupivacaine toxicity often presents as simultaneous neurotoxicity (seizures) and cardiotoxicity. Once bupivacaine is avidly bound to the cardiac conduction system, ventricular fibrillation and high-grade conduction block results. Resuscitation has been very difficult to achieve (approximately 70% mortality, half of survivors with long-term disability) (Box 2-3).

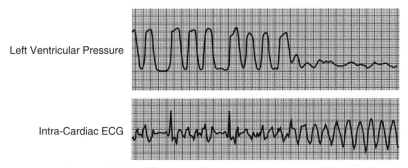

Left Ventricular Pressure

Intra-Cardiac ECG

Figure 2-7   Cardiac toxicity of bupivacaine. A rapid intravenous bolus of 150 mg of bupivacaine resulted in a fatal rapid decrease in left ventricular pressure (catheter tip transducer). Also ECG changed from a normal intracardiac quadripolar ECG pattern to that of ventricular tachycardia and subsequent ventricular fibrillation. (Redrawn from Nancarrow C: Acute toxicity of lignocaine and bupivacaine, PhD thesis, Flinders University of Southern Australia, 1986.)

Clinical Caveat: An Anesthesiologist's Nightmare

An epidural catheter in a term parturient in preparation for cesarean delivery. After receiving her fourth 5 mL bolus of 0.5% bupivacaine, the patient rapidly becomes agitated, and simultaneously suffers a seizure and ventricular fibrillation.

CPR is immediately begun with left uterine displacement. The patient receives 100 mg of IV succinylcholine and is rapidly intubated. Defibrillation and intravenous epinephrine are ineffective.

Emergency cesarean delivery is begun approximately 3.5 minutes after the onset of cardiac arrest. After receiving amrinone, defibrillation is successful. Fortunately, recovery of mother and neonate is complete.

Clinical Caveat: Avoiding Local Anesthetic Toxicity

The prudent anesthesiologist must be constantly aware of the risks of local anesthetic toxicity, and integrate multiple safety measures into his/her clinical practice. These include:

- Use of techniques that lessen the likelihood of intravascular injection of local anesthetic
- Aspiration of the needle before local anesthetic injection
- Giving small, fractionated doses of local anesthetic, and inquiring about symptoms that might reflect early CNS toxicity
- Be aware of recommended maximal local anesthetic dose, particularly with nerve blocks that result in high serum levels of local anesthetic
- Consider the addition of epinephrine to the local anesthetic: tachycardia suggests intravascular injection. In addition, epinephrine decreases systemic absorption of local anesthetics, resulting in lower serum blood levels
- Especially with large masses of local anesthetics delivered to highly vascular regions or for blocks with an increased risk of intravascular injection, consider using less cardiotoxic drugs, such as ropivacaine or *l*-bupivacaine
- Always have resuscitation equipment available
- Realize that sedation may lower seizure threshold, but it also attenuates the patient's ability to report symptoms of local anesthetic toxicity

Box 2-3   What Do I Do When I Suspect Systemic Local Anesthetic Toxicity?

Secure the airway and hyperventilate with 100% O_2. Acidosis worsens local anesthetic cardiotoxicity

Begin CPR. If the patient is pregnant with gestational age >24 weeks, emergency abdominal delivery is indicated. Abdominal delivery can be lifesaving for both the mother and baby: delivery relieves vena caval compression for the mother, and in-utero fetal blood flow is minimal during CPR, especially following intravenous epinephrine boluses

Amrinone (or milrinone), bretylium, and multiple doses of epinephrine have been associated with improved outcomes in animal models of bupivacaine cardiotoxicity. Bretlylium is no longer available, and it is unclear if amiodarone would achieve the same results

If available, initiation of femoral vein–femoral artery cardiopulmonary bypass has been lifesaving in a few case reports

CONCLUSIONS

With a thorough understanding of local anesthetic pharmacology, an anesthesiologist can rationally choose pharmacologic agents that are suited to particular surgical or obstetric objectives. Toxic reactions can be better prevented and treated with an in-depth knowledge of local anesthetic toxicology.

SUGGESTED READING

Benumof JL, Saidman LJ: *Anesthesia and Perioperative Complications*, Mosby, St. Louis, 1999.

Brown DL: *Atlas of Regional Anesthesia*, Second Edition, WB Saunders, Philadelphia, 1999.

Chestnut DH: *Obstetric Anesthesia: Principles and Practice*, Second Edition, Mosby, St. Louis, 2001.

Gabbe SG, Niebyl JR, Simpson JL: *Obstetrics: Normal and Problem Pregnancies*, Third Edition, Churchill Livingstone, New York, 1996.

Hahn MB, McQuillan PM, Sheplock GJ: *Regional Anesthesia: An Atlas of Anatomy and Techniques*, Mosby, St. Louis, 1996.

Stoelting RK, Miller RD: *Basics of Anesthesia*, Fourth Edition, Churchill Livingstone, Philadelphia, 2000.

CHAPTER 3

Local Anesthetic Additives

JOSEPH M. NEAL

INTRODUCTION

Additives enhance local anesthetic actions by prolonging block duration, limiting systemic uptake, acting as markers of intravascular injection, and improving anesthesia and analgesia. Some additives, such as epinephrine and clonidine, are capable of providing several of these actions, whereas others offer only a single benefit. Practitioners need to understand the pharmacology of local anesthetic additives and how their effects differ depending on the regional block procedure selected. Whether the additive is used centrally or peripherally also affects its side effect and complication profile. Besides pharmacologic effects, some additives are used to preserve or formulate local anesthetics. This chapter examines commonly used local anesthetic additives with emphasis on how they act centrally and peripherally. The neurotoxic profile of additives and preservatives is also discussed.

EPINEPHRINE

Since the early 1900s, epinephrine has been the most widely used local anesthetic additive. This versatile agent prolongs anesthesia and analgesia, increases block intensity, limits peak local anesthetic plasma concentrations (Fig. 3-1 on p. 26), acts as a test dose, and provides independent anesthesia and analgesia via α_2-adrenergic stimulation at the spinal cord (Box 3-1). Despite this plethora of desirable effects, epinephrine also causes side effects.

Neuraxial Effects

When deposited around the central neuraxis, epinephrine prolongs local anesthetic duration and intensifies its effects by causing vasoconstriction and stimulating spinal receptors. Vasoconstriction reduces clearance of local anesthetic from the subarachnoid and epidural spaces, thus prolonging spinal nerve root exposure to a higher local anesthetic concentration. Direct anesthesia and analgesia also occurs as a consequence of epinephrine's α_2-adrenergic agonist effects on the spinal cord. Subarachnoid epinephrine is historically delivered as a 200 μg dose, although doses as small as 50 μg are effective. Epidural epinephrine is usually administered as a 5 μg/mL dose, which also serves as an intravenous test dose. Although epinephrine increases the duration of all local anesthetics, it is most effective when combined with intermediate-acting, lipophobic agents such as lidocaine or mepivacaine, rather than bupivacaine and ropivacaine. This phenomenon occurs as a consequence of epinephrine's lipophobic properties and the already prolonged duration profile of bupivacaine and ropivacaine.

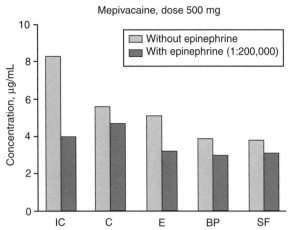

Mepivacaine, dose 500 mg

Figure 3-1   The effect of epinephrine on mean peak plasma concentrations of mepivacaine. Note that the magnitude of epinephrine's effects is largely determined by the site of injection. IC = intercostal; C = caudal; E = epidural, BP = brachial plexus; SF = sciatic and femoral. (Redrawn from Veering BT: Local anesthetics. In: Brown DL (ed), *Regional Anesthesia and Analgesia*, WB Saunders, Philadelphia, 1996, p. 193.)

Clinical Caveat: Epinephrine

Effective subarachnoid doses range from 50 to 200 μg
Effective epidural doses range from 1:500,000 to
    1:200,000 concentration (2-5 μg/mL)
Effective peripheral nerve doses range from 1:400,000
    to 1:200,000 (2.5-5 μg/mL)
Additive epinephrine is more effective with intermediate-acting, lipophobic rather than long-acting local anesthetics

Current Controversy: Epinephrine

Widespread clinical experience attests to the safety
    of adjuvant epinephrine in normal patients
In theory, however, epinephrine may exacerbate local
    anesthetic-induced neurotoxicity in the setting of:
    Altered spinal cord autoregulation
    Spinal or peripheral nerve trauma
    Vascular injury from diabetes or chemotherapy

Neuraxial epinephrine's side effects are both predictable and counterintuitive. Systemic vascular uptake of spinal epinephrine results in increased cardiac output and decreased peripheral resistance, primarily the result of its β2-adrenergic agonist actions. Particularly when given subarachnoid, epinephrine interferes with bladder

Box 3-1   Mechanism of Action: Additive Epinephrine

α1-adrenergic stimulation
    (vasoconstriction reduces local anesthetic clearance)
    Prolongs anesthesia and analgesia
    Increases block intensity
    Limits peak plasma concentration
α2-adrenergic stimulation
    Anesthesia and analgesia
β1-adrenergic stimulation
    Intravenous test dose

detrusor mechanisms and prolongs time to micturition. Fentanyl 10–20 μg is a good alternative additive for spinal anesthesia, because it provides similar increased block duration and intensity without prolonging time to void.

Spinal cord ischemia secondary to additive epinephrine is an unfounded myth, which is based on the notion that the extensive spinal vasculature is prone to epinephrine-induced vasoconstriction in the subarachnoid and epidural spaces (Fig. 3-2). However, spinal cord blood flow (SCBF) is highly autoregulated in response to metabolic requirements, and indeed exhibits minimal response to endogenous or exogenous vasoactive agents. Plain

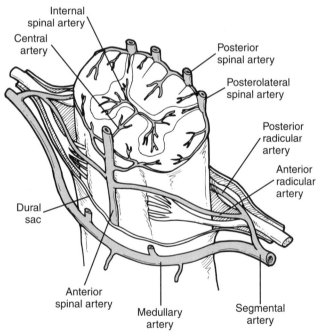

Figure 3-2   Arterial blood supply of the spinal cord. (Redrawn from Bridenbaugh PO, Greene NM, Brull SJ: Spinal (subarachnoid) neural blockade. In: Cousins MJ, Bridenbaugh PO (eds), *Neural Blockade in Clinical Anesthesia and Pain Management*, Third Edition, Lippincott-Raven, Philadelphia, 1998.)

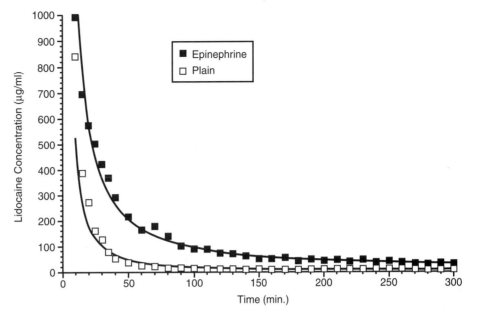

Figure 3-3 Epinephrine's effects on lidocaine concentrations at the superficial peroneal nerve, demonstrating a vasoconstrictive effect with resultant decreased clearance. (Redrawn from Bernards CM, Kopacz DJ: Effect of epinephrine on lidocaine clearance in vivo. A microdialysis study in humans, *Anesthesiology* 91:967, 1999.)

epinephrine has no effect on SCBF. When combined with local anesthetics, epinephrine normalizes the hyperemia induced by lidocaine and tetracaine, and has variable effects when added to bupivacaine. Vasoconstriction is indeed the mechanism for reduced clearance of neuraxial local anesthetics, but occurs in epidural fat and areolar tissues, and in the dura mater vessels, which do not supply the spinal cord. Epinephrine therefore does not adversely affect SCBF in normal patients. It is unclear if epinephrine reduces SCBF in patients with spinal cord injury or compromised blood flow, such as may occur with diabetes, chemotherapy, or atherosclerosis. Nevertheless, a century of use attests to the clinical safety of adjuvant neuraxial epinephrine.

Clincial Caveat: Local Anesthetic and Additive Dosing

1% solution = 1 g solute/100 mL solvent = 10 g/L = 10 mg/mL

1:1 solution = 1 g solute/g (mL) solvent

Thus, 1:1,000 = 1 g/1,000 mL = 1 mg/mL

1:100,000 = 0.01 mg/mL = 10 μg/mL

Peripheral Effects

Epinephrine is added to local anesthetics used for peripheral nerve block, where it increases block duration by 25–100% depending on the site of injection. Prolonged block duration is a direct consequence of reduced local anesthetic clearance at the injection site

(Fig. 3-3). Contrary to the neuraxis, peripheral epinephrine does not have significant α_2-adrenergic agonist effects. Epinephrine is much more effective when deposited at highly vascular sites, such as for intercostal block (Fig. 3-1 on p. 26). Furthermore, its effects are most apparent when combined with intermediate-acting agents, rather than long-acting drugs like bupivacaine, with its inherently prolonged duration.

Peripheral epinephrine has both systemic and local hemodynamic consequences. Systemic uptake of peripheral epinephrine causes tachycardia, which may be significant in patients with coronary artery disease. Epinephrine 1:200,000 (5 μg/mL) is typically used in peripheral blocks, but prolonged duration without tachycardia is possible with 1:400,000 dilution. Peripheral epinephrine significantly reduces peripheral nerve blood flow (PNBF), because extrinsic blood supply to peripheral nerve is under adrenergic control (Fig. 3-4). Indeed,

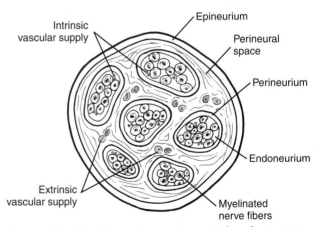

Figure 3-4   Blood supply to the peripheral nerve. The extrinsic vasculature is under adrenergic control. (Redrawn with permission from Mayo Clinic Foundation.)

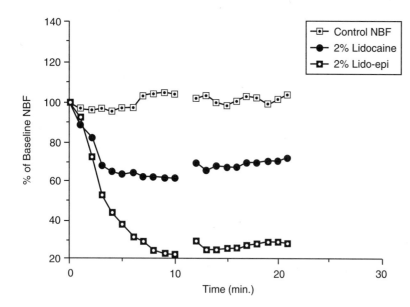

Figure 3-5 Epinephrine 1:200,000 plus 2% lidocaine reduces rat sciatic nerve blood flow (NBF) to 20% of normal. Washout occurs at 10 minutes. (Redrawn from Myers RR, Heckman HM: Effects of local anesthesia on nerve blood flow. Studies using lidocaine with and without epinephrine, *Anesthesiology* 71:760, 1989.)

when combined with 2% lidocaine, epinephrine 5 μg/mL reduces rat sciatic PNBF to 20% of normal (Fig. 3-5). Markedly reduced PNBF is apparently well tolerated in humans, as evidenced by the absence of peripheral nerve injury reported in large series. However, this may not be true if PNBF is compromised secondary to nerve injury (chemotherapy, intraneural injection) or disease processes (diabetes, atherosclerosis), either of which, in the presence of epinephrine, may worsen local anesthetic-induced neurotoxicity. Selecting epinephrine 1:400,000 is perhaps reasonable in these circumstances, because it initially causes PNBF to increase before returning to baseline.

Current Controversy: Epinephrine and Spinal Cord Ischemia

Subarachnoid epinephrine does not decrease spinal cord blood flow (SCBF)

When mixed with local anesthetic, subarachnoid epinephrine either normalizes SCBF or leaves it unchanged

Epinephrine reduces dural blood flow by a vasoconstrictive mechanism, but this does not affect SCBF

CLONIDINE

Clonidine is a selective α_2-adrenergic agonist with central and peripheral sites of action. Clonidine has undergone extensive neurotoxicity studies and is safe in humans. As with epinephrine, its neuraxial effects exhibit

a somewhat different profile as compared to its peripheral effects.

Neuraxial Effects

Clonidine exerts dose-dependent prolongation of neuraxial anesthesia and analgesia. Low-dose subarachnoid clonidine (≤ 100 μg) is equivalent to morphine for postoperative analgesia, yet higher doses are associated with hypotension, sedation, and bradycardia. Both epidural and subarachnoid clonidine produce analgesia for acute postoperative and labor-related pain, but their clinical usefulness is limited by the same side effect profile. Epidural clonidine (plain or with local anesthetic) is beneficial in the treatment of cancer pain, particularly neuropathic pain.

Peripheral Effects

Clonidine is a valuable additive for peripheral nerve block (Box 3-2). It prolongs anesthesia and analgesia as a consequence of peripheral α_2-adrenergic agonist actions and local anesthetic effects on nerve fibers. Block duration is increased in a dose-dependent manner, with 0.5 μg/kg prolonging mepivacaine anesthesia and analgesia by 50% as compared to placebo (Fig. 3-6 on p. 29). Like epinephrine, these effects are more apparent with intermediate-acting than with long-acting local anesthetics. Side effects (hypotension, bradycardia, and sedation) are dose dependent and generally do not occur at doses <1.5 μg/kg, to a maximum dose of 150 μg. Clonidine is not effective as a sole analgesic, does not affect tourniquet pain, and does not alter pain intensity once it occurs.

Clonidine is an effective peripheral additive to mepivacaine at the following doses:

0.1 μg/kg prolongs analgesia

0.5 μg/kg prolongs anesthesia

Side effects are absent at doses <1.5 μg/kg, or a maximum dose of 150 μg

OPIOIDS

Neuraxial adjuvant opioids are discussed in Chapters 9 and 10. Additive opioids for peripheral nerve block are largely without benefit, and their effectiveness for intra-articular application is controversial. Studies that control for systemic effects do not support opioid application for improving peripheral nerve blocks in terms of onset, intensity, or duration. Only the addition of the agonist–antagonist buprenorphine (0.3 mg) has been shown in one study to prolong the analgesic duration of a mepivacaine/tetracaine mixture.

PHENYLEPHRINE

Phenylephrine 5 mg is added to local anesthetics to prolong duration of spinal anesthesia. Its use is less common in modern practice, partially because phenylephrine lacks the significant analgesic effects associated with epinephrine or fentanyl. Furthermore, transient neurologic symptoms occur more frequently when subarachnoid tetracaine is combined with phenylephrine.

NEOSTIGMINE

Peripheral cholinergic stimulation modifies pain transmission; thus anticholinesterase drugs such as neostigmine are logical choices for use as additives. Indeed, neostigmine prolongs subarachnoid block in a dose-dependent fashion. Conversely, it has no beneficial effects when used for brachial plexus block. Because of its association with excessive nausea and vomiting, neostigmine is not an ideal additive for either central or peripheral blocks.

ALKALINIZATION OF LOCAL ANESTHETICS

The pH of a local anesthetic affects its diffusion through the cell membrane and surrounding tissues. In this process, the base (non-ionized) molecules preferentially diffuse across membranes, and once they reach the cytoplasm are converted to the protonated molecule that actually blocks sodium channels (Fig. 2-2 on p. 17). Local anesthetics are formulated at an acidic pH where protonated molecules dominate; thus it is logical that adjusting the pH towards a more alkaline solution with sodium

Figure 3-6   Clonidine added to mepivacaine for axillary block prolongs analgesia duration at 0.1 μg/kg and anesthesia duration at 0.5 μg/kg. (Redrawn from Singelyn FJ, Gouverneur J-M, Robert A: A minimum dose of clonidine added to mepivacaine prolongs the duration of anesthesia and analgesia after axillary brachial plexus block, *Anesth Analg* 83:1049, 1996.)

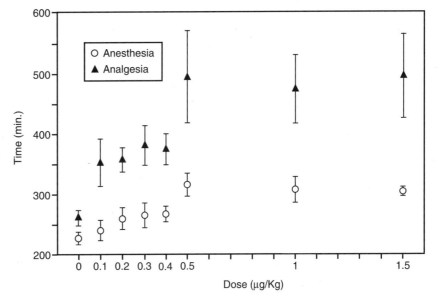

> **Box 3-3 Relative Effectiveness of Alkalinizing Local Anesthetics to Hasten Block Onset**
>
> Alkalinization is much more effective in hastening epidural block onset than it is with peripheral block onset times
>
> Alkalinization of commercially prepared local anesthetic/epinephrine mixtures is much more effective than adding sodium bicarbonate to either plain local anesthetic or freshly mixed local anesthetic/epinephrine combinations

bicarbonate would increase the base form and hasten block onset. The usefulness of this approach is highly dependent upon which regional technique is employed.

Alkalinization of local anesthetics administered into the epidural space hastens block onset by approximately 50% (e.g. 3–5 minutes faster onset for epidural lidocaine). This effect is most obvious when bicarbonate is added to a commercially prepared local anesthetic with epinephrine mixture, and least significant when added to plain local anesthetic (Box 3-3). This phenomenon is explained by the relatively greater change in pH that occurs when the more acidic commercial preparation is adjusted back towards the local anesthetic's pK_a. Clinically significant reduction of block onset time is more difficult to prove with peripheral blocks. Brachial plexus block onset is not hastened by the addition of bicarbonate to plain lidocaine or mepivacaine, or when epinephrine is freshly added to these local anesthetics. When commercial lidocaine with epinephrine is used, alkalinization results in an arguably insignificant reduction of onset time (1–2 minutes). Furthermore, animal models show that alkalinization of plain lidocaine significantly decreases block duration by 50% and intensity by 25%. In general, there is little advantage to admixing sodium bicarbonate with bupivacaine, particularly in the light of its propensity to precipitate with higher volumes of bicarbonate (Table 3-1). Alkalinization has no beneficial effect on block success rate or local anesthetic peak plasma concentration.

Table 3-1 Formula for Alkalinizing Local Anesthetics

Local Anesthetic	Sodium Bicarbonate:Local Anesthetic (mEq:mL)
2-Chloroprocaine	0.33:10
Lidocaine/mepivacaine	1:10
Bupivacaine	0.1:10

ADDITIVES FOR INTRAVENOUS REGIONAL ANESTHESIA

Several additives are beneficial for decreasing intraoperative tourniquet pain or prolonging analgesia after intravenous regional anesthesia (IVRA). Ketorolac 10–20 mg diminishes tourniquet pain and prolongs analgesia, but there have been concerns about associated hematoma formation. Alternatively, clonidine 1 μg/kg prolongs tourniquet tolerance and prolongs postoperative analgesia three-fold. Ketamine 0.1 mg/kg is superior to clonidine for attenuating tourniquet discomfort.

ANTIOXIDANTS, PRESERVATIVES, AND EXCIPIENTS

A variety of agents are added to local anesthetics for preservation, prolonging shelf life, or aiding in formulation. The potential of these agents to cause neurotoxicity has been inconsistently studied. Patient injury is known to occur, particularly when epidurally administered local anesthetics are unintentionally injected subarachnoid. For instance, in the 1980s motor, sensory, and sphincter injury occurred when epidural 2-chloroprocaine was unintentionally injected into the subarachnoid space. The combination of 2-chloroprocaine's antioxidant sodium bisulfite and the formulation's low pH was deemed responsible for these injuries. Some current 2-chloroprocaine formulations share a similar antioxidant profile. Back spasms have also been reported to occur upon the resolution of 2-chloroprocaine epidural block. This condition is not believed to reflect neurotoxicity, but rather is associated with higher doses of the drug and the preservative EDTA. Routinely used preservatives such as benzyl alcohol, benzethonium chloride, and methyl- and propylparaben have been poorly studied in humans. Similarly, the commonly used depot steroid excipient polyethylene glycol appears safe in humans, but has not been formally studied.

SUGGESTED READING

Bernards CM, Kopacz DJ: Effect of epinephrine on lidocaine clearance in vivo: a microdialysis study in humans, *Anesthesiology* 91:962–968, 1999.

Eisenach JC, De Kock M, Klimscha W: Alpha 2-adrenergic agonists for regional anesthesia. A clinical review of clonidine (1984–1995), *Anesthesiology* 85:655–674, 1996.

Hodgson PS, Neal JM, Pollock JE, et al.: The neurotoxicity of drugs given intrathecally (spinal). *Anesth Analg* 88:797–809, 1999.

Kennedy WF, Bonica JJ, Ward RJ, et al.: Cardiorespiratory effects of epinephrine when used in regional anesthesia, *Acta Anaesthesiol Scand* 23:320-333, 1966.

Neal JM, Hebl JR, Gerancher JC, et al.: Brachial plexus anesthesia: essentials of our current understanding, *Reg Anesth Pain Med* 27:402-428, 2002.

Neal JM: Effects of epinephrine in local anesthetics on the central and peripheral nervous systems: neurotoxicity and neural blood flow, *Reg Anesth Pain Med* 28:124-134, 2003.

Singelyn FJ, Gouverneur J-M, Robert A: A minimum dose of clonidine added to mepivacaine prolongs the duration of anesthesia and analgesia after axillary brachial plexus block, *Anesth Analg* 83:1046-1050, 1996.

REGIONAL ANESTHETIC TECHNIQUES

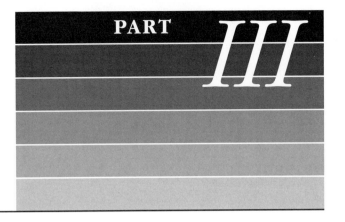

Providing Regional Anesthesia: Monitoring, Sedation, and Equipment

CHRISTOPHER M. VISCOMI

INTRODUCTION

Successful regional anesthesia practice requires adherence to basic safety guidelines and the ability to monitor patients, the provision of adequate sedation, and the availability of proper equipment. Despite the perception of being less risky, regional anesthesia demands the same level of safety precaution as would be afforded a patient undergoing general anesthesia. Further, patient care requires effective monitoring during block placement, as

well as intraoperatively. Even in the most skilled hands, instituting regional anesthesia involves some discomfort to the patient. While there is no substitute for practiced technique, the judicious use of sedation can improve patient comfort during block performance, as well as during the course of lengthy surgical procedures carried out under regional anesthesia. The safe provision of regional anesthesia also requires knowledge of the equipment necessary to perform the block, and to immediately treat any adverse reactions that are associated with block placement, resultant physiologic consequences, or sedation. This chapter addresses the following topics: (1) basic guidelines for the safe provision of regional anesthesia, (2) monitoring requirements during block placement and within the operating room, (3) principles of sedation, (4) equipment - including needles, catheters, and syringes, and (5) adjunctive devices to aid in nerve localization.

GUIDELINES FOR SAFELY PROVIDING AND MONITORING REGIONAL ANESTHESIA

Prior to beginning a regional anesthetic procedure, the anesthesiologist should verify the presence of a signed informed consent (both for surgery and anesthesia), the correct surgical site and sidedness (right versus left), and note any pre-existing neurological or vascular deficits that the patient may have. There must be immediate access to oxygen, suction, resuscitation equipment, and drugs for managing complications. At a minimum, pulse oximetry alone can be used to monitor heart rate and oxygenation during initial block placement. However, the use of more extensive monitoring is advisable whenever large volumes of local anesthetic or the anatomic location of placement make toxicity more likely (Box 4-1). The patient is monitored during the operation just as if

undergoing a general anesthetic, including temperature
monitoring (Box 4-2). Maintaining verbal communication
with a patient allows the anesthesiologist to assess level
of consciousness, appreciate early warning symptoms of
local anesthetic central nervous system (CNS) toxicity,
evaluate paresthesias, and assess other causes of discomfort. Standardized preparation and monitoring are necessary because anesthetic techniques may cause extreme
aberrations, such as total spinal anesthesia or seizures,
and rapid treatment is paramount for favorable outcome.
In addition to monitors and resuscitation equipment, the
following drugs should also be immediately available:

• *Succinylcholine.* Succinylcholine is essential for emergency intubation, as may become necessary with sedative overdose, local anesthetic-induced systemic toxicity
  (seizures or cardiac arrest), or total spinal anesthesia.
• *Atropine.* This anticholinergic agent is necessary for
  treatment of bradycardia secondary to high neuraxial
  block or vasovagal reactions to anesthetic procedures.
• *Thiopental or propofol.* These rapidly acting sedative-
  hypnotic drugs are used to treat local anesthetic-
  induced seizures.
• *Ephedrine.* This vasopressor treats hypotension caused
  by neuraxial anesthesia-induced sympathetic blockade.
• *Naloxone.* This antagonist reverses opioid-induced respiratory depression.
• *Flumazenil.* This antagonist reverses sedation and respiratory depression secondary to benzodiazepines.

SEDATION

Many patients will accept regional anesthesia only
with the proviso that they are comfortably sedated.
Sedative drugs are used to facilitate the placement of
regional anesthetic blocks, ease anxiety, and provide
comfort in the environs of a noisy operating room and
uncomfortable positioning (Box 4-3). Sedation during
block placement ideally provides anxiolysis, but is not so
deep as to obscure the patient's ability to appreciate a
paresthesia or similar warning sign. The anesthesiologist
is always mindful of the effects of over sedation, including respiratory depression and hemodynamic instability.
Ultimately, good sedation during regional anesthesia is an
art. Properly performed, it achieves patient comfort without dangerous blunting of protective airway reflexes. In
so doing, well-administered sedation will facilitate a positive patient experience, even when the regional block is
less than perfect. Commonly used sedative agents include
the following.

Midazolam

Midazolam is a benzodiazepine with effective amnestic
properties. It produces anxiolysis similar to barbiturates
and propofol, primarily via stimulation of central gamma

amino butyric acid (GABA) receptors. Midazolam also raises the seizure threshold, which may prevent or attenuate CNS toxicity following unintentional intravascular injection or high systemic uptake of local anesthetics. The extent to which midazolam or similar drugs are clinically effective in providing this margin of safety against systemic toxicity is uncertain; thus anesthesiologists should not alter local anesthetic dosing when using concomitant benzodiazepines. Like all sedative agents, excess amounts of midazolam can result in hypoventilation (particularly when combined with opioids) or hypotension. Even small amounts of midazolam will blunt the patient's ability to recognize the early symptoms of local anesthetic CNS toxicity, such as tinnitus or circumoral numbness, as would be observed during an epidural test dose. Midazolam is typically administered in intermittent boluses of ~0.02 mg/kg.

Opioids

Analgesia for a regional anesthetic procedure is commonly accomplished by using a short-acting opioid such as fentanyl (50–100 μg IV, ~1 μg/kg). Opioids can also facilitate the positioning of patients with painful injuries or lesions. Fentanyl is preferable to morphine or meperidine because of its faster onset, absence of histamine release, relative hemodynamic stability, and shorter duration of action. The latter characteristic is particularly important in ambulatory patients, for whom avoidance of respiratory depression is crucial. Opioid-induced respiratory depression is dose dependent and synergistic when combined with benzodiazepines. Hypotension and bradycardia are similarly accentuated by the combination of sedative drugs.

Propofol

Propofol is a non-barbiturate sedative-hypnotic that is frequently used as an adjuvant for monitored anesthesia care and regional anesthesia, because it provides reliable and titratable sedation, antiemetic properties, and rapid psychomotor recovery. Propofol primarily acts via the GABA receptor. It is administered either via intermittent 0.1–0.3 mg/kg boluses or as a continuous infusion of 20–100 μg/kg/minute.

Ketamine

Ketamine is an N-methyl-D-aspartate (NMDA) receptor antagonist that produces potent analgesia and dissociative anesthesia with minimal respiratory depression. Dissociative anesthesia refers to a functional disconnection between the thalamus and the limbic cortex, wherein patients appear awake, but are unable to process or respond to sensory input. The disadvantages of keta-mine include sympathetic stimulation (hypertension and tachycardia) and occasional delirium or unpleasant dreams. The latter side effects are largely inconsequential when small doses of ketamine are used and/or combined with benzodiazepines. In clinical use, ketamine is effective in 5–10 mg boluses that are repeated to the desired end point.

REGIONAL ANESTHESIA EQUIPMENT

As regional anesthesia becomes more advanced and specialized, an array of equipment has been developed to facilitate block placement, improve success rates, and reduce complications. This section examines various types of regional anesthesia equipment and the rationale for their development.

Induction Rooms

The provision of regional anesthesia is greatly facilitated by the presence of an induction room in the operating suite. These areas, which can range from a reserved space in the recovery room to a large dedicated room, provide the anesthesiologist with a defined workspace specifically designed for the efficient preoperative placement of peripheral nerve blocks and epidural anesthetics. Indeed, with appropriate care, subarachnoid blocks can also be placed prior to taking the patient into the operating room. Induction rooms also provide an area of privacy for patients that is typically quieter, less rushed, and warmer than an operating room. This ability to evaluate patients, place monitors, and perform regional techniques improves operating room efficiency and overall acceptance of regional anesthesia by surgeons and nursing personnel.

The ideal induction room contains all equipment necessary to perform regional blocks – local anesthetics, adjuvant drugs, and an assortment of needles, catheters, syringes, and block trays for specific procedures. Importantly, the induction room contains full resuscitative equipment and monitoring capabilities. Practices that perform a large volume of regional anesthesia often employ a dedicated induction room nurse who assists with patient preparation and block placement.

Needles

Spinal Needles

There are essentially two spinal needle designs – cutting tip and pencil-point (Fig. 4-1 on p. 38). Cutting needles have a sharp diamond-shaped bevel tip that allows easy insertion through non-osseous tissues. Despite ease of use and low cost, cutting tip needles are

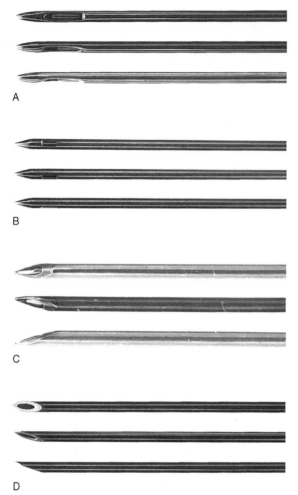

A

B

C

D

Figure 4-1   Frontal, oblique, and lateral views of common spinal needles. A, Sprotte needle. B, Whitacre needle. C, Greene needle. D, Quincke needle. (From Neal JM, McMahon DJ: Equipment. In Brown DL (ed), *Regional Anesthesia and Analgesia*, WB Saunders, Philadelphia, 1996, p. 167. By permission of the Mayo Foundation.)

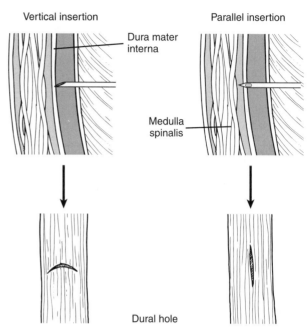

Figure 4-2   Types of needle insertion in lumbar puncture. In vertical insertion, the bevel of the spinal needle is inserted through the dura mater perpendicular, rather than parallel, to the longitudinal dural fibers. It is apparent that the number of fibers severed is greater using vertical insertion. (Redrawn from Raj PP: *Clinical Practice of Regional Anesthesia*, Churchill Livingstone, New York, 1991.)

Current Controversy: Needle Bevel Orientation

Older teachings suggest that orienting a cutting tip spinal or epidural needle parallel to dural fibers will decrease the incidence of PDPH. This admonition presumed that dural fibers coursed in a longitudinal, axial orientation (parallel to the axis of the vertebral spine). Electron microscopic studies have refuted this view of dural fiber orientation, discovering instead that fibers course in multiple longitudinal, transverse, and circumferential directions. Yet despite the dura's complex anatomic orientation, clinical studies still confirm the old adage – parallel oriented bevels result in fewer headaches.

infrequently selected for spinal anesthesia because their associated postdural puncture headache (PDPH) rate is much higher compared with pencil-point needles. Studies suggest that the increased headache rate is because cutting needles lacerate dural fibers during puncture, leaving behind a dural rent (hole). Conversely, pencil-point needles bluntly separate dural fibers, allowing them to re-approximate after needle removal. The degree of dural trauma varies with the orientation of the needle bevel relative to the dural fibers. During dural puncture with a cutting needle, the cutting bevel should be oriented parallel to the dural fibers (parallel to the long axis of the spine). This orientation lacerates fewer dural fibers as compared to a transverse orientation, and clinically results in less frequent PDPH (Fig. 4-2).

The most common cutting needle is the Quincke needle, which was one of the first needles designed for regional anesthesia. Quincke needles are typically reserved for patients over 60 years old, where PDPH risk is very low. There are several types of pencil-point needles (for example, the Whitacre or Sprötte designs) that vary in location and size of the injection port on the distal side of the needle. Among pencil-point needles of the same gauge, there is no difference in success rates or incidence of PDPH.

Cutting and pencil-point needles behave differently during local anesthetic injection. Quincke needles have an

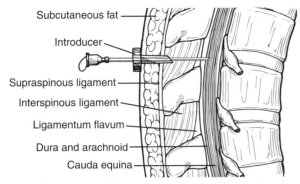

Subcutaneous fat
Introducer
Supraspinous ligament
Interspinous ligament
Ligamentum flavum
Dura and arachnoid
Cauda equina

Figure 4-3   Spinal block using a spinal needle placed through an introducer. (Redrawn from Brown DL: *Atlas of Regional Anesthesia*, Second Edition, WB Saunders, Philadelphia, 1999, p. 323.)

"end hole" that allows the injectate to exit in the same axis as the needle barrel. Dye studies indicate that injected local anesthetic rapidly admixes with CSF and swirls in both a caudal and cranial direction. In contrast, the lateral aperture of pencil-point needles directs the anesthetic at right angles to the needle axis. This characteristic can significantly influence block height and success rate. For instance, orienting the needle aperture cephalad directs local anesthetic – lipophilic opioid mixtures to their spinal cord site of action and improves block success. When unilateral spinal anesthesia is preferred, such as for knee surgery, directing a Whitacre needle aperture laterally towards the operative side improves the success of low-dose isobaric spinal anesthesia. Similarly, for perineal surgery, caudad orientation of a pencil-point needle aperture may aid in limiting spinal anesthesia to the sacral dermatomes.

Introducer needles (Fig. 4-3) are commonly used with smaller gauge (smaller than 24 gauge) spinal needles. With cutting tip needles, tissue resistance against the bevel angle causes the spinal needle to deviate away from the bevel. The use of an introducer needle minimizes this deviation. The blunter tips of pencil-point needles bring about increased resistance to needle advancement through tissues. An introducer needle helps to bypass these areas of resistance and thus aids in placing the spinal needle tip closer to the target site.

Epidural Needles

Epidural needles are specifically designed to identify the epidural space and facilitate the subsequent passage of an epidural catheter. Two main designs are used – the sharper Crawford needle and the curved tip Tuohy or Hustead needles (Fig. 4-4). Crawford needles were designed for paramedian insertion. Using a 45° cephalad and medial trajectory, the bevel of the Crawford epidural needle can be oriented so that it enters the epidural space with the needle bevel parallel to the plane of the dura mater (Fig. 4-5 on p. 40), theoretically reducing the risk of dural puncture. For the midline approach, many anesthesiologists prefer curved tip epidural needles such as the Tuohy or Hustead needles. Their blunt, rounded tip helps prevent tissue plugs from

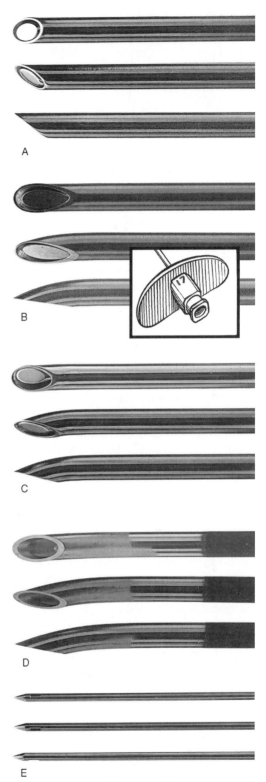

A

B

C

D

E

Figure 4-4   Frontal, oblique, and lateral views of common epidural needles. A, Crawford needle. **B,** Tuohy needle; the inset shows a winged hub assembly common to winged needles. **C,** Hustead needle. **D,** Curved, 18-G epidural needle. **E,** Whitacre 27-G spinal needle. (From Neal JM, McMahon DJ: Equipment. In Brown DL (ed), *Regional Anesthesia and Analgesia*, WB Saunders, Philadelphia, 1996, p. 168. By permission of the Mayo Foundation.)

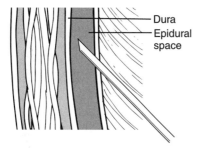

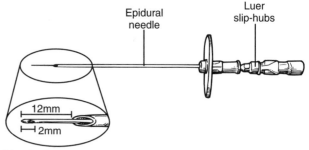

"Needle through needle"

Figure 4-6 Combined spinal and epidural needle as used for the combined spinal–epidural technique. (Redrawn from Bridenbaugh PO, Greene NM, Brull SJ: Spinal (subarachnoid) blockade. In Cousins MJ, Bridenbaugh PO (eds), *Neural Blockade in Clinical Anesthesia and Management of Pain*, Lippincott-Raven, Philadelphia, 1988, pp. 203–242.)

Figure 4-5 Crawford needle shown entering the epidural space with the needle bevel parallel to the plane of the dura mater to reduce the risk of dural puncture.

occluding the epidural needle and interfering with loss-of-resistance. Rounded tips also aid in identification of the ligamentum flavum, because they do not cut through it easily. The rounded needle tips also help to direct the epidural catheter along the axis of the epidural space and away from the dura. Tuohy and Hustead needles also work well for paramedian approaches.

Many epidural needle modifications exist. Fixed or detachable wings near the needle hub aid in gripping the needle. Guiding devices attach to the needle hub to assist with threading a catheter into the epidural needle. Epidural needles also have markings etched along their side to help quantify depth of needle insertion.

Combined Spinal–Epidural Needles

The use of combined spinal–epidural (CSE) analgesia and anesthesia has increased significantly, because it combines the faster onset and better sacral block of spinal anesthesia with the epidural component's ability to provide prolonged analgesia. This technique typically involves placing an epidural needle in the L2–5 region, and then using it as a long "introducer needle" for a spinal needle (Fig. 4-6). After being used for subarachnoid injection, the spinal needle is removed and a catheter is threaded via the epidural needle into the epidural space. Needles used for CSE must be appropri-

ately paired so that the spinal needle protrudes at least 1 cm beyond the tip of the epidural needle, which compensates for "tenting" of the dura as it is pushed away by the spinal needle. One can combine a standard 25–27 gauge 5 inch spinal needle with a $3\frac{1}{2}$ inch epidural needle for this technique, or use specially designed needle sets. One such needle set has a separate "back eye" opening for the spinal needle (Fig. 4-7). Others use a parallel and separate needle barrel for the spinal needle that permits initial placement of an epidural catheter and test dosing prior to initiatin subarachnoid block. Some sets allow locking of the spinal needle to the epidural needle so that both hubs do not have to be held separately. No studies demonstrate the superiority of any particular CSE set.

Peripheral Block Needles

Although significant effort has focused on needle designs that purportedly lower the risk of intraneural injection, there is no credible clinical evidence that needle design has a direct impact on nerve injury (see

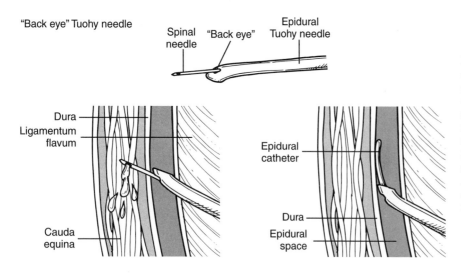

Figure 4-7 Tuohy needle with a "back eye" that permits placement of the spinal needle directly into the subarachnoid space (left panel) and subsequent threading of the epidural catheter into the epidural space following removal of the spinal needle. (Redrawn from Bridenbaugh PO, Greene NM, Brull SJ: Spinal (subarachnoid) blockade. In Cousins MJ, Bridenbaugh PO (eds), *Neural Blockade in Clinical Anesthesia and Management of Pain*, Lippincott-Raven, Philadelphia, 1988, pp. 203–242.)

Chapter 14). A conventional hypodermic needle (Fig. 4-8) has a long, sharp tip with a 14° bevel. The advantage of sharp needles is that they pass smoothly through tissue with relatively less pain. However, some studies suggest that sharp needles more easily impale peripheral nerves than blunt needles. Some clinicians therefore prefer needles with a short, blunt bevel ("B"-bevel). The primary advantage of blunt needles is that the operator can appreciate the "feel" of tissues as they offer resistance to needle passage. Although blunt needles are less likely to penetrate nerves, when they do, they cause more damage which takes longer to heal as compared with using sharp needles. Needle length should be compatible with the expected distance from the skin to the target nerve or plexus. Needles in excess of this length may result in unintentional entry into vascular or neuraxial structures.

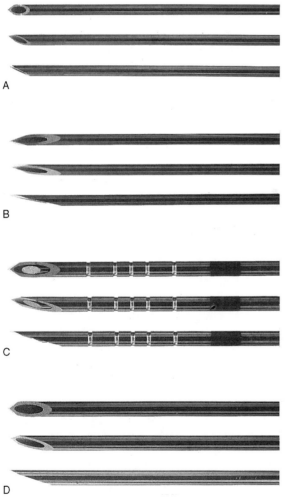

Figure 4-8   Frontal, oblique, and lateral views of regional block needles. A, Blunt-beveled, 25 gauge axillary block needle. **B,** Long-beveled, 25 gauge ("hypodermic") block needle. **C,** Ultrasound "imaging" needle. **D,** Short-beveled, 22 gauge regional block needle. (From Neal JM, McMahon DJ: Equipment. In Brown DL (ed), *Regional Anesthesia and Analgesia,* WB Saunders, Philadelphia, 1996, p. 170. By permission of the Mayo Foundation.)

Needle gauge should balance patient comfort with the ability to aspirate and inject solutions. This balance seems optimal with 22 to 25 gauge needles. For procedures where the target site is distant from the skin (for example, celiac plexus or lumbar sympathetic blocks), larger gauge needles (20-22 gauge) give the operator better control over needle bending and less resistance to injection.

Catheters

Epidural Catheters

An epidural catheter should display high tensile strength and resistance to shearing, be biochemically inert, have depth indicators, and be pliable enough to minimize vascular puncture. Several epidural catheter designs are available. Multiorifice catheters typically have openings in the distal 1.5 cm of the catheter, while single-orifice designs have only a hole at the catheter tip (Fig. 4-9). Many anesthesiologists prefer multiorifice to single-orifice catheters, because the multiorifice design is associated with fewer unilateral blocks and better ability to detect intravascular catheter placement. Metal stylets were previously used to facilitate catheter advancement into the epidural space, but have lost favor because they were associated with a higher rate of cannulation of epidural veins and an increased frequency of paresthesiae.

Peripheral Catheters

Continuous peripheral nerve blocks are accomplished by passing a catheter through a needle and properly situating it near the target neural structure. An insulated regional block needle is often employed to facilitate catheter placement. The insulated needle is attached to a peripheral nerve stimulator to confirm perineural placement of the needle tip (see discussion on the use of the nerve stimulator later in this chapter) and is then followed by blind passage of a non-stimulating catheter alongside the nerve. Recently, electrically insulated nerve stimulating catheters have been developed. They utilize an internal wire that is connected to the nerve stimulator after perineural location of the needle is confirmed. The distal end of the catheter has an external contact point where the current exits the catheter, allowing more precise placement of the catheter next to the target nerve.

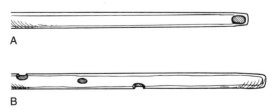

Figure 4-9   Epidural catheter designs. A, Single distal orifice. **B,** Closed tip with multiple side orifices. (Redrawn from Brown DL: *Regional Anesthesia and Analgesia,* WB Saunders, Philadelphia, 1996. By permission of the Mayo Foundation.)

This arrangement promises to increase the success of continuous blockade, although clinical studies have yet to confirm this potential advantage.

Syringes

Well-constructed syringes facilitate both neuraxial and peripheral nerve block procedures. In addition to the epidural needle and catheter, epidural anesthesia requires a reliable loss-of-resistance syringe (see Chapter 9). Commonly made of polished glass, these syringes are now available in a low-friction plastic–Teflon combination. The latter is much less expensive than the older glass varieties and is ideally suited for single-use settings. Low friction between the syringe barrel and plunger is essential so that loss-of-resistance upon entering the epidural space can be optimally appreciated. For peripheral blocks, a three-ring syringe allows the anesthesiologist to aspirate easily on the needle and/or refill the syringe, which enhances one's ability to perform regional anesthesia without an assistant.

Clinical Controversy: Air versus Saline for Epidural Loss-of-Resistance Technique

As a needle is advanced toward the epidural space, the loss-of-resistance technique identifies when the needle tip emerges from the ligamentum flavum. The basics of this technique involve attaching a low-resistance syringe, filled with either normal saline or air, to an epidural needle. Since the ligamentum flavum is a very dense tissue, a needle advancing within it encounters substantial resistance to injection of air or saline. When the needle exits the ligamentum flavum and enters the highly compliant epidural space, injection occurs easily. Anesthesiologists have long debated the superiority of using normal saline or air for loss-of-resistance.

Advantages of using air:
Limitless supply
No foreign particles from opening glass vials
Fluid aspirated from the epidural needle or catheter is likely CSF, rather than saline
Advantages of using saline:
Air injection is associated with patchy blocks
Air injection into the CSF can cause pneumocephalus, which is accompanied by severe headache
A higher rate of intravenous epidural catheter placement occurs with the air technique compared with a saline technique. The explanation for this observation is unclear, but may be due to saline displacing the epidural veins by creating a pocket of fluid that accommodates the epidural catheter before it encounters a vein

Regional Anesthesia Trays

Most contemporary spinal, epidural, and peripheral block procedures involve the use of a block-specific, prefabricated equipment tray. These sterile trays have in common components such as sterile drapes, antiseptic solution, local anesthetic for skin infiltration, and basic syringes and needles. Basic trays are then customized for a specific use. For example, spinal needles and local anesthetic agents are packaged for subarachnoid block trays; and epidural needles, catheters, and loss-of-resistance syringes for epidural trays. Manufacturers frequently customize block trays for individual anesthesiology departments, thus reducing costs by facilitating bulk purchase of custom, yet standardized, regional anesthesia trays.

AIDS TO NERVE LOCALIZATION

Peripheral Nerve Stimulators

Peripheral nerve stimulators (PNS) are valuable adjuncts to block performance, albeit they are not a substitute for anatomic knowledge or meticulous technique. Special stimulating needles have an insulating covering except for the distal 1 mm of the needle tip. The PNS cathode (negative) lead is affixed to the stimulating

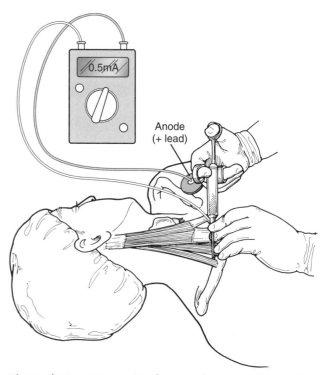

Figure 4-10 Nerve stimulator technique. (Redrawn from Brown DL: *Atlas of Regional Anesthesia*, Second Edition, WB Saunders, Philadelphia, 1999, p. 10.)

needle and the anode (positive) lead is attached to a surface ECG patch away from the limb to be blocked (Fig. 4-10 on p. 42). Applying a 1.5 mA, 2 Hz current to the stimulating needle and seeking an appropriate motor response (muscle twitch) localizes the nerve. Once obtained, the motor response is optimized down to a current of ≤0.5 mA prior to injection of local anesthetic. In theory, this technique affords an objective measure that nerve and needle tip are close together without actually being in contact. However, because paresthesias can occur prior to a motor response, perineural contact is possible before motor neurons are stimulated. This information reinforces the enhanced safety of only performing nerve blocks in patients who are awake or lightly sedated, except under special circumstances (pediatric patients, mentally challenged adults) where the benefits are thought to outweigh the risks. In these cases, frank discussion and thorough documentation are essential risk management strategies.

Ultrasound

Ultrasound can be useful for perivascular nerve blocks, such as femoral or axillary blocks. Whereas nerves are not always as clearly delineated, ultrasound does allow easy localization of arterial and venous structures, thus directing accurate placement of block needles close to these structures and their nerve counterparts. Ultrasound appears to be most useful as a teaching tool or in patients with challenging anatomy (for example, obese patients). There is no evidence that ultrasound improves block success rates or outcomes in normal patients.

Fluoroscopy

Fluoroscopy is routinely performed in pain management to facilitate accurate needle placement. Facet blocks, sympathetic nerve blocks, neurolytic plexus blocks, and diagnostic nerve root injections are commonly placed using fluoroscopic guidance. Based on the knowledge that surface landmarks (such as the iliac crest) do not accurately predict vertebral interspace levels, fluoroscopy improves the accuracy of injectate deposition next to a particular source of neuraxial pathology. Nonetheless, fluoroscopy has not found a routine use in perioperative regional anesthesia, in part because of its requirement for cumbersome and expensive radiographic equipment in poorly shielded induction rooms. While fluoroscopy may help to guide deeper blocks, such as approaches to the sciatic nerve or epidural placement in morbidly obese patients, there is no clinical evidence that its routine use is mandated in these settings. Indeed, some studies have shown routine fluoroscopy not to be of practical benefit in certain circumstances, such as during placement of psoas compartment blocks.

CONCLUSIONS

The safety of regional anesthesia depends on the proper use of appropriate monitors to allow early detection of adverse events like intravascular local anesthetic injection and hypotension accompanying neuraxial blockade. The success of regional techniques requires technical skill and familiarity with the equipment that can best facilitate each technique coupled with the judicious use of sedation to promote patient comfort. This chapter has given a broad overview of how best to combine monitoring, sedation, and regional anesthetic equipment for safety and success.

SUGGESTED READING

American Society of Anesthesiologists: Standards for Basic Anesthetic Monitoring, 2003, Available at http://www.asahq.org/publications And Services/standards/02.pdf#2 (last accessed November 27, 2003).

Brown DL: *Atlas of Regional Anesthesia*, Second Edition, WB Saunders, Philadelphia, 1999.

Hahn MB, McQuillan PM, Sheplock GJ: *Regional Anesthesia: An Atlas of Anatomy and Techniques*, Mosby, St. Louis, 1996.

Neal JM, McMahon D: Equipment. In: Brown DL (ed), *Regional Anesthesia and Analgesia*, WB Saunders, Philadelphia, 1996, pp. 159-175.

CHAPTER 5

Head and Neck Blocks

JAMES P. RATHMELL

INTRODUCTION

Regional anesthetic techniques for the head and neck have a long and successful history. They remain the main-stays for performing ophthalmologic and dental proce-dures. With improvements in availability and safety of general anesthesia, regional techniques have been largely supplanted for many operations on the head and neck. Nonetheless, successful anesthesia and analgesia for a number of procedures can be accomplished with the dili-gent application of these techniques. Because of the close proximity of many nervous and vascular structures in this region, there are a number of complications that are unique to regional anesthesia carried out within the head and neck (Box 5-1). This chapter reviews the anatomy relevant to regional blocks of the head and neck and highlights examples for the use of each technique in cur-rent practice.

TRIGEMINAL (GASSERIAN) GANGLION BLOCK

Clinical uses. Gasserian ganglion block is used almost solely for treatment of trigeminal neuralgia, a common and devastating form of neuropathic facial pain. Patients with trigeminal neuralgia typically present with the spontaneous onset of pain in one or more divisions of the trigeminal nerve. The most common presentation involves both V_2 and V_3; however, any or all divisions may be involved. Patients report paroxysmal lancinating pain in the face that is often severe. The pain usually has a spe-cific area of trigger – pressure on this trigger area elicits the pain. Patients who present with new symptoms sug-gestive of trigeminal neuralgia should undergo a thor-ough neurologic evaluation, including imaging studies to rule out intracranial pathology. The majority of patients with trigeminal neuralgia will respond to oral neuro-pathic medications; carbamezapine remains the agent of choice. Neural blockade is usually reserved for those with trigeminal neuralgia that does not respond to phar-macologic therapy. Local anesthetic block of the trigemi-nal ganglion and its primary divisions is often used as a diagnostic test to predict response to neural blockade prior to proceeding with neurolysis.

Anatomy. The trigeminal nerve, the fifth cranial nerve, supplies the majority of sensory innervation to the face (Fig. 5-1 on p. 45). Preganglionic fibers exit the brainstem and travel anteriorly to synapse with second-order neu-rons within the trigeminal (Gasserian) ganglion. The ganglion lies within the cranial vault at the base of the petrous portion of the temporal bone in a dural invagina-tion containing cerebrospinal fluid known as Meckel's

Box 5-1 Specific Complications Associated with Head and Neck Blocks

Subarachnoid or epidural placement of local anesthetic may lead to high-spinal and brain stem anesthesia

Generalized seizures may occur with the injection of even small intra-arterial volumes of local anesthetic (0.5 mL or less) as the arterial blood flow continues directly from the arteries in the head and neck to the brain

Hematoma formation may lead to airway compromise

Respiratory distress may result from block of the phrenic or recurrent laryngeal nerves, pneumothorax, or loss of sensory or motor function of the nerves to the airway

Rapid and complete absorption of topical anesthetics from the oral mucosa can lead to unexpected systemic toxicity

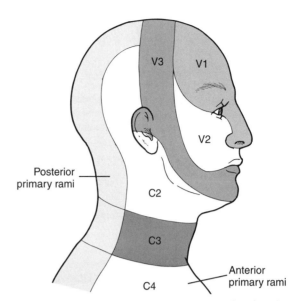

Figure 5-1   Cutaneous innervation of the head and neck. (Redrawn from Cousins MJ, Bridenbaugh PO: *Neural Blockade in Clinical Anesthesia and Management of Pain*, Third Edition, Lippincott-Raven, Philadelphia, 1998, p. 491.)

cave. Postganglionic fibers exit the ganglion to form the ophthalmic (V_1), maxillary (V_2), and mandibular (V_3) nerves. The three divisions of the trigeminal nerve and the functions they serve are detailed in Box 5-2. The first division, the ophthalmic nerve, is discussed in detail in the section below on anesthesia for eye surgery.

The second division of the trigeminal nerve, the maxillary nerve, exits the middle cranial fossa via the foramen rotundum. Outside the cranial vault, the maxillary nerve sends pterygopalatine branches to the pterygopalatine ganglion, zygomatic nerve, and the infraorbital nerve. The pterygopalatine branch supplies the pterygopalatine ganglion which, in turn, supplies sensory branches to the nasal septum, the lateral nasal wall, and the soft and hard palates. The zygomatic nerve supplies sensory innervation surrounding the zygomatic arch (zygomaticotemporal and zygomaticofacial nerves; Fig. 5-2 on p. 46). The infraorbital nerve sends sensory branches to the upper teeth (superior

alveolar nerves) and terminates in a small sensory branch over the maxillary prominence (infraorbital nerve; Fig. 5-2 on p. 46).

The third division of the trigeminal nerve, the mandibular nerve, exits the middle cranial fossa via the foramen ovale and divides into anterior and posterior divisions. The anterior division supplies motor innervation to the masseter muscle and other muscles involved in mastication and a small terminal sensory branch to the cheek (the buccal nerve; Fig. 5-2 on p. 46). The posterior division divides into the auriculotemporal nerve (cutaneous sensation in front of the ear; Fig. 5-2 on p. 46), the lingual nerve (sensation to the tongue), and the inferior alveolar nerve (sensation to the lower teeth). The inferior alveolar nerve terminates in

Box 5-2 The Trigeminal Nerve and its Branches

		DIVISIONS	
	OPHTHALMIC (V_1)	**MAXILLARY (V_2)**	**MANDIBULAR (V_3)**
Function	Sensory	Sensory	Sensory; motor: muscles of mastication
Route of exit from the skull	Superior orbital fissure	Foramen rotundum	Foramen ovale
Terminal branches	Nasociliary, lacrimal, frontal (supraorbital; supratrochlear)	Zygomatic, infraorbital, superior alveolar, sphenopalatine	Inferior alveolar (mental), anterior branch (motor), lingual, posterior branch (auriculotemporal, buccal)
Cutaneous distribution	Eye, forehead	Midface, upper jaw	Lower jaw

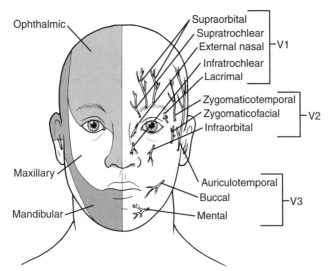

Figure 5-2   Cutaneous innervation of the face. (Redrawn from Cousins MJ, Bridenbaugh PO: *Neural Blockade in Clinical Anesthesia and Management of Pain,* Third Edition, Lippincott-Raven, Philadelphia, 1998, p. 491.)

a small cutaneous nerve supplying sensation to the chin (the mental nerve; Fig. 5-2).

The anatomy relevant to individual regional techniques is reviewed along with each technique in the sections that follow.

Block technique. Block of the Gasserian ganglion is performed with the patient in the supine position. Location of the foramen ovale is facilitated by the use of fluoroscopic guidance. When fluoroscopy is used, the c-arm is angled so that the axis of the x-ray beam is aligned to reveal the foramen ovale (oblique and caudal angulation). A skin wheal of local anesthetic is raised 2–3 cm lateral to the corner of the mouth and a 22 gauge, 10 cm spinal needle is advanced upward toward the mandibular condyle in a plane in line with the pupil (Fig. 5-3). The surface of the greater wing of the sphenoid bone is typically contacted at a depth of 4–6 cm and the needle is withdrawn and redirected in a more posterior direction until the foramen ovale is entered. Once the needle enters the foramen, it is advanced

an additional 1–1.5 cm. As the foramen is entered, a paresthesia in the mandible is usually elicited. As the advancement continues, paresthesiae in the maxilla and orbit are also typically reported. An injection volume of 1.0 mL is usually sufficient to produce dense analgesia. Paresthesiae in the effected division is sought to guide needle placement prior to neurolysis.

Complications. Complications associated with local anesthetic block of the trigeminal ganglion include direct intravascular injection into the carotid artery, persistent paresthesia, and total spinal anesthesia due to local anesthetic deposition within the cerebrospinal fluid over the ventral surface of the brainstem. Complications associated with neurolysis are more common. Facial numbness occurs in nearly all patients, and may be profound. Other complications include anesthesia dolorosa (pain and numbness), reduced corneal reflex, abolition of the corneal reflex, keratitis, and masticatory weakness. Percutaneous trigeminal neurolysis (using either glycerol or radio frequency lesioning) remains an effective, minimally invasive treatment for patients with trigeminal neuralgia.

REGIONAL ANESTHESIA FOR EYE SURGERY

Clinical use. Ophthalmologic surgery has changed dramatically in recent years. The most common method for removal of cataracts is now through a small self-sealing incision using phacoemulsification. It is no longer essential to ensure complete akinesia and methods for peribulbar and topical anesthesia that do not result in paralysis of the extraocular muscles have evolved. Self-sealing incisions have also reduced the need for maintaining very low intraocular pressures.

Anatomy. Regional anesthesia for the eye, orbit, and periorbital structures requires a detailed knowledge of the innervation of these structures, which are largely supplied by the first division of the trigeminal nerve and its terminal branches. The face is innervated primarily by terminal branches of the trigeminal nerve and the

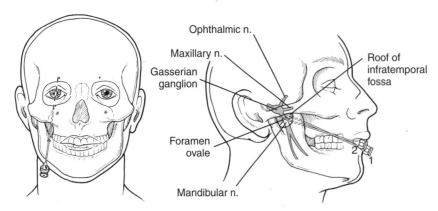

Figure 5-3   Trigeminal (Gasserian) ganglion block. The needle is placed through the skin 2–3 cm lateral to the lateral margin of the mouth and advanced toward the mandibular condyle and toward the ipsilateral pupil until bone is contacted (1). The needle is then withdrawn and redirected more posteriorly until the foramen ovale is entered (2). (Redrawn from Brown DL: *Regional Anesthesia and Analgesia,* WB Saunders, Philadelphia, 1996, p. 242.)

anterior primary division of the second cervical nerve (Fig. 5-1 on p. 45). The first division of the trigeminal nerve (cranial nerve V_1 or the ophthalmic nerve) supplies the forehead, eyebrow, upper eyelid, and the nose. The ophthalmic nerve traverses anteriorly through the superior orbital fissure and enters the orbit to supply the orbital contents and sensory branches to the ethmoid sinuses. The ophthalmic nerve ramifies into numerous peripheral branches that supply the face (supratrochlear, supraorbital, infratrochlear, external nasal, and lacrimal nerves) (Fig. 5-2 on p. 46). The intraorbital branches and the terminal branches are blocked by retrobulbar (peribulbar) block performed for ophthalmologic surgery.

Topical Anesthesia

Technique. The most commonly used topical anesthetic for corneal surgery is 0.4% oxybuprocaine due to its intermediate duration of action (30 minutes) and low corneal toxicity. Tetracaine (0.5%) and amethocaine (1%) are also used often, but their duration of action is brief (20 minutes). Lidocaine (4%) and bupivacaine (0.75%) have longer duration (45 minutes), but have been associated with corneal toxicity. The aim of topical anesthesia is to block the nerves that supply the superficial cornea and conjunctiva: the long and short ciliary, nasociliary, and lacrimal nerves. The application is simple, but the patient should be warned that application of the drops onto the surface of the cornea will sting. Visual perception is maintained.

Complications. There have been no reported side effects associated directly with topical application of local anesthetic solutions prepared for ophthalmic surgery. High concentrations of local anesthetic can lead to direct cellular damage of the corneal epithelium.

Intraocular Lidocaine

Technique. Recently, the use of preservative-free lidocaine (0.3 mL of a 1%, isobaric solution) injected into the anterior chamber has been advocated. Use of this technique results in complete anesthesia within 10 seconds and often obviates the need for any supplemental intravenous sedation. It also preserves the ability of the patient to cooperate during surgery.

Complications. Lidocaine can cause transient retinal toxicity if the posterior capsule is not intact and the agent is injected toward the posterior aspect of the anterior chamber of the eye.

Retrobulbar Block

Technique. The aim of this technique is to block the branches of the oculomotor nerve before they enter the

four rectus muscles in the posterior intraconal space. Some activity often remains in the superior oblique muscle due to the extraconal course of the abducens nerve. The patient is asked to rest the eye in the position of primary gaze. This positions the optic nerve directly behind the globe and toward the medial side of the midsagittal plane, out of the path of the advancing needle. The site of injection is just above the inferior orbital rim midway between the lateral canthus and the lateral limbus (the lateral most extent of the cornea where it joins the conjunctiva). A 25 or 27 gauge needle not more than 31 mm in length is used to avoid puncturing the optic nerve. A sharp needle is typically used as it is less painful and results in less tissue distortion. With the globe in the position of primary gaze, the lower eyelid is pulled down and the needle placed just over the lateral, inferior orbital rim halfway between the lateral canthus and the lateral limbus (Fig. 5-4). The needle is passed posteriorly in a plane parallel to the plane of the orbital floor until the tip is past the equator of the globe (Fig. 5-5 on p. 48). The needle is then directed slightly upward and medially so that it approaches, but does not cross, the midsagittal plane of the globe. When the hub of the needle reaches the plane of the iris, the needle tip should be within the intraconal space, 4-5 mm behind the globe. After aspiration, 2-4 mL of local anesthetic solution is injected. Common local anesthetic combinations include 0.5-0.75% bupivacaine mixed 1:1 with 2% lidocaine and containing 150 IU of hyaluronidase. Hyaluronidase is thought to break down connective tissue, allowing the local anesthetic to permeate into the tissues more effectively; its use reduces the volume of local anesthetic required and speeds the

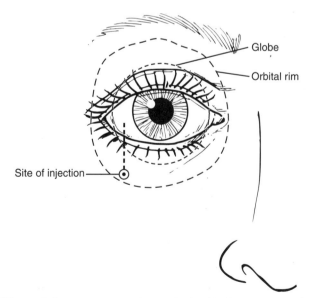

Figure 5-4 Injection site for retrobulbar block lies just over the inferior orbital rim halfway between the lateral canthus and the limbus (Redrawn from Sanderson Grizzard W: *Ann Ophthalmol* 21:265–294, 1989.)

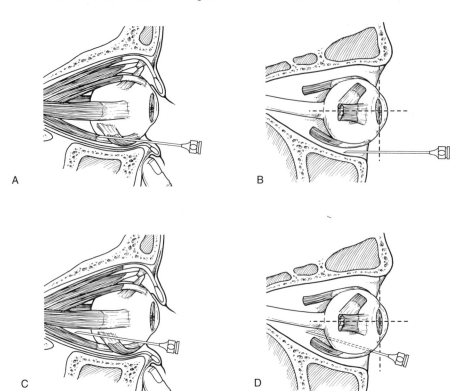

Figure 5-5   Retrobulbar block. A, Sagittal view demonstrating initial needle entry over the inferior orbital rim in a plane parallel to the orbital floor (approximately 10 degrees from the horizontal plane). **B**, Axial view from above demonstrating initial needle entry lateral to the globe and directly posterior until the needle is advanced beyond the equator of the globe. **C**, Sagittal view demonstrating final needle position within the muscle cone behind the globe. **D**, Axial view from above demonstrating final needle position within the muscle cone behind the globe. (Redrawn from Hamilton RC: *Br J Anaesth* 75:88–92, 1995.)

onset of anesthesia. Retrobulbar block produces excellent anesthesia with akinesia; the majority of patients will lose visual perception during the duration of the block.

Complications. Complications occur in 1% or less of cases and include retrobulbar hemorrhage, ocular perforation, subarachnoid and intradural injection with resultant generalized seizure, optic nerve contusion, and retinal vascular occlusion.

Peribulbar Block

Technique. The principle of this technique is to instill the local anesthetic outside of the muscle cone, thus avoiding proximity to the optic nerve. As compared with retrobulbar block, larger volumes of local anesthetic are required, onset of anesthesia is slower, and the quality of resultant anesthesia is less assured. Complete paralysis of the extraocular muscles is not assured with this technique. A 25 or 27 gauge needle 25 mm in length is used. The insertion site is identical to that for retrobulbar block (Fig. 5-4 on p. 47). The needle is advanced over the inferior orbital rim parallel to the orbital floor and 5–7 mL of local anesthetic is deposited at a depth of 25 mm (Fig. 5-6 on p. 49). After 5 minutes, the amount of akinesia is assessed. Often a second injection is required to obtain paralysis of the superior oblique muscle. A 25 gauge 25 mm needle is inserted between the medial canthus and the caruncle (Fig. 5-7 on p. 50) and directed immediately posteriorly. At a depth of 1.5 cm, an additional 5 mL of local anesthetic

solution is deposited. The same local anesthetic solutions employed for retrobulbar block are used.

Complications. The risks of complications associated with peribulbar block are similar to those for retrobulbar block, but are lower because attempts are made to avoid penetrating the muscle cone. Ptosis occurs in about 5% of patients with both retrobulbar and peribulbar blocks and may persist for up to 90 days (Box 5-3).

REGIONAL ANESTHESIA FOR INTRAORAL SURGERY

Clinical use. Regional anesthetic techniques using local anesthesia are the primary method of pain control for intraoral dental procedures. Injections within the oral cavity can be used to anesthetize the maxillary and mandibular nerves and their major divisions with the exception of the auriculotemporal branch of the mandibular nerve. Local anesthetics for use in dentistry are typically supplied in stable, epinephrine-containing solutions in pre-filled cartridges containing 2 or 3 mL. Epinephrine produces vasoconstriction and significantly prolongs the duration of the local anesthetic effect. Intravascular injection of epinephrine and the resultant tachycardia ("palpitations") is the most common adverse reaction resulting from regional anesthesia for dentistry. This adverse reaction is among the most common problems identified by patients coming for surgery as an "allergy" to local anesthetic.

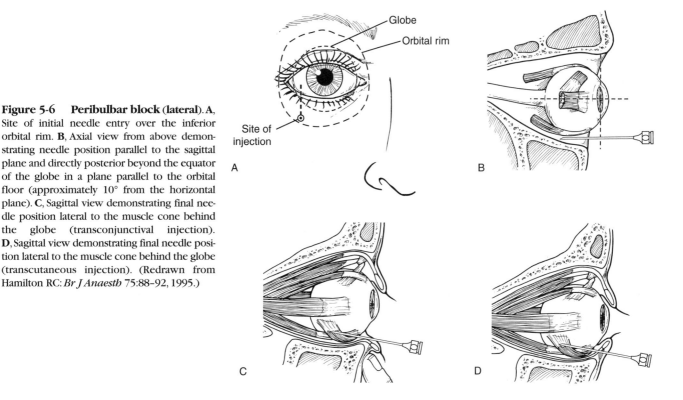

Figure 5-6 **Peribulbar block** (lateral). **A,** Site of initial needle entry over the inferior orbital rim. **B,** Axial view from above demonstrating needle position parallel to the sagittal plane and directly posterior beyond the equator of the globe in a plane parallel to the orbital floor (approximately 10° from the horizontal plane). **C,** Sagittal view demonstrating final needle position lateral to the muscle cone behind the globe (transconjunctival injection). **D,** Sagittal view demonstrating final needle position lateral to the muscle cone behind the globe (transcutaneous injection). (Redrawn from Hamilton RC: *Br J Anaesth* 75:88–92, 1995.)

Careful questioning about the symptoms that ensued following the injection can usually clarify this mistake and obviate the need to avoid local anesthetics or pursue further testing for allergies.

Clinical Caveat: Does the Patient Who Reports "Allergy to All the Caines" After a Reaction at the Dentist Have a True Local Anesthetic Allergy?

It is not uncommon for a patient arriving in the operating room for an elective surgical procedure to report an allergy to local anesthetics. When questioned further, the majority of these patients can relate enough details about the circumstances surrounding their "allergy" to allow the anesthesiologist to proceed comfortably with the use of local anesthetics. The most common report is that of "palpitations" or a "racing heart" or even a "heavy sensation in my chest" following local anesthetic injection for a dental procedure. The majority of local anesthetic solutions used in dentistry contain epinephrine as a vasoconstrictor to prolong the duration of the block. Intravascular injection of even small quantities of an epinephrine containing solution will result in a predictable rise in heart rate and these associated symptoms. There is no need to avoid local anesthetics after this type of reaction. True allergy to local anesthetics is exceedingly rare and is associated with symptoms typical of other hypersensitivity reactions (pruritic rash, urticaria, and bronchospasm).

Blockade of the Maxillary Nerve and its Terminal Intraoral Branches

Anatomy. The maxillary nerve exits the middle cranial fossa through the foramen rotundum to enter the pterygopalatine fossa. The nerve then divides into several branches (Fig. 5-8 on p. 50): (1) short descending branches that enter the pterygopalatine ganglion and emerge as numerous terminal branches that innervate portions of the ethmoid and sphenoid sinuses, the orbit, the nasal mucosa, and the hard and soft palates; (2) the zygomatic nerve, supplying sensation to the skin over the zygoma and the anterior temporal region; (3) the posterior superior alveolar nerve, supplying the posterior wall of the maxillary sinus and the posterior maxillary alveolar process; and (4) the infraorbital nerve, which supplies sensory innervation to the anterior, upper teeth via the middle and anterior alveolar nerves and sensation to the skin over the inferior orbital rim via its terminal branch.

Technique. Maxillary nerve block anesthetizes the entire maxilla and surrounding structures of the midface on one side. The nerve is anesthetized within the pterygopalatine fossa by inserting a needle through the greater palatine foramen. The foramen is located in the lateral aspect of the posterior hard palate adjacent to the second and third molars (Fig. 5-8 on p. 50) and can be identified by a small depression in the palatal mucosa. After applying topical anesthesia, a small needle is advanced through the foramen in a superior and posterior direction

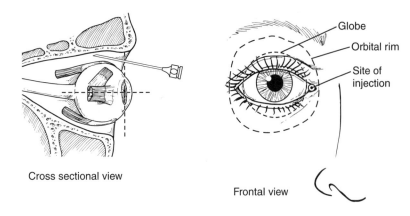

Cross sectional view

Frontal view

Globe
Orbital rim
Site of injection

Figure 5-7 Peribulbar block (medial). The globe is positioned in primary gaze. The needle is placed through the conjunctiva at the extreme medial side of the palpebral fissure. The needle is advanced into the orbit in a plane slightly medial to the sagittal plane and toward the medial orbital wall. (Redrawn from Hamilton RC: *Br J Anaesth* 75:88–92, 1995.)

and a total of 1.5 to 2.0 mL of local anesthetic solution is deposited.

The nasopalatine nerve supplies sensation to the anterior third of the hard palate. The greater palatine nerve innervates the posterior two-thirds (Fig. 5-8). The nasopalatine nerve enters the hard palate through the incisive foramen, located under the incisive papilla (a midline soft tissue prominence of the anterior palate, 5–10 mm posterior to the central incisors). The needle is inserted just lateral to the incisive papilla, 5–10 mm posterior to the central incisors, and advanced until the foramen is entered or bone is contacted. An amount of 0.25 mL of anesthetic solution is deposited. The greater palatine nerve emerges onto the hard palate via the greater palatine foramen. Blockade is best accomplished by injection just anterior to the foramen, unless anesthesia of the soft palate is also required. The needle is advanced just anterior and medial to the third molar and advanced until

bone is contacted and 0.25 to 0.5 mL of local anesthetic is deposited.

Infraorbital Nerve Block

Anatomy. The infraorbital nerve supplies sensation to the skin over the cheek, the lateral surface of the nose, and the upper lip. The nerve emerges from the orbit through the infraorbital foramen located along the infraorbital rim directly inferior to the midpoint of the pupil (Fig. 5-9 on p. 51). The depression surrounding the foramen can be palpated in most individuals.

Technique. The infraorbital nerve can be anesthetized by placing a needle directly in the vicinity of the foramen through the skin. More typical for dental procedures, the needle can be advanced from an intraoral location. The upper lip is retracted and a needle is inserted adjacent to the second premolar and advanced in a superior

Box 5-3 Retrobulbar versus Peribulbar Block

Retrobulbar block produces excellent anesthesia with paralysis of the extraocular muscles and better immobility of the eye during surgery; the majority of patients will lose visual perception during the duration of the block. This technique carries a small but larger risk of hemorrhage, ocular perforation, subarachnoid and intradural injection, generalized seizure, optic nerve contusion, and retinal vascular occlusion than does peribulbar block

Often a second injection is required to obtain paralysis of the superior oblique muscle following peribulbar block via a lateral approach. The risk of complications with this technique is lower as attempts are made to avoid penetrating the muscle cone

Ptosis occurs in about 5% of patients with both retrobulbar and peribulbar blocks and may persist for up to 90 days

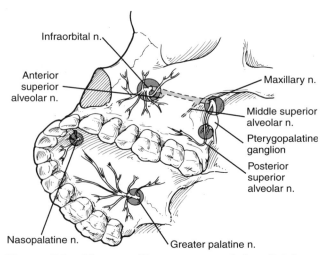

Infraorbital n.
Anterior superior alveolar n.
Maxillary n.
Middle superior alveolar n.
Pterygopalatine ganglion
Posterior superior alveolar n.
Nasopalatine n.
Greater palatine n.

Figure 5-8 The maxillary nerve and its divisions. Shaded areas indicate the typical site for anesthetizing each branch. (Redrawn from Yagiela JA: Regional anesthesia for dental procedures, *Int Anesthesiol Clin* 27:68–82, 1989.)

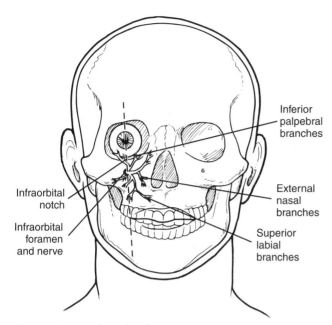

Figure 5-9   Infraorbital nerve. The infraorbital nerve can be anesthetized directly through the skin over where the infraorbital foramen is palpable along the inferior rim of the orbit. This nerve can also be anesthetized using a transoral approach (see further description in the text). (Redrawn from Yagiela JA: Regional anesthesia for dental procedures, *Int Anesthesiol Clin* 27:68–82, 1989.)

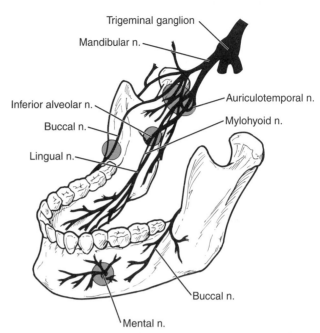

Figure 5-10   The mandibular nerve and its terminal branches. Shaded areas indicate the typical site for anesthetizing each branch. (Redrawn from Yagiela JA: Regional anesthesia for dental procedures, *Int Anesthesiol Clin* 27:68–82, 1989.)

direction until reaching the foramen. A total of 1 mL of local anesthetic solution is used.

Blockade of the Mandibular Nerve and its Terminal Intraoral Branches

Anatomy. The mandibular nerve and its terminal branches can be readily blocked to provide anesthesia for a number of intraoral procedures (Fig. 5-10). The mandibular division of the trigeminal nerve exits the middle cranial fossa via the foramen ovale to enter the infratemporal fossa where it divides into numerous terminal sensory and motor branches. The anterior root gives off several motor branches to the muscles of mastication and terminates in the buccal nerve, supplying sensation to the lateral buccal mucosa overlying the mandible and the gingiva of the mandibular molars. The posterior root gives off three branches. The auriculotemporal nerve traverses laterally behind the mandible to provide sensation to the temporomandibular joint and the skin over the lateral cheek and parts of the external ear. The lingual nerve descends anteriorly to provide sensation to the anterior two-thirds of the tongue, the lingual mucosa, and the floor of the mouth. The inferior alveolar nerve enters the mandible through the mandibular foramen and supplies sensation to the mandible, and the mandibular teeth. The inferior alveolar nerve terminates as the mental nerve, which exits the mandible anteriorly via the mental

foramen to provide sensation to the labial mucosa and the skin of the lower lip and chin.

Technique. The standard method for providing anesthesia for the mandibular teeth and the surrounding bony structures and soft tissue is to deposit local anesthetic adjacent to the inferior alveolar and lingual nerves over the posterior and superior portion of the mandible. The oral mucosa is typically first anesthetized with topical anesthetic. The needle is then inserted over the posterior and superior portion of the mandible, just inferior to the condyle of the mandible and advanced until bone is contacted. A total of 1.5 to 2.0 mL of local anesthetic is deposited and then the needle is withdrawn slightly where an additional 0.5 mL of solution is placed to ensure anesthesia of the lingual nerve, which lies more anterior and medial. The mandibular nerve itself can be anesthetized over the posterior portion of the condyle of the mandible using an intraoral approach. This technique is used less often as it typically results in anesthesia in the auriculotemporal branch of the mandibular nerve (numbness in the lateral cheek and a portion of the pinna of the ear).

OCCIPITAL NERVE BLOCK

Clinical use. Occipital nerve block is most often used in the diagnosis and treatment of occipital neuralgia and cervicogenic headache. True occipital neuralgia typically follows blunt trauma to the nerves over the occiput and is characterized by pain in the distribution of the occipital nerves. Cervicogenic headache is more ill-defined, insidious in onset, and characterized by pain in the same distribution. Many patients with cervicogenic headaches have associated spondylosis of the cervical facet joints. When the pain is limited to the region overlying the occiput, occipital nerve blocks may be of some benefit in reducing the associated pain.

Anatomy. The greater occipital nerve arises from the posterior primary ramus of the second cervical nerve root (Fig. 5-11). It travels deep to the cervical paraspinous musculature and becomes superficial just inferior to the superior nuchal line and lateral to the occipital protuberance of the skull; at this point, the nerve is just lateral to the occipital artery. The lesser occipital nerve and greater auricular nerve are terminal branches of the superficial cervical plexus (see further discussion below). Both arise from the posterior primary ramus of the second and third cervical nerve roots, travel through the cervical paraspinous musculature, and become superficial over the inferior nuchal line of the skull, just superior and medial to the mastoid and just inferior to the tragus of the ear, respectively.

Technique. Occipital nerve block is typically performed with the patient in the sitting position with the head and neck held in the flexed position. The occipital protuberance and mastoid process are identified, and an imaginary line connecting these two landmarks is made. The occipital artery is often palpable about a third of the distance from midline to the mastoid process and is the site of greater occipital nerve block. The lesser occipital nerve is blocked at a distance two-thirds of the way from the mid-

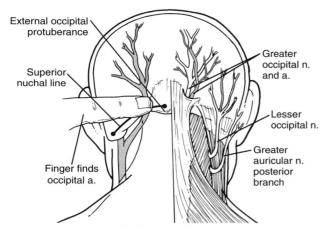

Figure 5-11 Occipital nerve block. The occipital artery is palpated and a skin wheal is raised extending laterally from the site of the artery along a line between the occipital protuberance and the mastoid process. The greater occipital nerve typically lies one-third of the distance from the occipital protuberance to the mastoid while the lesser occipital nerve is more lateral, approximately two-thirds of this distance. (Redrawn from Brown DL: *Atlas of Regional Anesthesia*, Second Edition, WB Saunders, Philadelphia, 1999, p. 145.)

line to the mastoid process along this imaginary line. The block can be carried out using a single skin entry point midway between the mastoid process and the occipital protuberance. An amount of 3 to 5 mL of local anesthetic is infiltrated medially along this line and another 3 to 5 mL laterally along this line. An effective block can also be achieved by using two separate skin entry sites one-third and two-thirds along this line. The local anesthetic is deposited within the skin and subcutaneous tissues in a fanwise fashion to create a subcutaneous wall along the imaginary line. A 25 or 27 gauge $1\frac{1}{2}$ inch needle is used.

Complications. There are few complications associated with occipital nerve blocks. The local anesthetic itself creates a significant mass within the scalp and the patient should be warned that this swelling is normal. Puncture of the occipital artery is not uncommon. Notify the patient that simple pressure should be applied and warn that a painless hematoma may form in this area. Those patients with a history of blunt trauma to the area or prior posterior fossa intracranial surgery may be left with a significant defect in the bony cranium; in such cases, direct entry into the cranial vault may produce total spinal anesthesia.

Case Study: Occipital Neuralgia

A 35-year-old man is struck over the occiput during an altercation. He subsequently develops chronic, intermittent lancinating pains that extend from the occiput toward the vertex associated with sensitivity to light touch (allodynia) in the same distribution. He is referred for diagnostic occipital nerve block for suspected occipital neuralgia.

CERVICAL PLEXUS BLOCK

Clinical uses. Cervical plexus blocks can be used as the sole anesthetic to carry out both superficial and deep operations in the neck and superclavicular fossa. The most common procedure where cervical plexus block is used is for performing carotid endarterectomy.

Anatomy. Cervical plexus block can be divided into superficial and deep techniques. The cervical plexus is comprised of the anterior primary rami of the first through fourth cervical nerves and provides both motor and sensory functions within the neck. The terminal sensory branches emerge in close proximity to one another along the posterior border of the sternocleidomastoid muscle midway between the mastoid process and the clavicle. The terminal branches of the cervical plexus are shown in Fig. 5-12 on p. 53. As described earlier for occipital nerve block, the lesser occipital nerve supplies the scalp over the lateral occiput and the mastoid process, while the greater

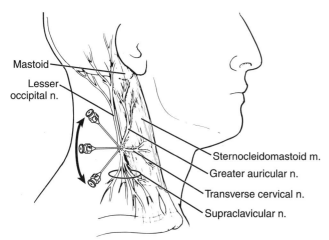

Mastoid
Lesser occipital n.
Sternocleidomastoid m.
Greater auricular n.
Transverse cervical n.
Supraclavicular n.

Figure 5-12   Superficial cervical plexus block. Block of the superficial cervical plexus is performed with a 25 gauge, $1\frac{1}{2}$ inch needle inserted along the posterior border of the sternocleidomastoid midway between the clavicle and the mastoid process. A small volume (2–3 mL) of local anesthetic is placed just deep to the posterior border of the muscle, the needle is then directed superiorly and inferiorly along the posterior border of the muscle and an additional 2–3 mL of local anesthetic is deposited in each direction. (Redrawn from Brown DL: *Atlas of Regional Anesthesia*, Second Edition, WB Saunders, Philadelphia, 1999, p. 185.)

occipital nerve supplies the skin inferior to the external ear. Both have contributions from the second and third cervical nerves. There is no cutaneous sensory innervation provided by C1. Moving inferiorly, the transverse cervical nerve supplies sensation over the midportion of the neck and below the jaw, comprised of primarily fibers from C3. Finally, the supraclavicular nerve, comprised primarily of fibers from C4, supplies the inferior neck and supraclavicular region.

Current Controversies: Is Regional Anesthesia Safer Than General Anesthesia for Carotid Endarterectomy?

There remains no definitive answer to this question; however, there are many vocal advocates for the use of either regional anesthesia or general anesthesia. The primary advantage of regional anesthesia is that it allows repeated neurologic evaluation of the patient during the course of surgery. Regional anesthesia requires a surgeon who is accustomed to operating on the awake, lightly sedated patient. One to three minutes after initial occlusion of the carotid artery, if no neurologic deficit occurs, the surgeon proceeds with endarterectomy. If a new neurologic deficit is detected, the clamp is released and an alternative approach is devised: either through insertion of a shunt or conversion to general anesthesia. The disadvantages of this technique include the need for patient cooperation, loss of patient cooperation if a new deficit appears, panic, seizure, and the inability to control the airway should any of these occur.

Technique. Block of the superficial cervical plexus takes advantage of the close proximity of all of the sensory branches as they emerge from behind the sternocleidomastoid muscle (Fig. 5-12). A 25 gauge, $1\frac{1}{2}$ inch needle is inserted along the posterior border of the sternocleidomastoid midway between the clavicle and the mastoid process. A small volume (2–3 mL) of local anesthetic is placed just deep to the posterior border of the muscle, the needle is then directed superiorly and inferiorly along the posterior border of the muscle and an additional 2–3 mL of local anesthetic is deposited in each direction. Deep cervical plexus block is a paravertebral block of the cervical nerve roots as they emerge from the intervertebral foramina at the C2 through C4 levels. The nerves exit the intervertebral foramina in a somewhat anterior and caudad direction, traversing through a sulcus within the transverse process just posterior to the vertebral artery. Deep cervical plexus block is typically carried out at three discrete levels (Fig. 5-13 on p. 54). A line is drawn connecting the mastoid process with the lateral process of C6 (Chassaignac's tubercle); this will lie just posterior to the posterior border of the sternocleidomastoid muscle. The lateral processes are then palpated, starting with the transverse process of C2 which is located just inferior to the mastoid process. The transverse processes of C3 and C4 lie inferiorly along this line at approximately 1 cm intervals. To perform the block, three separate 22 gauge $1\frac{1}{2}$ inch needles are directed in a somewhat medial, anterior, and caudad direction. Maintaining this direction of advance keeps the plane of the needle out of the plane of the exiting nerve root, and makes direct entry through the intervertebral foramen less likely. The needle is advanced until bone is contacted and 3 to 4 mL of local anesthetic are deposited. The cervical nerve roots are tightly invested within fascia at the level of the transverse processes and lie in close proximity to one another. Injection at a single level is often sufficient to produce a block of the entire cervical plexus.

Complications. Complications associated with superficial cervical plexus block are uncommon as the injection is quite superficial and uses only small volumes of local anesthetic. Direct arterial injection into the carotid artery, which lies just posterior to the sternocleidomastoid muscle, is possible with deep needle penetration. Deep cervical plexus block carries significant risk of direct intra-arterial injection into the vertebral artery, which lies within the bony foramen transversarum of the cervical vertebrae just anterior to the exiting nerve root. Careful aspiration before injection is essential to avoid this complication. Direct intra-arterial injection of even small volumes of local anesthetic (0.1 mL) may produce generalized seizure and even transient blindness following direct delivery of the undiluted anesthetic to the cerebral circulation. The advancing needle may also enter the vertebral canal via the intervertebral foramen leading to epidural or intrathecal placement of the local

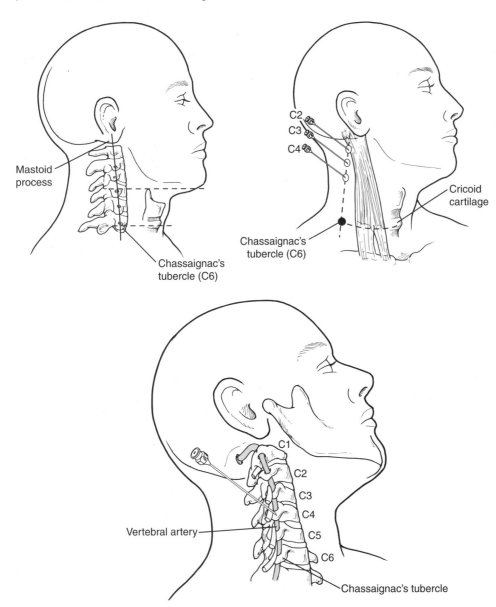

Figure 5-13 Deep cervical plexus block. Deep cervical plexus block is typically carried out at three discrete levels. A line is drawn connecting the mastoid process with the lateral process of C6 (Chassaignac's tubercle); this will lie just posterior to the posterior border of the sternocleidomastoid muscle. The lateral processes are then palpated, starting with the transverse process of C2 which is located just inferior to the mastoid process. The transverse processes of C3 and C4 lie inferiorly along this line at approximately 1 cm intervals. To perform the block, three separate 22 gauge, $1\frac{1}{2}$ inch needles are directed in a somewhat medial, anterior, and caudad direction. The needle is advanced until bone is contacted and 3 to 4 mL of local anesthetic is deposited. (Redrawn from Cousins MJ, Bridenbaugh PO: *Neural Blockade in Clinical Anesthesia and Management of Pain*, Third Edition, Lippincott-Raven, Philadelphia, 1998, p. 508.)

anesthetic and resultant high epidural or total spinal block. Direct injury to the spinal cord has also been reported. Advancing the needle in a plane aiming somewhat anteriorly and caudad keeps the plane of the needle out of the plane of the exiting nerve roots, and makes entry through the foramen less likely. The deep cervical plexus also provides branches to the phrenic nerve, and phrenic nerve paralysis occurs when this block is performed; this leads to unilateral paralysis of the diaphragmatic musculature, thus the block must never be performed bilaterally. Finally, blockade of the sympathetic chain, which lies over the anterolateral margin of the prevertebral fascia, may occur if local anesthetic spreads slightly anteriorly. The deep cervical plexus lies deep to the prevertebral fascia, thus spread anteriorly will occur only if the local anesthetic has been deposited anterior to the prevertebral fascia. This may

also result in block of the recurrent laryngeal nerve and result in hoarseness (Box 5-4).

BLOCKS FOR REGIONAL ANESTHESIA OF THE AIRWAY

Clinical uses. There are many situations when the anesthesiologist is called on to secure an airway in less than ideal circumstances. Expertise with regional anesthesia of the airway allows intubation in awake patients with suspected difficult intubation, upper airway trauma, or cervical spine fractures.

Anatomy. There are three major neural pathways supplying sensation to airway structures (Fig. 5-14 on p. 55). Terminal branches of the ophthalmic and maxillary divisions of the trigeminal nerve supply the nasal cavity

Box 5-4   Complications of Cervical Plexus Block

Superficial cervical plexus block
  Complications are uncommon with superficial
    cervical plexus block as this involves infiltration
    into only the superficial tissues; however, direct
    injection into the underlying carotid artery or
    jugular vein is always a danger when the position
    of the needle tip is not watched closely
Deep cervical plexus block
  Generalized seizures: intra-arterial injection into the
    adjacent carotid or vertebral arteries
  Epidural or spinal anesthesia: needle advancement
    directly through the intervertebral foramen into
    the epidural or subarachnoid space
  Direct trauma to the exiting spinal nerve root or
    the spinal cord
  Dyspnea: local anesthetic spread to the adjacent
    phrenic nerve (diaphragmatic paralysis) or recur-
    rent laryngeal nerve
  Hoarseness: recurrent laryngeal nerve
  Horner's syndrome: ipsilateral miosis, ptosis, and
    anhydrosis due to local anesthetic spread to
    the adjacent sympathetic chain

Case Study: Regional Anesthesia for Awake, Nasotracheal Intubation

A 23-year-old man suffered an acute hyperflexion injury of the cervical spine resulting in bilateral facet dislocation and comes to the operating room for posterior spinal fixation. He remains neurologically intact and is receiving continuous cervical traction to maintain bony alignment of his cervical spine. Because of the instability of his cervical spine, awake nasotracheal intubation is planned prior to induction of general anesthesia. The patient is brought to the operating room and monitors placed; light sedation is administered using fentanyl and midazolam. Topical anesthesia of the nasal cavity is achieved using a cotton swab soaked with 5% lidocaine directed first posteriorly to anesthetize sphenopalatine branches and then superiorly to block the ethmoidal nerve; the swab is left in each position for 1–2 minutes (Fig. 5-15 on p. 56). His tongue is then anesthetized with topical 5% lidocaine spray and a glossopharyngeal nerve block placed bilaterally using a 22 gauge $3\frac{1}{2}$ inch needle to place 5 mL of 2% lidocaine solution submucosally at the caudal aspect of the posterior tonsillar pillar (Fig. 5-17 on p. 57). The superior laryngeal nerve is then blocked bilaterally below the greater cornu of the hyoid bone using a 25 gauge $\frac{3}{4}$ inch needle and 1 mL of 2% lidocaine on each side (Fig. 5-18 on p. 57). Finally, the subglottic structures are anesthetized by placing a 20 gauge styletted Teflon intravenous catheter through the cricothyroid membrane, removing the stylette, and injecting 3 mL of 2% lidocaine directly into the trachea (Fig. 5-19 on p. 58). Nasotracheal intubation using a flexible fiberoptic bronchoscope is carried out with the patient cooperative and responding to commands throughout the procedure; general anesthesia is induced after the airway is secured.

and turbinates. The oropharynx and posterior third of the tongue are supplied by the glossopharyngeal nerve. Branches of the vagus nerve innervate the epiglottis and more distal airway structures.

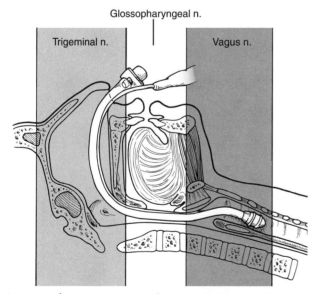

Figure 5-14   Innervation of airway structures. Simplified innervation of the airway structures is illustrated showing regions of the airway whose sensation is supplied by branches of the trigeminal, glossopharyngeal, and vagus nerves. (Redrawn from Brown DL: *Atlas of Regional Anesthesia*, Second Edition, WB Saunders, Philadelphia, 1999, p. 197.)

Block of the Nasal Septum and Lateral Wall of the Nasal Cavity

Anesthesia of the nasal septum and the lateral wall of the nasal cavity facilitates nasotracheal intubation. Sensation to the superior portions of both the septum and lateral wall of the nasal cavity is supplied by the anterior ethmoidal nerve, a terminal branch of the ophthalmic division of the trigeminal nerve. The inferior portions of the septum and the lateral wall of the nasal cavity are innervated by branches arising from the sphenopalatine ganglion. These terminal branches lie superficially just beneath the nasal mucosa and can be anesthetized by direct topical application of local anesthetic (Fig. 5-15 on p. 56).

Glossopharyngeal Nerve Block

The oropharynx, soft palate, posterior portion of the tongue, and pharyngeal surface of the epiglottis are

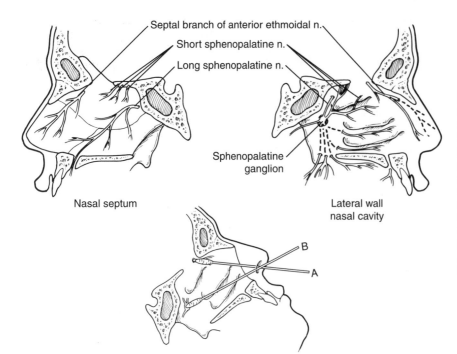

Figure 5-15 Topical anesthesia of the nasal septum and lateral wall of the nasal cavity. A cotton swab soaked with local anesthetic solution is advanced (A) first toward the anterior and superior most portion of the nasal cavity, and then (B) directly posteriorly to the posterior most aspect of the nasal cavity. The swab is left in position for several minutes to allow the topical anesthetic to penetrate the nasal mucosa. (Redrawn from Cousins MJ, Bridenbaugh PO: *Neural Blockade in Clinical Anesthesia and Management of Pain*, Third Edition, Lippincott-Raven, Philadelphia, 1998, p. 499.)

innervated by the glossopharyngeal nerve. Block of the glossopharyngeal nerve facilitates endotracheal intubation by blocking the gag reflex associated with direct laryngoscopy as well as facilitating passage of a nasotracheal tube through the posterior pharynx. The glossopharyngeal nerve emerges through the jugular foramen just posterior to the styloid process. The nerve lies in close proximity to the carotid artery, the vagus nerve, and the spinal accessory nerve in this location (Fig. 5-16). The glossopharyngeal nerve can be anesthetized using either intraoral or extraoral (peristyloid) approaches (Fig. 5-16 and Fig. 5-17 on p. 57). For the intraoral approach, the mouth is opened and the tongue is anesthetized with topical anesthetic. A 22 gauge $3\frac{1}{2}$ inch needle is used to place 5 mL of local anesthetic solution submucosally at the caudal aspect of the posterior tonsillar pillar (palatopharyngeal fold). To perform the peristyloid approach to the glossopharyngeal block, the patient is placed supine and a line is drawn between the angle of the mandible and the mastoid process. Using deep

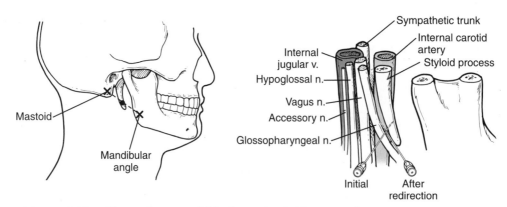

Figure 5-16 Glossopharyngeal block, peristyloid approach. Using deep pressure, the styloid process is palpated just posterior to the angle of the jaw along this line and a short, small-gauge needle is seated against the styloid process. The needle is then withdrawn slightly and directed posterior off of the styloid process. As soon as bony contact is lost, 5 to 7 mL of local anesthetic solution is injected after careful aspiration for blood. (Redrawn from Brown DL: *Atlas of Regional Anesthesia*, Second Edition, WB Saunders, Philadelphia, 1999, p. 207.)

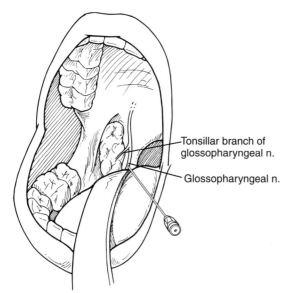

Figure 5-17   Glossopharyngeal block, intraoral approach. The mouth is opened and the tongue is anesthetized with topical anesthetic. A 22 gauge, $3\frac{1}{2}$ inch needle is used to place 5 mL of local anesthetic solution submucosally at the caudal aspect of the posterior tonsillar pillar (palatopharyngeal fold). (Redrawn from Brown DL: *Atlas of Regional Anesthesia*, Second Edition, WB Saunders, Philadelphia, 1999, p. 206.)

pressure, the styloid process is palpated just posterior to the angle of the jaw along this line and a short, small-gauge needle is seated against the styloid process. The needle is then withdrawn slightly and directed posteriorly off of the styloid process. As soon as bony contact is lost, 5 to 7 mL of local anesthetic solution is injected after careful aspiration for blood. Both approaches involve deposition of local anesthetic in close proximity to the carotid artery, and careful aspiration before injection is essential.

Superior Laryngeal Nerve Block

The vagus nerve supplies innervation of the larynx. The laryngeal surface of the epiglottis and the laryngeal inlet down to the vocal folds are supplied by the internal laryngeal branch of the vagus nerve, which reaches the larynx by piercing the thyrohyoid membrane (Fig. 5-18). This branch can be blocked by anesthetizing the parent nerve, the superior laryngeal nerve, below the greater cornu of the hyoid bone rendering the laryngeal mucosa insensitive down to the vocal cords.

Transtracheal Block

Below the vocal cords, the recurrent laryngeal nerve innervates the larynx and trachea. Although the recurrent laryngeal nerve can be blocked directly, anesthesia below the vocal cords is usually administered topically, either by direct "transtracheal" application through the cricothyroid membrane (Fig. 5-19 on p. 58) or using inhaled, aerosolized local anesthetic. The recurrent laryngeal nerve also supplies motor function to all of the intrinsic muscles of the larynx except the cricothyroid muscle, thus bilateral block produces loss of ability to phonate and close the glottis.

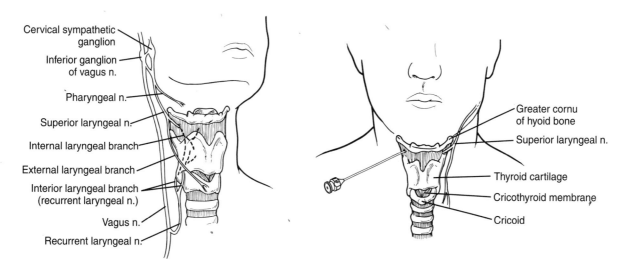

Figure 5-18   Laryngeal nerve supply and technique of superior laryngeal nerve block. The superior laryngeal nerve is anesthetized using a 25 gauge, $\frac{3}{4}$ inch needle and depositing 1-2 mL of local anesthetic below the greater cornu of the hyoid bone. (Redrawn from Brown DL: *Atlas of Regional Anesthesia*, Second Edition, WB Saunders, Philadelphia, 1999, p. 198.)

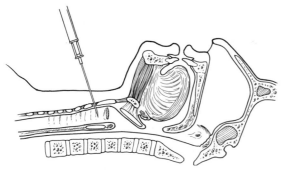

Figure 5-19   Transtracheal nerve block. After anesthetizing the overlying skin and subcutaneous tissues, a 20 gauge, $1\frac{1}{2}$ inch styletted flexible intravenous catheter attached to a syringe containing local anesthetic is inserted directly through the cricothyroid membrane. Intratracheal location is assured by aspirating air. The stylette is removed and 2–3 mL of local anesthetic solution is injected; the patient will inevitably cough as the local anesthetic is injected. Removing the stylette prior to injection minimizes the risk of tracheal injury. (Redrawn from Mulroy MF: *Regional Anesthesia*, Little, Brown, Boston, 1989, p. 209.)

SUMMARY

Successful anesthesia and analgesia for a number of procedures performed on the head and neck can be carried out with application of regional anesthesia.

Practitioners having familiarity with the anatomy and block techniques will have a wider range of choices.

SUGGESTED READING

Hamilton RC: Techniques of orbital regional anaesthesia, *Br J Anaesth* 75:88–92, 1995.

Murphy TM: Somatic blockade of head and neck. In: Cousins MJ, Bridenbaugh PO (eds), *Neural Blockade in Clinical Anesthesia and Management of Pain*, Third Edition, Lippincott-Raven, Philadelphia, 1998, pp. 489–514.

Sanderson Grizzard W: Ophthalmic anaesthesia, *Ann Ophthalmol* 21:265–294, 1989.

Tucker JH, Flynn JF: Head and neck regional blocks. In: Brown DL (ed), *Regional Anesthesia and Analgesia*, WB Saunders, Philadelphia, 1996, pp. 204–253.

Yagiela JA: Regional anesthesia for dental procedures, *Int Anesthesiol Clin* 27:68–82, 1989.

Upper Extremity Blocks

JOSEPH M. NEAL

INTRODUCTION

Upper extremity blocks performed at the brachial plexus or individual nerves are the most common peripheral nerve blocks in the anesthesiologist's armamentarium. Brachial plexus anesthesia presents many options of approaches and techniques. Upper extremity blocks can be used for surgical procedures from the shoulder to the hand, and are particularly useful for postoperative analgesia using long-acting local anesthetics or continuous catheter techniques. This chapter reviews upper extremity anatomy pertinent to brachial plexus anesthesia; describes commonly used approaches for blocking the plexus and individual nerves; discusses the major complications associated with upper extremity regional block; and compares techniques for improving block quality.

BASIC ANATOMY

The anatomic structure of the brachial plexus and its peripheral branches is complex. By understanding a few basic principles, the anesthesiologist can successfully select an appropriate approach for a specific surgery; understand which nerves require supplemental block; and accurately assess the block prior to incision. Knowledge of important anatomic structures adjacent to the brachial plexus is essential to avoid complications.

Anatomy of the Brachial Plexus

The brachial plexus originates as the ventral rami of the fifth cervical through the first thoracic nerves, with variable contributions from C4 and T2. As the nerves traverse laterally toward the axilla, they undergo a complex grouping and re-grouping as trunks, divisions, cords, and ultimately end as five main terminal nerves (Fig. 6-1 on p. 60). It is not essential for the anesthesiologist to memorize the various segments of the brachial plexus, but a general understanding of brachial plexus layout builds the conceptual basis for what to expect from approaching the plexus at a specific level and how to interpret the subsequent paresthesia or motor response (Table 6-1). For instance, interscalene blocks are performed high in the plexus at the level of the roots and trunks, thus one should expect initial stimulation of the superior trunk (shoulder and upper arm movement), but a tendency towards incomplete anesthesia of the inferior

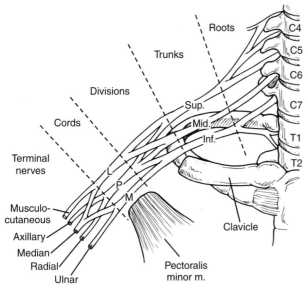

Figure 6-1 Anatomical layout of the brachial plexus.
L = lateral; P = posterior; M = medial. (Redrawn from Urmey WF: Upper extremity blocks. In Brown DL (ed), *Regional Anesthesia and Analgesia*, WB Saunders, Philadelphia, 1996, p. 255, Fig. 16-1.)

muscles; here the interscalene groove becomes the key surface landmark for performing interscalene block. The subclavian artery is useful for supraclavicular approaches, as the brachial plexus lies posterior and lateral to it. The coracoid process is an easily palpable structure for facilitating infraclavicular block. The axillary artery serves as the primary surface landmark for axillary block and the reference point around which the terminal nerves predictably lie.

The extent of upper extremity anesthesia must be assessed prior to incision to allow timely reinforcement of an incomplete block. Block assessment of the upper extremity is deceptively difficult, because its cutaneous innervation consists of overlapping contributions from many nerve fibers (Fig. 6-2 on p. 61). A simple means of assessing upper extremity block – push, pull, pinch, pinch – utilizes specific functions to evaluate individual terminal nerves.

trunk (ulnar distribution). As blockade is performed more distally towards the relatively loose terminal nerves, it is intuitive that multiple stimulation or injection techniques will be more successful than the single injection techniques used proximally where the plexus is more compact.

Appreciating surface landmarks and major structures adjacent to the plexus facilitates learning brachial plexus anesthetic procedures. For example, brachial plexus roots travel laterally between the anterior and middle scalene

---

Clinical Caveat: Assessing Upper Extremity Block

PUSH – Patient extends the forearm against resistance (radial nerve)
PULL – Patient flexes the forearm against resistance (musculocutaneous nerve)
PINCH – Anesthesiologist pinches palmar base of index finger (median nerve)
PINCH – Anesthesiologist pinches palmar base of little finger (ulnar nerve)

Table 6-1 Brachial Plexus Stimulation: Expected Motor Response

Approach	Stimulated Portion of the Brachial Plexus	Expected Motor Response
Interscalene	Superior trunk	Shoulder abduction, elbow flexion
Supraclavicular	Middle and inferior trunk	Hand movement
Infraclavicular	Lateral cord	Forearm flexion, hand pronation (pinkie moves lateral)
	Posterior cord	Wrist extension (pinkie moves posterior)
	Medial cord	Finger flexion, thumb opposition (pinkie moves medial)
Axillary/mid-humeral	Musculocutaneous nerve	Forearm flexion, hand supination
	Median nerve	Forearm pronation, wrist flexion
	Ulnar nerve	Finger flexion, thumb opposition
	Radial nerve	Wrist extension

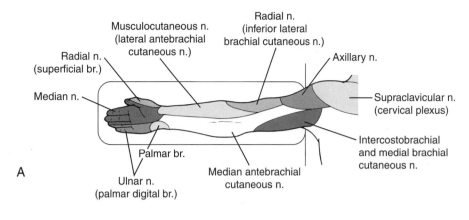

Figure 6-2   Upper extremity cutaneous innervation. A = palmar, B = dorsal surfaces. (Redrawn from Brown, DL: *Atlas of Regional Anesthesia*, WB Saunders, Philadelphia, 1992, pp. 16, 17, Figs. 2-2, 2-4.)

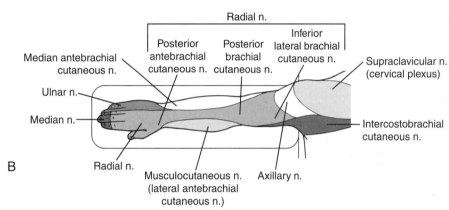

Peripheral Nerves Supplying the Chest, Shoulder, and Upper Extremity That Lie Outside the Brachial Plexus

Nerves that are not a part of the brachial plexus innervate several regions of the upper extremity. Depending on the incision location, blocking these nerves separately may be necessary. For example, the supraclavicular approach is usually made too distal in the brachial plexus to anesthetize consistently the supraclavicular nerves (C3–C4), which supply the skin over the upper shoulder and chest; or the suprascapular nerve, which innervates the majority of the shoulder joint. The intercostobrachial nerve (T1–2) supplies the medial portion of the upper arm and requires separate anesthesia for surgery in this region. Anesthetizing the intercostobrachial nerve is also important to facilitate pain relief when an upper arm tourniquet is used.

The Axillary Sheath

The clinical importance of the axillary sheath is an ongoing controversy. The prevertebral fascia that separates the anterior and middle scalene muscles forms the sheath. One concept of the axillary sheath holds that it is a dense tubular structure extending from the vertebral column to the terminal nerves and virtually encasing the neurovascular bundle. Based on this concept, a single injection of sufficient volume should fill the sheath and anesthetize all nerves within it. In contrast, some experts hold that the sheath is not contiguous, but instead a multi-compartmental structure with distinct fibrous septae. Based on this concept, multiple small-volume injections are necessary to overcome flow limitation imposed by the septae. Although cryomicrotome analysis does not delineate a defined sheath (Fig. 6-3 on p. 62), other anatomic studies are conflicting. Clinical studies demonstrate a high degree of success in blocking the brachial plexus using either single or multiple injection techniques.

Current Controversy: The Sheath

Is the fibrous sheath that emanates from the prevertebral fascia a dense, continuous tubular structure that extends to the terminal nerves; or a flimsy, multi-compartmental structure with multiple septae?

Anatomic studies are conflicting. The few studies that show high success with single-injection axillary techniques support the tubular concept. Conversely, more studies demonstrate higher success with multiple injection techniques, which supports the concept of a multi-compartmental, poorly organized structure.

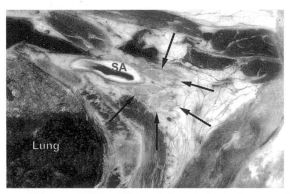

Figure 6-3 **Cryomicrotome of the brachial plexus at the supraclavicular level.** The arrows point out the brachial plexus. Note the absence of a clearly delineated sheath, the proximity of the lung, and that the plexus lies posterior and lateral to the subclavian artery (SA). (Original cryomicrotome from Quinn H Hogan, MD. Reproduced from Neal JM, Hebl JR, Gerancher JC, Hogan QH: Brachial plexus anesthesia: essentials of our current understanding, *Reg Anesth Pain Med* 27:404, 2002, Fig. 5.)

APPROACHES TO THE BRACHIAL PLEXUS

Plexus Blocks

Interscalene Block

Patient selection. The interscalene block (ISB) is ideally suited for shoulder and upper arm surgery (Fig. 6-4). Because local anesthetic is deposited high along the brachial plexus at the level of the distal roots and trunks, the ISB consistently provides anesthesia to the proximal upper extremity, but anesthesia within the ulnar nerve distribution is less predictable. The major surface landmark for performing ISB is the interscalene groove, where the brachial plexus exits between the anterior and middle scalene muscles (Fig. 6-5 and Fig. 6-6 on p. 63).

Block technique. When placing an interscalene block, the anesthesiologist turns the patient's head 30° towards the contralateral side and identifies the interscalene groove at the C6 level (cricoid cartilage). The interscalene groove is palpable just deep and posterior to the posterior border of the sternocleidomastoid muscle. With two fingers firmly in the groove, a ≤1.5 inch needle or stimulating needle is passed perpendicular to all planes, with a slightly caudad inclination. A paresthesia or motor response to the anterior shoulder or the arm signals adequate needle proximity to the brachial plexus. Diaphragmatic movement indicates phrenic nerve stimulation and the needle being too anterior (Fig. 6-6 on p. 63), whereas trapezius movement signals needle placement that is too posterior. Aspiration is followed by a 1 mL test injection to rule out intra-arterial or subarachnoid placement. Marked pain on injection should alert the operator to possible intraneural injection and prompt slight withdrawal of the needle prior to deposition of 30–40 mL local anesthetic in divided doses. When placing a continuous catheter via the interscalene approach, it is often helpful to angle the needle more caudad, thereby lessening the angle the catheter must turn to pass alongside the plexus.

Complications. The interscalene approach may lead to significant complications and side effects (Box 6-1). As noted in Fig. 6-5 on p. 63, neighboring anatomy includes the carotid artery, epidural space, subarachnoid space, and the spinal cord. The proximity of these structures leads to several nuisance side effects, including Horner's syndrome (ipsilateral ptosis, miosis, and anhydrosis) and recurrent laryngeal nerve block causing hoarseness. Epidural and subarachnoid anesthesia may occur with deep needle placement, as the vertebral column is only 35 mm from the skin. The proximity of the phrenic nerve and high cervical nerve roots results in 100% of all ISBs causing ipsilateral hemidiaphragmatic paresis (Fig. 6-7 on p. 64). This

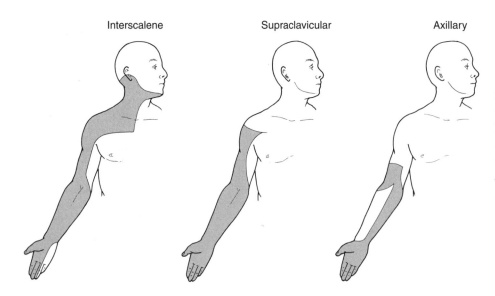

Interscalene   Supraclavicular   Axillary

Figure 6-4 Typical sensory anesthesia patterns of three common approaches to the brachial plexus. (Redrawn from Urmey WF: Upper extremity blocks. In: Brown DL (ed), *Regional Anesthesia and Analgesia*, WB Saunders, Philadelphia, 1996, p. 259, Fig. 16-5.)

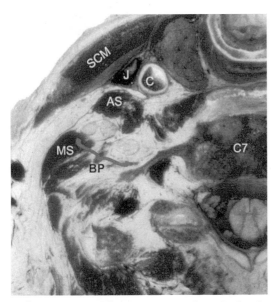

Figure 6-5   Cryomicrotome of the neck at the level of the seventh cervical vertebra (C7). Note the brachial plexus (BP) between the anterior scalene (AS) and middle scalene (MS) muscles. Also note the proximity of the internal jugular vein (J), the carotid artery (C), the sternocleidomastoid muscle (SCM), and the epidural and subarachnoid spaces. (Original cryomicrotome from Quinn H Hogan, MD. Reproduced from Neal JM, Hebl JR, Gerancher JC, Hogan QH: Brachial plexus anesthesia: essentials of our current understanding, *Reg Anesth Pain Med* 27:403, 2002, Fig. 3.)

phenomena can be associated with subjective dyspnea and up to 30% diminution in pulmonary function in a significant number of patients, thus ISB is relatively contraindicated in patients unable to tolerate these changes. A complication unique to ISB is a 13 to 24% incidence of

sudden severe hypotension and bradycardia when awake patients are undergoing shoulder surgery in the sitting position (Fig. 6-8 on p. 65). This phenomenon is believed to occur secondary to exogenous epinephrine and possibly the Bezold–Jarisch reflex. This reflex occurs when ventricular mechanoreceptors are activated by forceful contraction of an empty ventricle, causing reflex bradycardia. The frequency of hypotensive/bradycardic events can be decreased with prophylactic metoprolol, but not glycopyrrolate. Finally, as with all brachial plexus approaches, there is significant risk of intravascular injection or soft tissue local anesthetic absorption with subsequent systemic toxicity (Table 6-2). Intra-arterial injection is particularly relevant to ISB because even 1 mL of local anesthetic injected directly into the vertebral artery can cause immediate seizure. Conversely, toxicity from local anesthetic tissue uptake may be delayed for up to an hour.

Clinical Caveat: Local Anesthetic Plasma Concentrations

Unintended intravascular injection immediately causes high peak plasma concentrations of local anesthetic

In the absence of intravascular injection, local anesthetic uptake from tissues around the brachial plexus may not manifest peak plasma concentration for 15 to 30 minutes, or upwards of 60 minutes if epinephrine has been added

Figure 6-6 Interscalene anatomy. Note the brachial plexus exiting through the interscalene groove, and how the phrenic nerve lies on top of the anterior scalene muscle (inset). (Redrawn from Brown DL: *Atlas of Regional Anesthesia*, Second Edition, WB Saunders, Philadelphia, 1999, p. 26, Fig. 3-2.) (See colour inserts, Plate 1.)

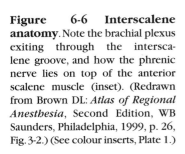

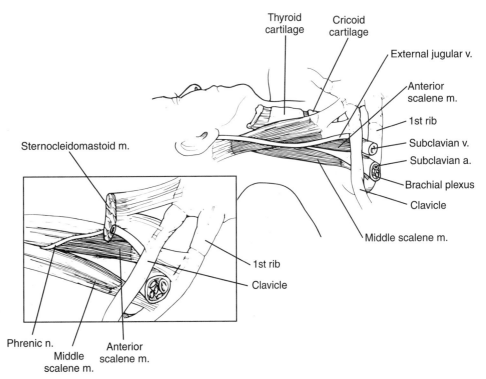

Box 6-1 Complications and Side Effects of Interscalene Block

Hemidiaphragmatic paresis (100% incidence)
Hypotensive/bradycardic events (13–24% incidence in awake patients)
Intra-arterial (vertebral, carotid, subclavian) local anesthetic injection
Epidural or spinal anesthesia
Cervical sympathetic block (Horner's syndrome)
Recurrent laryngeal nerve block (hoarseness)

Table 6-2 Seizure Frequency as a Function of Brachial Plexus Approach

Brachial Plexus Approach	Seizures per 1,000 Patients
Axillary block	1.3
Interscalene block	7.6
Supraclavicular block	7.9

Data adapted from Brown DL, Ransom DM, Hall JA, et al.: Regional anesthesia and local anesthetic-induced systemic toxicity: seizure frequency and accompanying cardiovascular changes, *Anesth Analg* 81:321–328, 1995.

Supraclavicular Block

Patient selection. The supraclavicular approach can be used for almost any surgery on the arm or shoulder (Fig. 6-4 on p. 62). One reason for this universality is because it is here that the brachial plexus is most compact as it dips under the clavicle and crosses the first rib (Fig. 6-9 on p. 65). Shoulder surgery may require supplemental superficial cervical plexus block to anesthetize the supraclavicular nerves (C3-C4).

Block technique. At least five variations of the supraclavicular block (SCB) have been described. A popular one is the "plumb-bob" approach. The anesthesiologist turns the patient's head 30° to the contralateral side and positions a 1.5 inch needle or stimulating needle alongside the lateral border of the sternocleidomastoid muscle's clavicular head just superior to the clavicle. The needle is directed straight downward, just as a brick mason's plumb-bob would point (Fig. 6-10 and Fig. 6-11 on p. 66). The needle is advanced until paresthesia or motor response is achieved. If hand surgery is planned, the ideal response is in the middle trunk distribution (hand movement or paresthesia). If a paresthesia or motor response is not elicited on the first pass, then the needle is swept up to 20° cephalad in the parasagittal plane, followed by up to 20° in the caudad direction (Fig. 6-12 on p. 66). If the subclavian artery is entered, the needle should be redirected posteriorly and laterally (Fig. 6-3 on p. 62). Once the desired response is obtained, a slow 1 mL injection is performed to rule out subclavian artery or intraneural needle placement, followed by incremental injection of 30–40 mL of local anesthetic.

Complications. Pneumothorax is the most worrisome complication of SCB, although its incidence in contemporary practice has probably decreased as a consequence of lung-avoiding techniques such as the plumb-bob or first rib palpation approaches. Most pneumothoraces will present with dyspnea or pleuritic chest pain 6 to 12 hours after SCB placement. These symptoms should prompt an expiratory chest radiographic to rule out pneumothorax. The natural history of SCB-induced pneumothorax suggests that careful consideration be given prior to selecting this block for outpatients. Like interscalene block, patients undergoing SCB may experience hemidiaphragmatic paresis (Fig. 6-7), although the incidence is less (50%) and pulmonary function is not altered in healthy patients. Nevertheless, SCB is relatively contraindicated in patients with pulmonary disease. Unintended anesthesia of the cervical sympathetic chain and recurrent laryngeal nerve can also occur (Box 6-2).

Infraclavicular Block

Patient selection. The infraclavicular block (ICB) is appropriate for surgery of the arm and hand. As compared to the axillary block, it is placed more proximally along the brachial plexus at the cord level (Fig. 6-13 on p. 67), and therefore more reliably produces anesthesia in the axillary and musculocutaneous nerve distributions. Conversely, ICB is performed distal to the interscalene and supraclavicular insertion sites, and thus causes little

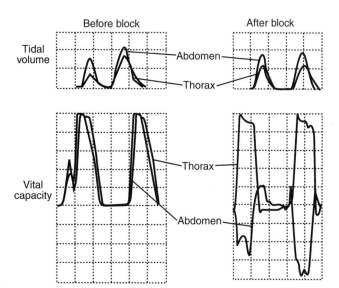

Figure 6-7 Plethysmograph before and after interscalene or supraclavicular block. Negative abdominal excursion indicates hemidiaphragmatic paresis. (Redrawn from Neal JM, Moore JM, Kopacz DJ, et al.: Quantitative analysis of respiratory, motor, and sensory function after supraclavicular block, *Anesth Analg* 86:1241, 1998, Fig. 2.)

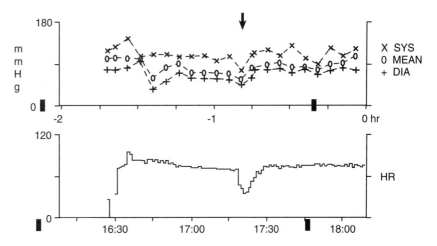

Figure 6-8   Hypotension and bradycardia after interscalene block. Blood pressure and heart rate trendlines illustrating a sudden hypotensive/bradycardic event (arrow) that occurred nearly 60 minutes following interscalene block placement. (Redrawn from Liguori GA, Kahn RL, Gordan J, et al.: The use of metoprolol and glycopyrrolate to prevent hypotension/bradycardic events during shoulder arthroscopy in the sitting position under interscalene block, *Anesth Analg* 87:1320, 1998, Fig. 1.)

or no embarrassment of pulmonary function and is less likely to cause pneumothorax.

Block technique. While several techniques for ICB exist, the coracoid approach is based on straightforward surface landmarks. In the supine patient, the anesthesiologist identifies the lateral portion of the coracoid process and then marks a point 2 cm medial and 2 cm caudad (Fig. 6-13 on p. 67). A 4 inch stimulating needle is directed posteriorly, perpendicular to all planes. Pectoralis muscle contraction will be noted first, followed by lateral cord stimulation (Table 6-1). Hand contraction is ultimately sought, which may require caudad redirection of the needle tip, taking care to remain in the parasagittal plane (medial redirection will increase the risk of pneumothorax). Once appropriate motor response is achieved, a small test injection is made to rule out intraneural or intravascular needle placement, followed by deposition of 30–40 mL of local anesthetic. Whether a single injection technique is superior to multiple injections during the coracoid infraclavicular approach is unclear. The technique's perpendicular approach can make threading a catheter problematic.

Complications. Complications of the coracoid infraclavicular block are not as well reported as those from the interscalene or supraclavicular approaches. Because local anesthetic is placed more distal in the brachial plexus, the incidence of hemidiaphragmatic paresis, recurrent laryngeal block, and cervical sympathetic block is likely to be less frequent. Since the needle is theoretically directed lateral to the thoracic cage, the incidence of pneumothorax will be less than that seen with supraclavicular block. Intravascular injection may occur.

Axillary Block

Patient selection. The axillary block is the workhorse of upper extremity regional anesthesia. It is suitable for surgery of the hand, forearm, and elbow (Fig. 6-4 on p. 62). The popularity of this approach is partially based on its easily identified landmark – the axillary artery. All axillary approaches ultimately use this landmark to guide initial needle placement. Understanding the orientation of the

four terminal nerves surrounding the axillary artery is key to successful anesthesia. The four terminal nerves (the axillary nerve has already exited the plexus) lie in close proximity to the artery in a predictable, quadrant-like fashion (Fig. 6-14 on p. 67). Significant anatomic variation exists with the arrangement of terminal nerves and the axillary artery, the most common of which is the radial nerve lying more superficial than the ulnar nerve. At this level, the musculocutaneous nerve resides within the belly of the coracobrachialis muscle and requires supple-

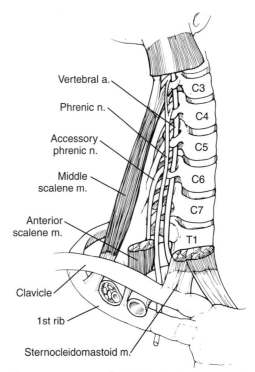

Figure 6-9   Relationship of the brachial plexus to the interscalene groove, clavicle, first rib, and subclavian artery. Note the compactness of the plexus at this level. (Redrawn from Brown DL: *Atlas of Regional Anesthesia*, Second Edition, WB Saunders, Philadelphia, 1999, p. 20, Fig. 2-9.) (See colour inserts, Plate 2.)

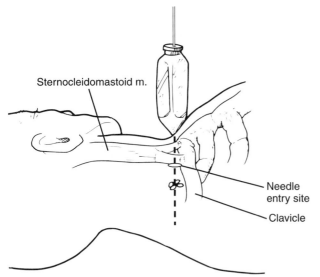

Figure 6-10   Supraclavicular approach, illustrating the plumb-bob concept of needle entry. (Redrawn from Brown DL: *Atlas of Regional Anesthesia*, Second Edition, WB Saunders, Philadelphia, 1999, p. 38, Fig. 4-6C.)

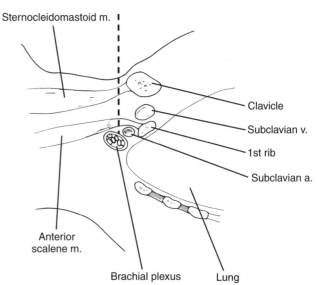

Figure 6-11   Plumb-bob technique to supraclavicular block. The true vertical needle path of the plumb-bob approach should contact the brachial plexus at a position cephalad to the lung. (Redrawn from Brown DL: *Atlas of Regional Anesthesia*, Second Edition, WB Saunders, Philadelphia, 1999, p. 38, Fig. 4-6A.)

mental injection for successful anesthesia. It is best anesthetized by fanning 5 mL of local anesthetic into the belly of the coracobrachialis muscle while directing the needle towards the coracoid process.

Block technique. A number of techniques for axillary block have been described (Box 6-3). The transarterial technique is highly successful and can be performed with either a single injection anterior or posterior to the axillary artery, or with a double injection technique. The perivascular technique deposits small volumes of local anesthetic through a constantly moving needle. About

15 mL of local anesthetic is placed superior to the artery in three passes, followed by another 15 mL deposited inferior to the artery in three passes (Fig. 6-15 on p. 68). Paresthesia-seeking techniques rely on eliciting one or more paresthesias, preferably corresponding with the cutaneous anesthesia requirements of the specific surgery. Peripheral nerve stimulation is yet another technique suitable for axillary block. Regardless of what technique is chosen, initial injection should be given slowly. Any discomfort voiced by the patient must be interpreted as possible intraneural injection, prompting

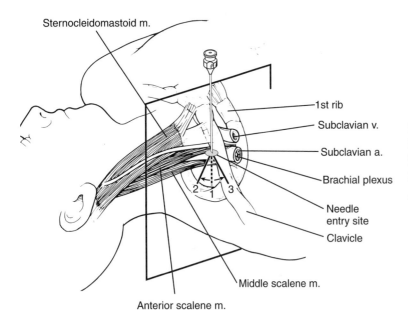

Figure 6-12   Plumb-bob approach. Note how the limited 20° cephalad and caudad needle traverse is made strictly within the parasagittal plane. (Redrawn from Brown DL: *Atlas of Regional Anesthesia*, Second Edition, WB Saunders, Philadelphia, 1999, p. 39, Fig. 34-7.) (See colour inserts, Plate 3.)

Box 6-2 Complications and Side Effects of Supraclavicular Block

Pneumothorax (0.5–6%) with "classic" approaches
Intravascular local anesthetic injection
Hemidiaphragmatic paresis (50%; 95% CI 14–86%)
Cervical sympathetic chain anesthesia – Horner's
 syndrome (20–90%)
Recurrent laryngeal nerve anesthesia – hoarseness (1%)

slight needle withdrawal prior to continuing. Axillary block requires 30–40 mL of local anesthetic.

Clinical Caveat: Why Axillary Blocks Fail

Relying on "fascial clicks"
Single-injection techniques (with rare exceptions)
Depositing local anesthetic too deep (behind the
 neurovascular bundle)
Neglecting to supplement the musculocutaneous nerve

Complications. Minor complications after axillary block are common and include bruising, axillary discomfort, and residual numbness (Fig. 6-16 on p. 69). Intravascular injection is possible in this highly vascular area and is best prevented with frequent aspiration. Damage to the axillary artery may occur from injection into the arterial wall. As with all peripheral blocks, nerve injury is a worrisome complication. This topic is discussed fully in Chapter 14.

Mid-humeral Block

Patient selection. The mid-humeral approach can be thought of as an extremely distal axillary block. Here the four terminal nerves are widely spaced, thus requiring separate stimulation and injection. Proponents of this

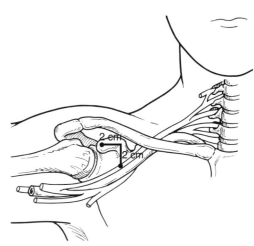

Figure 6-13   Coracoid infraclavicular block. The brachial plexus is blocked at the level of the cords. Note the needle entry point is 2 cm medial and 2 cm caudad to the lateral border of the coracoid process. (Redrawn from Mulroy MF: *Regional Anesthesia. An Illustrated Procedural Guide*, Third Edition, Lippincott Williams & Wilkins, Philadelphia, 2002, p. 169, Fig. 12.9.)

approach believe that its multiple injections provide a more complete and successful block as compared to the axillary or coracoid infraclavicular approaches. Studies to support this claim are often flawed in their design. Nevertheless, the mid-humeral approach is unique in its ability to deposit selectively different local anesthetics on individual nerves to custom design block characteristics. For instance, by placing lidocaine on the radial and musculocutaneous nerves, and bupivacaine on the median and ulnar nerves, one is able to extend analgesia without prolonging motor block.

Block technique. To perform the mid-humeral block, the anesthesiologist abducts the patient's arm to 80° and then identifies the brachial artery pulsation at the junction of the upper and middle thirds of the arm. The four terminal nerves are anesthetized sequentially (Fig. 6-17 on p. 69). Placing a stimulating needle superior to the brachial artery and directing it towards the

Figure 6-14   Axillary anatomy, illustrating the concept of functional quadrants of four terminal nerves surrounding the axillary artery. M = median nerve; Mc = musculocutaneous nerve; R = radial nerve; U = ulnar nerve. (Redrawn from Brown DL: *Atlas of Regional Anesthesia*, Second Edition, WB Saunders, Philadelphia, 1999, p. 52, Fig. 6-1.)

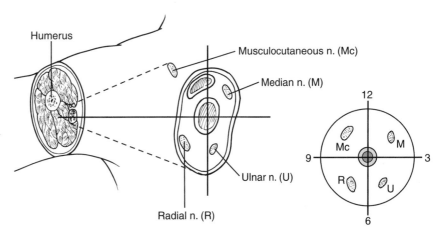

Box 6-3 Axillary Block Techniques

Transarterial
Perivascular infiltration
Paresthesia-seeking
Peripheral nerve stimulation

axilla seeks the median nerve. When the median nerve is encountered (Table 6-1), 5 mL of local anesthetic is injected after negative aspiration. Care is used to avoid intraneural injection. A similar process is repeated for the remaining three nerves, identifying each by their characteristic motor response (Table 6-1). Placing the needle inferior to the artery and directing posteriorly finds the ulnar nerve. Identifying the radial nerve requires directing the needle inferior to the artery and perpendicular to the skin. If the humerus is encountered, the needle is redirected more inferior. The musculocutaneous nerve is sought by placing the needle superior to the artery and directing it under the biceps and into the belly of the coracobrachialis muscle.

Complications. Complications of the mid-humeral approach include intravascular injection, bruising, hematoma, and nerve injury.

Selective Nerve Blocks

Selective block of individual nerves plays a limited role in upper extremity regional anesthesia. One's preference should be to perform a plexus block, as this approach is more reliable, generally less painful, faster, and allows the use of a tourniquet. Moreover, there is the poorly defined risk of performing supplemental selective nerve blocks in the setting of partial anesthesia secondary to an incomplete plexus block. The risk involves the patient's impaired ability to detect an intraneuronal injection. Suprascapular and intercostobrachial nerve blocks do not present this concern.

Suprascapular Nerve Block

Patient selection. The suprascapular nerve innervates the majority of the shoulder joint. Anesthetizing this nerve is a valuable adjunct to general anesthesia for shoulder arthroscopy, or as a method to provide prolonged analgesia after total shoulder replacement. Suprascapular block has less impact if combined with an interscalene block, particularly for non-arthroscopic shoulder surgery.

Block technique. The block is performed by tracing out the scapular spine, then bisecting it with a second line drawn parallel to the vertebral spine. In the upper outer quadrant, a third line is drawn at a 45° angle and a point marked 1 inch along this line (Fig. 6-18 on p. 69). The block is completed by injecting 10 mL of local anesthetic near the suprascapular notch.

Complications. A needle that is placed too deeply through the suprascapular notch can lead to pneumothorax. This can be avoided by placing the needle back onto the scapula to confirm the location and depth of the suprascapular notch.

Clinical Caveat: Suprascapular Nerve Block

For arthroscopic shoulder surgery or that involving the posterior joint (such as total shoulder arthroplasty), a suprascapular nerve block is a valuable adjunct to interscalene block, because it anesthetizes the posterior two-thirds of the shoulder joint.

Intercostobrachial Nerve Block

Patient selection. The intercostobrachial nerve consists of T1 and T2 terminal nerve roots, which are not part of the brachial plexus. Therefore, surgeries involving the upper medial arm or high axilla require supplemental intercostobrachial block. A common misperception is that this block

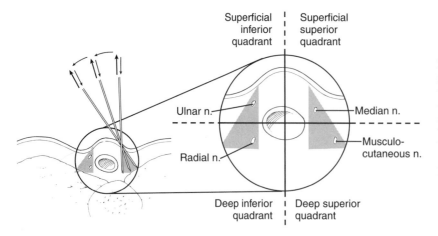

Figure 6-15 Typical arrangement of the four terminal nerves in quadrants around the axillary artery. The perivascular technique deposits local anesthetic by fanning the needle away from the axillary artery. (Redrawn from Thompson GE, Brown DL: The common nerve blocks. In: Nunn JF, Utting JE, Brown BR (eds), *General Anaesthesia*, Fifth Edition, Butterworths, London, 1989, p 1068, Figs. 23-5 and 23-6.)

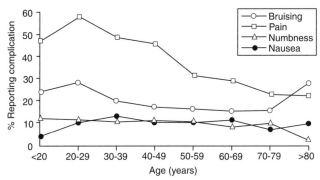

Figure 6-16　Minor complications of axillary block. (Redrawn from Cooper K, Kelly H, Carrithers K: Perceptions of side-effects following axillary block used for outpatient surgery, *Reg Anesth* 20:214, 1995, Fig. 1.)

also prevents tourniquet pain. However, while anesthetizing the intercostobrachial nerve will prevent tourniquet *sensation* within its cutaneous distribution, there is no evidence that *ischemic tourniquet pain* is mediated through the intercostobrachial nerve.

Block technique. Intercostobrachial block is easily accomplished by subcutaneous injection of 5 mL of local anesthetic placed across the axilla.

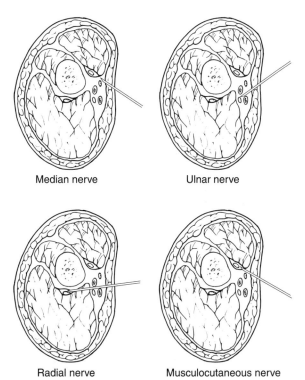

Figure 6-17　Mid-humeral approach. Note the needle orientation and its relationship to the brachial artery as each individual nerve is sought. (Redrawn from Mulroy MF: *Regional Anesthesia. An Illustrated Procedural Guide*, Third Edition, Lippincott Williams & Wilkins, Philadelphia, 2002, p. 173, Fig. 12.13.)

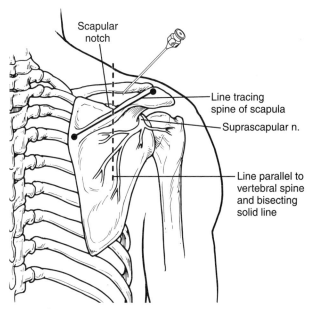

Figure 6-18　Suprascapular nerve block. (Redrawn from Moore DC: *Regional Block*, Fourth Edition, Charles C. Thomas, Springfield, IL, 1965, p. 300, Fig. 205.)

Selective Blocks at the Elbow

When surgery is facilitated by motor block, selective blocks at the elbow are preferable to those placed at the wrist. At the elbow, the radial nerve is relatively deep, while the median and ulnar nerves are superficial (Fig. 6-19). The median nerve is blocked by inserting a needle just ulnar (medial) to the brachial artery, at the level of the epicondyles (Fig. 6-20 on p. 70). Local anesthetic (5 mL) is either injected alongside the artery, or at the point of paresthesia or motor response. The radial nerve is identified by inserting a needle 1.5 cm radial (lateral) to the biceps tendon, in the plane of the

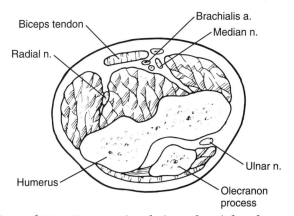

Figure 6-19　Cross-sectional view of peripheral nerves at the elbow. (Redrawn from Brown DL: *Atlas of Regional Anesthesia*, Second Edition, WB Saunders, Philadelphia, 1999, p. 59, Fig. 7-1.)

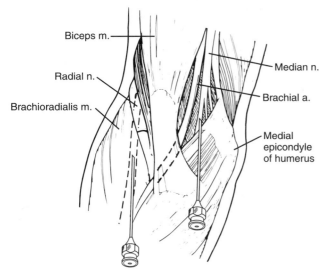

Figure 6-20 Technique of median and radial nerve block at the elbow. (Redrawn from Brown DL: *Atlas of Regional Anesthesia*, Second Edition, WB Saunders, Philadelphia, 1999, p. 60, Fig. 7-2.)

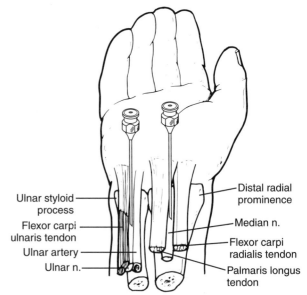

Figure 6-21 Technique of median and ulnar nerve block at the wrist. (Redrawn from Brown DL: *Atlas of Regional Anesthesia*, Second Edition, WB Saunders, Philadelphia, 1999, p. 63, Fig. 7-5.)

epicondyles. Paresthesia can be sought or 5 mL of local anesthetic simply fanned alongside the tendon (Fig. 6-20). The ulnar nerve is blocked in the ulnar groove, where no more than 3 mL of local anesthetic is placed to prevent compression injury in this tight area. The lateral antebrachial cutaneous nerve provides sensory innervation to the radial forearm. It is easily blocked by subcutaneous infiltration of 5–10 mL of local anesthetic placed at the middle of the antecubital fossa and directed towards the lateral epicondyle.

Selective Blocks at the Wrist

Selective nerve blocks at the wrist are useful for minor hand surgery or postoperative analgesia. The ulnar nerve is blocked by directing a small-gauge needle between the flexor carpi ulnaris tendon and the ulnar artery, at the level of the ulnar styloid process (Fig. 6-21). Three to five mL of local anesthetic is sufficient via infiltration or after a paresthesia is obtained. The median nerve is blocked by a perpendicular needle placed between the palmaris longus and flexor carpi radialis tendons at the level of the ulnar and radial styloid processes. Local anesthetic (5 mL) is deposited with or without paresthesia guidance (Fig. 6-21). The radial and superficial radial nerves are blocked by infiltration of 5 mL of local anesthetic in two injections. The first injection places 2 mL of local anesthetic just lateral to the radial artery, about 2 cm proximal to the radial styloid process. The needle is then redirected dorsally and further lateral, where the remaining anesthetic solution is injected subcutaneously (Fig. 6-22).

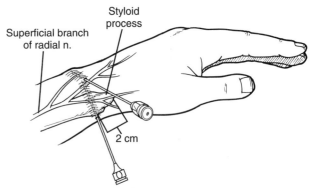

Figure 6-22 Technique of radial nerve block at the wrist. (Redrawn from Urmey WF: Upper extremity blocks. In: Brown DL (ed), *Regional Anesthesia and Analgesia*, WB Saunders, Philadelphia, 1996, p. 274, Fig. 16-22.)

INTRAVENOUS REGIONAL ANESTHESIA

Patient selection. Intravenous regional anesthesia (IVRA or Bier block) is commonly used for upper extremity anesthesia. Its use is limited to hand and forearm surgery that is expected to last only 30 to 45 minutes, due to ischemic tourniquet pain. Some surgeons find the oozing inherent to IVRA to be objectionable.

Block technique. This rather simple procedure involves exsanguinating the arm by wrapping it tightly with an elastic band, followed by inflation of an upper arm tourniquet to 100 mmHg above systolic blood pressure, and then injecting 50 mL of 0.5% lidocaine into a hand vein. Anesthesia is most likely accomplished by a combination of local anesthetic block of large nerve trunks and small nerve terminals. When tourniquet pain occurs, the use of a double tourniquet allows the operator to inflate the distal cuff over an area of anesthetized skin, followed by deflating the proximal cuff.

Complications. There are two critical times when local anesthetic systemic toxicity can occur during IVRA. If the tourniquet fails or injection pressure exceeds tourniquet pressure, large volumes of local anesthetic can enter the systemic circulation. This is best avoided by slow (90 second) injection into a distal vein. The second critical period occurs at the time of tourniquet deflation, which allows an immediate systemic release of local anesthetic followed by a washout period that can last for 30 minutes or more. The tourniquet should not be deflated until at least 30 minutes have passed. If <45 minutes have elapsed since local anesthetic injection, some experts recommend cycling the tourniquet as a means of limiting systemic uptake. The effectiveness of a cycling deflation/re-inflation sequence is controversial; but if elected, two cycles are adequate, provided the deflation phase does not exceed 10 seconds.

TECHNIQUES FOR IMPROVING UPPER EXTREMITY BLOCK

Which Approach for Which Surgery?

The question of which approach is best for a specific surgery has received little prospective, controlled study. For elbow surgery, a single retrospective study showed that axillary block was more successful than either interscalene or, perhaps surprisingly, supraclavicular block. There is no consensus regarding hand surgery. The axillary, infraclavicular, and mid-humeral approaches have been variously compared, but study results are difficult to interpret because the number of stimulations or injections was not held constant.

Local Anesthetic Selection and Dosing

The choice of local anesthetic for an upper extremity block is based primarily on the desired duration of anesthesia and analgesia. Short-acting agents such as 2-chloroprocaine facilitate rapid block resolution (about an hour), but provide inconsistent anesthesia. In general, the intermediate-acting agent profile is one of faster onset and greater consistency, but shorter duration as compared to the long-acting local anesthetics. Lidocaine and mepivacaine are ideal for intermediate needs, as each provides analgesia for upwards of 6 to 8 hours when epinephrine is added. For longer-acting blocks or infusions, bupivacaine and *l*-bupivacaine last slightly longer than ropivacaine, pro-

viding 10 to 18 hours of analgesia depending on the approach used. There is a paucity of evidence to support the practice of combining a short-acting with a long-acting local anesthetic in an attempt to create faster onset and longer duration. The resultant block is more like that obtained with an intermediate-acting agent.

The concept of "dose is duration" applies well to spinal anesthesia, but not so with brachial plexus anesthesia. The total mass (concentration $\times$ volume) of local anesthetic delivered to the brachial plexus has relatively little effect on block success, onset, or duration. The only well-performed studies in this area involved a catheter-dosed axillary block technique, which may have limited applicability to the majority of clinical situations. Nevertheless, varying the volume of mepivacaine between 20 and 80 mL, the dose between 200 and 600 mg, and the concentration between 0.5 and 1.5% had very little effect on block quality. Thus, the accurate placement of local anesthetic in close proximity to the nerve appears to be of primary importance. Using higher volumes, concentrations, or doses of local anesthetic is much more likely to cause local anesthetic toxicity than to improve block success.

Clinical Controversy: Local Anesthetic Dosing

- Despite the logical tendency to increase local anesthetic dose, concentration, or volume as a means of improving block quality, there is little evidence to support the effectiveness of this practice
- High local anesthetic concentration contributes to neurotoxicity, while high volume and dose contributes to systemic toxicity

Single versus Multiple Injection

Interscalene and supraclavicular blocks are successfully performed as single-injection techniques, which may explain the lack of comparative studies of single versus multiple injections for these two approaches. However, as one moves distally down the brachial plexus, the superiority of single versus multiple stimulation or injection techniques becomes more controversial, particularly for axillary block. Transarterial axillary block has high success rates with both single (one study only) and double injections made anterior and posterior to the axillary artery. Most studies demonstrate higher success and more rapid onset with two or three paresthesias or motor responses, as compared to a single paresthesia, motor response, or fascial "click." Four stimulations add time to block performance without improving success. When seeking individual nerve responses, an ulnar response is least important, while a musculocutaneous response is important only if the surgery includes its distribution. Whether to perform single or multiple stimulations with the coracoid infraclavicular approach remains controversial.

Clinical Caveat: Single versus Multiple Injections

A single injection is adequate for interscalene and supraclavicular blocks

For transarterial axillary block, one or two injections are effective

For paresthesia or nerve stimulator axillary block technique, two or three injections are better than one or four

---

Clicks, Paresthesias, Nerve Stimulation, and Ultrasound

Reliance on the tactile sensation of a "fascial click" is an inferior technique for axillary block, although one study has shown reasonable success when it is used for a single-injection coracoid infraclavicular block. For axillary block, success is comparable with transarterial, paresthesia, or peripheral nerve stimulation techniques. In general, success is higher when multiple paresthesias or injection techniques are compared to single-injection, paresthesia, or "fascial click" techniques. There is no significant difference in success between paresthesia-seeking and peripheral nerve stimulation techniques. The use of ultrasound to aid needle guidance during brachial block holds promise, especially in patients with difficult anatomy. However, technical difficulties in visualizing nerves, combined with the lack of outcome studies proving benefit, makes it difficult to recommend ultrasound for routine practice.

Physical Manipulations

A variety of manipulations designed to limit the spread of local anesthetic to unintended destinations have been described. The use of digital pressure proximal or distal to the injection site has been proposed as a means of limiting hemidiaphragmatic paresis or adjusting a block's sensory distribution pattern. Multiple studies have proven these maneuvers to be without merit (Fig. 6-23). Similarly, adducting the arm to 0° after axillary block increases central spread without affecting block success or overall sensory anesthesia.

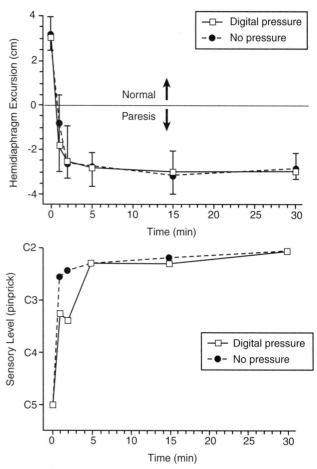

Figure 6-23   Digital pressure during interscalene block does not reduce hemidiaphragmatic paresis or limit sensory spread. (Redrawn from Urmey WF, Grossi P, Sharrock NE, et al.: Digital pressure during interscalene block is ineffective in preventing anesthetic spread to the cervical plexus, *Anesth Analg* 83:368, 1996, Figs. 1 and 2.)

SUGGESTED READING

Benumof JL: Permanent loss of cervical spinal cord function associated with interscalene block performed under general anesthesia, *Anesthesiology* 93:1541-1544, 2000.

Bouaziz H, Narchi P, Mercier FJ, et al.: Comparison between conventional axillary block and a new approach at the midhumeral level, *Anesth Analg* 84:1058-1062, 1997.

Brown DL: *Atlas of Regional Anesthesia*, Second Edition, WB Saunders, Philadelphia, 1999.

Brown DL, Cahill DR, Bridenbaugh LD: Supraclavicular nerve block: anatomic analysis of a method to prevent pneumothorax, *Anesth Analg* 76:530-534, 1993.

Neal JM, Hebl JR, Gerancher JC, et al.: Brachial plexus anesthesia: essentials of our current understanding, *Reg Anesth Pain Med* 27:402-428, 2002.

Thompson GE, Rorie DK: Functional anatomy of the brachial plexus sheaths, *Anesthesiology* 59:117-122, 1983.

Winnie AP: Interscalene brachial plexus block, *Anesth Analg* 49:455-466, 1970.

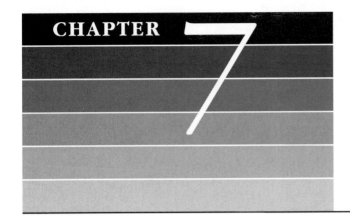

CHAPTER 7

Regional Anesthesia of the Trunk

JAMES P. RATHMELL

INTRODUCTION

Anesthesiologists think of peripheral nerve blocks first for providing anesthesia in the extremities. When choosing regional techniques to provide anesthesia and analgesia for the trunk, most will turn reflexively to spinal and epidural blockade. Nonetheless, there are a number of peripheral regional techniques ranging from field infiltration of the breast to specialized methods like interpleural block, in which local anesthetic is placed within the chest cavity, that can provide effective anesthesia and analgesia for the chest and abdomen. While the usefulness of these techniques has largely been supplanted by the widespread use of epidural anesthesia, familiarity with them can prove useful in a number of specific circumstances.

BREAST BLOCK

Anatomy. The breast and surrounding structures lying over the superior and anterior chest wall derive their sensory innervation from the distal branches of the lower cervical and upper thoracic nerve roots (Fig. 7-1 on p. 74). The glandular tissue and overlying skin are supplied by the lateral and anterior cutaneous divisions of the first through sixth intercostal nerves (T1-T6). The supraclavicular nerve, part of the superficial cervical

plexus, is primarily comprised of nerve fibers from C4, and supplies sensation to the skin in the supraclavicular fossa, overlying the clavicle and the superior portion of the breast. The axilla is innervated by the brachial plexus (C5-T1), and the intercostobrachial nerve (T2-T3).

Clinical uses. Surgical procedures carried out on the breast vary tremendously in scope and complexity, and regional anesthesia can be employed for many of these procedures. Simple needle or excision biopsies will rarely require anything more than local anesthetic infiltration. Excision of larger lesions (lumpectomy), partial mastectomy, and some simple plastic surgical procedures on the breast can be accomplished using field blocks. Regional anesthesia can also be used as an adjunct to general anesthesia to reduce anesthetic requirements and improve postoperative analgesia for more extensive procedures such as mastectomy with axillary lymph node dissection or reduction mammoplasty. Some centers have also employed thoracic epidural anesthesia for more extensive procedures (see Chapter 9).

Block technique. Regional anesthesia for procedures on the breast involves infiltration along the terminal branches of the numerous nerves that supply this region. Simple incision or excision biopsies are best performed with local anesthetic infiltration limited to the direct operative site. However, injecting local anesthetic directly into the glandular tissue of the breast itself results in inconsistent anesthesia because local anesthetic placed directly into the ducts of the breast will provide only topical anesthesia. Excision of larger lesions and simple mastectomy can be carried out using a series of field blocks (Fig. 7-1 on p. 74). Because of the large area that must be infiltrated, it is best to use a small-gauge (25 g Quincke), spinal needle that is $3\frac{1}{2}$ to 4 inches in length. The inferolateral portion of the breast can be anesthetized by placing local anesthetic within the retromammary space in a fanwise fashion through a single skin entry site inferolateral to the breast. The anterior branches of the intercostal

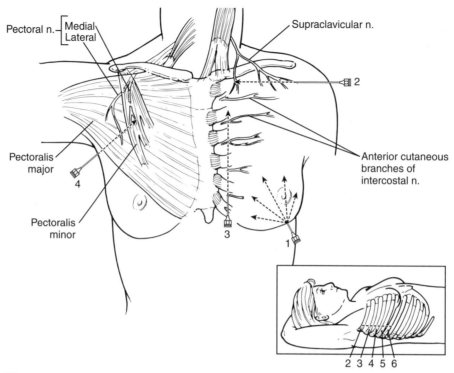

Figure 7-1 **Breast block**. Breast block can be accomplished in multiple ways and the approach must be matched to the magnitude of the surgery that is planned. (1) For simple excision biopsy or lumpectomy, infiltration behind the breast over the anterior chest wall within the pectoralis muscle will suffice. For more extensive procedures (reduction or augmentation mammoplasty, simple mastectomy), the other points of innervation must be anesthetized. This can be accomplished by placing (2) a subcutaneous line of local anesthetic from the sternoclavicular junction laterally to the acromion process, just inferior to the clavicle (supraclavicular branch of the superficial cervical plexus); (3) a second subcutaneous line of local anesthetic along the sternal border extending from the manubrium to the xiphoid process overlying the costosternal junctions (anterior cutaneous branches of the intercostal nerves); and (4) infiltrating within the superior portion of the pectoralis muscles where the anterior axillary fold meets the chest wall (medial and lateral pectoral nerves). Extensive anesthesia of the anterior chest wall can also be achieved using multiple intercostal nerve blocks placed over the lateral chest wall (inset). (Redrawn from Brown DL: *Regional Anesthesia and Analgesia*, WB Saunders, Philadelphia, 1996, p. 299.)

nerves supply the medial portion of the breast and are blocked using a single line of subcutaneous local anesthetic extending from the sternal notch to the xiphoid process overlying the costochondral junctions. The superior portion of the breast in anesthetized by placing a subcutaneous line of local anesthetic along the inferior margin of the clavicle extending from the sternal notch to the acromion process. If the surgical procedure will extend to the pectoral muscles, they can be anesthetized by infiltrating within the superolateral portion of the pectoralis muscles near the insertion of the pectoralis minor.

Complications. In the process of placing the numerous field blocks required to anesthetize the breast, large volumes of dilute local anesthetic are required (40–120 mL of 0.25–1% lidocaine or 0.125–0.25% bupivacaine). Close attention should be paid to the total dose of local anesthetic used as the volumes required can eas-

ily exceed those that produce toxic blood levels. For the same reason, bilateral procedures can rarely be accomplished using regional anesthesia alone without significant risk of local anesthetic toxicity. Other complications, including pneumothorax, are rare.

INTERCOSTAL NERVE BLOCK

Anatomy (Fig. 7-2 on p. 76). The intercostal nerves arise from the anterior primary rami of the first through twelfth thoracic nerve roots. The thoracic nerve roots exit the intervertebral foramina to enter the paravertebral space. The paravertebral space is bounded by the pleura anteromedially, the vertebral body medially, and the transverse spinous processes and paravertebral musculature posteriorly. The ribs traverse this space where they form two articulations with the vertebral bodies:

Clinical Caveat: Breast Block

The various injections that comprise this block must be tailored to supply appropriate analgesia for the planned procedure.

Inferior/lateral breast: Local anesthetic infiltration within the retromammary space from the inferolateral margin of the breast supplies sufficient anesthesia for biopsy or excision of small lesions within the glandular tissue of the breast. Extensive lesions and those more superior and medial within the breast should be supplemented.

Superior/medial breast: A line of subcutaneous local anesthetic extending from the manubrium to the xiphoid process overlying the costochondral junctions will anesthetize the anterior divisions of the intercostal nerves where they become superficial to supply sensation over the anteromedial chest wall.

Superior breast: A line of subcutaneous local anesthetic extending from the manubrium to the acromion process just inferior to the clavicle will anesthetize the descending supraclavicular branches of the superficial cervical plexus that supply sensation to the superior chest in the infraclavicular region.

Pectoralis muscles, including the anterior axillary fold: Local anesthetic is placed where the pectoralis muscles that form the anterior axillary fold first join the anterior chest wall in the superolateral quadrant of the breast. This will block sensory nerves to the pectoralis muscles, producing anesthesia of the anterior axilla and the deeper tissues of the chest wall.

the costotraverse articulation where the rib contacts the transverse process, and the costovertebral articulation where the head of the rib meets the vertebral body. The thoracic spinal nerve root exits the intervertebral foramen and ramifies into anterior and posterior branches – the anterior branch forms the intercostal nerve. The intercostal nerve traverses laterally to lie in the subcostal groove, a shallow notch along the inferior margin of each rib. Within this groove, the intercostal vein and artery lie in close proximity, just superior to the nerve. This accounts for the high plasma levels of local anesthetic produced with intercostal nerve blocks. The costal groove becomes shallow and ceases to exist some 5–8 cm lateral to the posterior midline. The intercostal nerve may lie immediately below the rib margin or closer to the midpoint between ribs as it traverses laterally. The lateral branch of the intercostal nerve arises over the posterolateral chest wall anterior to the posterior axillary line (an imaginary line extending directly inferior from the posterior axillary fold). This is an important factor to understand, as intercostal nerve blocks performed anterior to the posterior axillary line may not anesthetize this branch and may produce incomplete truncal anesthesia. The nerves continue anteriorly around the chest wall, ending in the anterior branches. These terminal branches supply sensation to the anterior chest wall and are described in the previous section on breast block.

Clinical uses. Prior to the widespread adoption of the thoracic epidural approach to provide analgesia following major thoracic and abdominal surgery, multiple intercostal nerve blocks were frequently used to provide postoperative pain control for common abdominal operations such as open cholecystectomy. The use of intercostal blocks has also been described for repair of small umbilical hernias, extracorporeal shock wave lithotripsy, and pacemaker insertion. Use of one or two level blocks remains an excellent means of providing anesthesia for chest tube insertion. Intercostal nerve block is a simple and effective means for relieving the pain of rib fractures, albeit limited to the duration of local anesthetic effect. Intercostal neurolytic blocks using phenol or alcohol have also proven effective for treating painful, isolated metastatic lesions involving the ribs.

Block technique. The intercostal nerves can be blocked anywhere along their course from the paravertebral region to the anterior chest wall. To obtain complete anesthesia along the trunk within the distribution of a given intercostal nerve, the nerve must be blocked before the lateral branch arises (posterior to the posterior axillary line). Posterior access to the intercostal nerves is blocked by the overlying scapula above the level of T6 over the posterior chest wall. While intercostal blocks can be performed with the patient in nearly any position, the simplest way to perform multiple intercostal blocks is with the patient fully prone. The shoulder can be easily abducted, placing the forearm over the head in order to swing the scapula laterally and gain access to the upper ribs. The flat portion of each rib is easily palpated several centimeters from midline, and the inferior margin of each rib is marked. Six or seven levels (T5 to T11 or T12) are anesthetized for abdominal surgery, while only the levels adjacent to the planned incision need be anesthetized for thoracic surgery.

The block is then carried out at each marked level (Fig. 7-3 on p. 77). A skin wheal of local anesthetic is placed over each marked site to provide anesthesia of the skin and subcutaneous tissues. The skin over each rib is then retracted superiorly and a 22 gauge, $1\frac{1}{2}$ inch needle attached to a syringe containing local anesthetic is advanced to contact the inferior margin of the rib. Use of smaller-gauge needles is advocated by some experts, but detecting contact with bone is more difficult as less rigid needles bend easily. Using a control syringe with three round holes for two fingers and the thumb makes aspiration and injection with one hand much easier (Fig. 7-3 on p. 77). The needle is angled

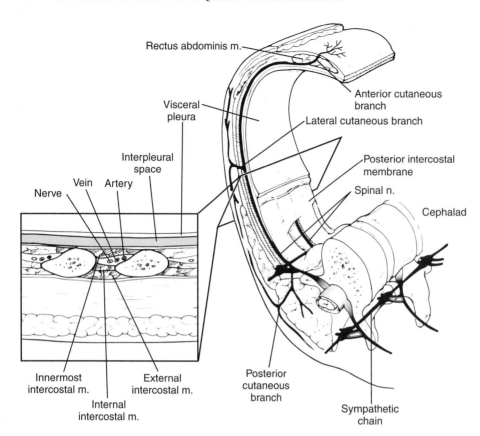

Figure 7-2   Anatomy of the intercostal nerve. The thoracic spinal nerve root exits the intervertebral foramen and divides into anterior and posterior rami. The posterior branch supplies motor innervation to the spinal erector muscles and terminates in the posterior cutaneous branch which supplies sensation to the skin overlying the spinous processes. The anterior ramus of the spinal nerve traverses laterally in the paravertebral space, inferior to the transverse process where it enters the subcostal groove inferior to the intercostal vein and artery. The lateral cutaneous branch arises somewhat anterior to the posterior axillary line and supplies sensation to the lateral chest wall. The intercostal nerve terminates as the anterior cutaneous branch which courses both medially and laterally as it becomes superficial, supplying sensation to the anterior torso. (Redrawn from Brown DL: *Regional Anesthesia and Analgesia*, WB Saunders, Philadelphia, 1996, p. 498.)

slightly cephalad and walked off the inferior margin of the rib maintaining the slight cephalad angulation, allowing the needle to slip beneath the rib and into the intercostal groove. Once the needle walks beneath the rib margin, it is advanced 2 to 3 mm further. The needle should be moved slightly (about 1 mm) in and out during the course of the injection to decrease the possibility that all of the local anesthetic will be given directly intravascularly, and that some of the agent will be placed in close proximity to the nerve. The same procedure is carried out for adjacent levels. The small distance between the rib's inferior margin and the pleura must be emphasized; advancing the needle more than a few millimeters beyond the bony margin may result in pneumothorax.

Complications. Because of the close proximity of vascular structures to the intercostal nerves, there is a significant risk of direct intravascular injection and vascular uptake during each block. Intercostal nerve blocks result in plasma concentrations of local anesthetic greater than any other peripheral nerve block (see Fig. 2-5 on p. 22). Thus, close attention must be paid to the total local anesthetic dose delivered and to adequate monitoring, intravenous access, and ready availability of resuscitation equipment and drugs.

Pneumothorax can occur, but the incidence is low. Centers with extensive experience using intercostal nerve blocks for postoperative analgesia have reported significant pneumothorax in 0.073% of a series of 10,000 intercostal nerve blocks performed by physicians at various levels of training. The incidence of clinically insignificant, but radiographically demonstrable pneumothorax is somewhat higher (0.42%). Treatment of most pneumothoraces should be conservative, with observation and administration of oxygen, which will aid reabsorption. Needle aspiration or chest tube drainage are rarely necessary and should be reserved only for those with symptomatic pneumothoraces.

Clinical Caveat: Intercostal Nerve Block

A common mistake while performing intercostal nerve block is placing the block too anteriorly along the rib margin. The lateral cutaneous branch of the intercostal nerve arises anterior to the posterior axillary line (a line extending directly inferior from the posterior axillary fold). This branch supplies sensation to a variable and often extensive area over the lateral chest wall. Thus, for complete anesthesia of the chest wall, intercostal block should be performed posterior to the posterior axillary line before the lateral cutaneous branch arises.

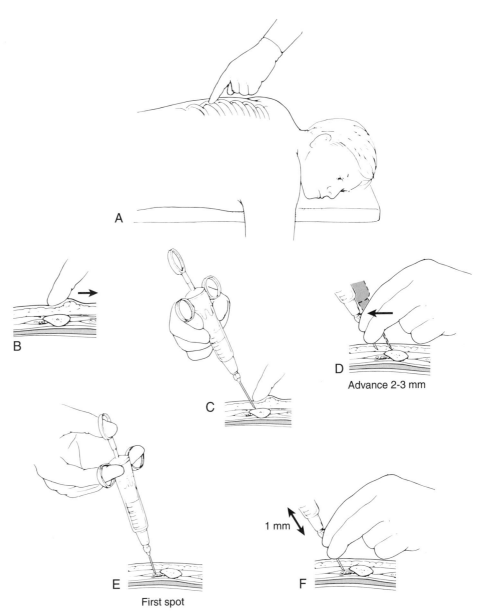

Figure 7-3   Technique for intercostal nerve block. A, The patient typically lies prone (although the block can be carried out anywhere along the course of each intercostal nerve). The illustrations demonstrate the technique for a right-handed person. **B,** The left index finger is used to palpate the rib margin and pull the skin and subcutaneous tissues upward over the rib. **C,** Using a control syringe in the right hand, the needle is placed through the skin with a slight cephalad angulation and into contact with the inferior margin of the rib. **D,** The left hand is then moved to grasp the needle at the point of skin entry and the needle is walked off the inferior margin of the rib while maintaining the slight cephalad angulation and advanced 2 to 3 mm beyond the inferior margin of the rib. **E,** Local anesthetic (3–5 mL) is then injected. **F,** The needle tip is moved 1 mm in and out throughout the injection to minimize the chance that the entire volume will be placed intravascularly. (Redrawn from Brown DL: *Regional Anesthesia and Analgesia,* WB Saunders, Philadelphia, 1996, p. 302.)

Advance 2-3 mm

First spot

1 mm

INTERPLEURAL BLOCK

Anatomy. The pleural space is a potential space between two thin connective tissue layers: the parietal pleura and the visceral pleura. The visceral pleura adheres tightly to the lung itself, following the fissures of the lung. The parietal pleura extends along the surface of the chest wall, mediastinum, and diaphragm. The pleura extend from the cupola of the lung in the supraclavicular fossa to the diaphragm at about the level of L1. It has been long recognized that various fluids accumulate between the pleural layers in traumatic and pathologic conditions (hemothorax, pneumotho-

rax, etc.). Investigators recognized that the parietal pleura form only a thin connective tissue barrier overlying the thoracic nerve roots and intercostal nerves, the thoracic sympathetic chain, and the splanchnic nerves. They found that placing local anesthetic solution within the pleural space can provide effective analgesia via diffusion of the local anesthetic through the thin pleural barrier to the adjacent neural structures (Fig. 7-4 on p. 78).

Clinical uses. The use of interpleural block has gained only limited popularity, largely due to the fear of pneumothorax and toxicity from the large doses of local anesthetic required to maintain continuous analgesia. Thoracic epidural infusions have largely

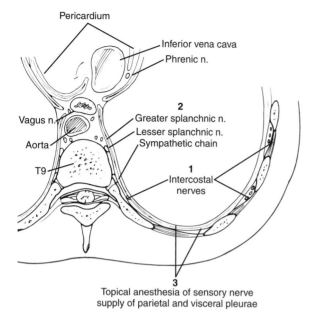

Pericardium

Inferior vena cava
Phrenic n.

2
Greater splanchnic n.
Lesser splanchnic n.
Sympathetic chain

Vagus n.

Aorta

T9

1
Intercostal
nerves

3
Topical anesthesia of sensory nerve
supply of parietal and visceral pleurae

Figure 7-4   Anatomy of the pleura and the theoretical basis for success of interpleural analgesia. Local anesthetic placed between the visceral and parietal pleura can easily penetrate to anesthetize adjacent neural structures. (1) Local anesthetic can reach the intercostal nerves anywhere along their course from the paravertebral space to the anterior chest wall. (2) Visceral fibers descending from the thoracic sympathetic chain via the splanchnic nerves lie just beneath the pleura over the anterolateral aspect of the inferior thoracic vertebral bodies. (3) Local anesthetic may also provide direct topical anesthesia to the pleural surfaces themselves. The predominant effect of the local anesthetic solution likely has much to do with the patient's position during the initial interpleural placement of the local anesthetic solution. For instance, if anesthesia is required for the lower intercostal segments following cholecystectomy, the patient should be placed with the head slightly elevated and the operative side tilted upward about 45°. The local anesthetic will pool inferiorly over the exiting nerve roots and provide extensive analgesia limited to the lower thoracic nerve roots. (Adapted from Brown DL: *Regional Anesthesia and Analgesia*, WB Saunders, Philadelphia, 1996, p. 304.)

supplanted the use of interpleural catheters for postoperative pain control. The technique is best suited for unilateral procedures in the upper abdomen and lower thorax such as open cholecystectomy, renal surgery, and unilateral breast procedures. The usefulness of this technique is limited for thoracotomy – the degree of analgesia appears to be compromised when the parietal pleura has been breached, and when the thoracostomy drainage tube promotes loss of the infused local anesthetic.

Interpleural anesthesia also provides an effective method for producing sympathetic blockade of the upper extremity (inferior cervical ganglion, superior thoracic ganglia), the torso (thoracic paravertebral sympathetic chain), and intra-abdominal structures (greater, lesser, and least splanchnic nerves).

Block technique. Interpleural catheters are most commonly placed with the patient in the lateral position (Fig. 7-5 on p. 79). The point of entry is 8 to 10 cm from the posterior midline near the posterior axillary line. Entry from this position will ensure that the catheter preferentially travels posteriorly toward the exiting nerve roots. Placing local anesthetic solution close to the nerve roots assures the most effective analgesia. Depending on the region where analgesia is needed, the entry is made in the fifth through tenth intercostal space. The skin and subcutaneous tissues are first anesthetized overlying the superior margin of the rib. A 16 or 18 gauge Tuohy needle is then advanced to contact the superior margin of the rib. The stylette is removed and replaced with a typical glass loss-of-resistance syringe containing a small volume of air or saline. The needle bevel is oriented in the direction in which the catheter is intended to travel. The needle is then walked over the superior margin of the rib and slowly advanced until the fluid in the syringe is drawn inward. The patient will often experience a brief localized painful twinge as the needle penetrates the parietal pleura. The use of loss of resistance to positive pressure is unnecessary and can be misleading. The negative interpleural pressure will reliably draw the fluid inward when the pleura is penetrated. At this point, local anesthetic solution or, more typically, a catheter for continuous infusion is placed through the Tuohy needle and the needle is removed. As during epidural placement, local anesthetic should be given in divided doses to assure that intravascular cannulation has not occurred. An amount of 20 to 30 mL of local anesthetic is usually required for effective analgesia (0.25–0.5% bupivacaine). As the interpleural space is continuous from top to bottom, the patient must be positioned properly to produce analgesia in the desired region. The most effective position for extensive analgesia of the chest or abdominal wall is with the effected side raised 45° to allow the local anesthetic to pool over the exiting nerve roots.

Complications. The most common complication associated with interpleural block is pneumothorax. The reported incidence is approximately 2% and is most common in patients who are receiving mechanical ventilation or when an active loss-of-resistance technique is employed. Pneumothorax occurring during this block is often due to sudden patient movement during the procedure.

Plasma levels of local anesthetic after interpleural block are similar to or greater than those that occur during intercostal block, and are not affected by addition of epinephrine. The intensity of the local anesthetic block is not as dense as that found with intercostal blocks and the duration is shorter.

The appearance of Horner's syndrome (ptosis, miosis, and anhidrosis) on the side of interpleural block is

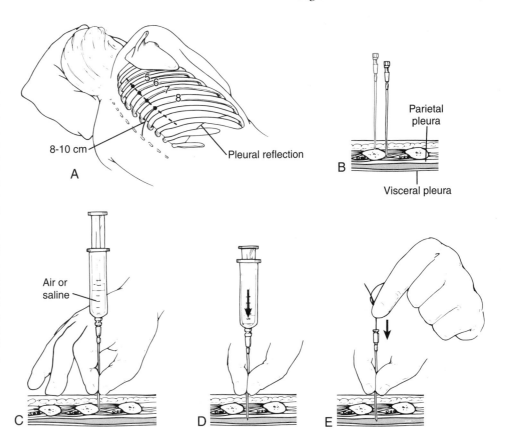

Figure 7-5 Interpleural block. A, The patent is placed in the lateral decubitus position and the ribs are palpated 8 to 10 cm from midline. B, A skin wheal is raised and a Tuohy needle is advanced to contact the superior margin of the rib. C, The needle is grasped at the point of skin entry and a glass syringe filled with 3 to 5 mL of air or saline is attached. D, The needle is advanced until the pleura is penetrated and the fluid in the syringe is drawn inward. E, Using caution to prevent the entry of air, a catheter is inserted through the needle and advanced 8 to 10 cm to lie over the exiting nerve roots. (Redrawn from Brown DL: *Regional Anesthesia and Analgesia*, WB Saunders, Philadelphia, 1996, p. 305.)

common and stems from blockade of the stellate ganglion over the head of the first rib. Phrenic nerve paralysis can also occur due to the close proximity of this nerve to the medial pleural reflection.

Clinical Caveat: Limitations of Interpleural Block

One of the most useful settings that can be imagined for applying interpleural block is for managing post-thoracotomy pain. What could seem easier to perform and potentially more useful? The pleural cavity is open and a catheter can be placed directly over the exiting thoracic nerve roots in the best location to anesthetize the surgical incision. There is no risk of pneumothorax, as the chest has been open and a thoracotomy drainage tube will be in place. However, the continuous suction needed to maintain lung inflation and prevent pneumothorax in the early hours after surgery also results in loss of the infused local anesthetic. Indeed, adequate analgesia cannot be maintained in most patients following thoracotomy without turning the thoracostomy suction off for 20–30 minutes after a bolus of local anesthetic is placed to allow time for the agent to penetrate the pleura and anesthetize the nerve roots.

THORACIC PARAVERTEBRAL NERVE BLOCK

Anatomy. Thoracic paravertebral block is essentially a proximal intercostal block that anesthetizes the exiting nerve root just outside the intervertebral foramen within the paravertebral space. The thoracic spinal nerve roots exit the vertebral foramina just below the pedicle where it meets the transverse process (Fig. 7-6 on p. 80). Anterior to the foramen lies the medial pleural reflection and the lung. The proximal portion of the rib lies just superior to the foramen and articulates with the transverse process (costotransverse articulation) and the vertebral body (costovertebral articulation). The thoracic paravertebral space is contiguous with the epidural space as well as adjacent thoracic segments. Local anesthetic injected at one level will extend partially into the lateral epidural space via the intervertebral foramen and to adjacent segments within the paravertebral space. The transverse processes of the thoracic vertebrae serve as the bony landmark for performing thoracic paravertebral block and they are variable in size: small in the lower thoracic region and more pronounced in the upper thoracic region. The exiting nerve roots lie just caudad and anterior to the transverse processes.

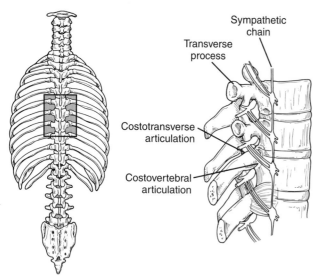

Figure 7-6   Anatomy of the thoracic nerve roots. The rib articulates with the transverse process and the vertebral body just superior to the pedicle and the intervertebral foramen. The thoracic spinal nerve root exits the vertebral foramen where the posterior cutaneous branch arises; the nerve then traverses laterally where it enters the subcostal groove as the intercostal nerve.

Clinical uses. Thoracic paravertebral block is analogous to a proximal block of the intercostal nerve and can be substituted for intercostal nerve block. This block is rarely sufficient as the sole anesthetic for anything but simple, brief procedures. It has been combined with general anesthesia to reduce anesthetic requirements and provide early postoperative analgesia for a number of thoracic and abdominal surgeries. Like intercostal nerve blocks, thoracic paravertebral blocks can be used to treat pain associated with rib fractures, chronic postthoracotomy pain, and herpes zoster involving the thoracic dermatomes. Because agents injected into the thoracic paravertebral space tend to spread to adjacent nerve roots as well as proximally to involve the lateral epidural space, use of this technique is favored for intercostal neurolysis when metastatic lesions of the chest wall involve several adjacent ribs. In this instance, neurolysis at a single level can be used to produce analgesia in adjacent affected levels.

Block technique. Thoracic paravertebral block can be performed with the patient in the prone, lateral, or sitting position (Fig. 7-7). The spinous processes are palpated in the midline. Because of the large overlying

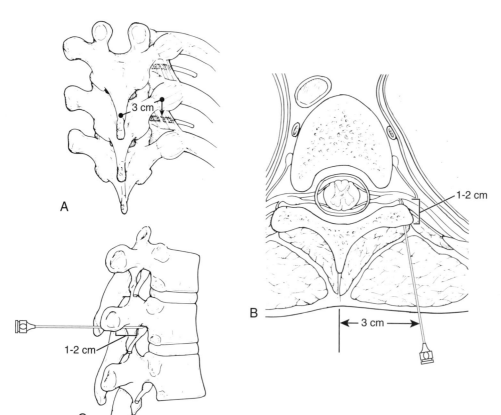

Figure 7-7   Thoracic paravertebral block. **A**, A skin wheal is raised 3 cm lateral and 1 cm superior to the spinous process overlying the transverse process. **B**, The needle is advanced perpendicular to the skin's surface except for a slight (5–10°) medial angulation. Note the proximity of the sympathetic chain and pleura to the needle's final location. **C**, The transverse process is contacted at a depth of 2 to 5 cm and the needle is walked caudad. The needle is then advanced 1 to 2 cm anterior to the transverse process to lie adjacent to the exiting nerve root outside of the intervertebral foramen. (Redrawn from Brown DL: *Regional Anesthesia and Analgesia*, WB Saunders, Philadelphia, 1996, p. 308.)

spinal erector muscles, the transverse processes can rarely be palpated, even in slender individuals. They lie approximately 3 cm lateral and slightly superior to the spinous processes. A skin wheal is raised 3 cm lateral and 1 cm superior to the caudal tip of the spinous process. A 3 to $3\frac{1}{2}$ inch needle is directed slightly medially (10° from the sagittal plane) and perpendicular to the skin in the cephalad to caudad direction. The needle should contact the transverse process at a depth of 2 to 5 cm. If the needle does not contact bone by a depth of 5 cm, the needle should be removed and the point of skin entry moved slightly cephalad to contact the transverse process. The needle is then walked off the caudal margin of the transverse process and advanced 1 to 2 cm to lie within the intervertebral foramen. After aspiration, 6 to 8 mL of local anesthetic is deposited adjacent to each nerve root.

Complications. Pneumothorax is uncommon, but the exact incidence is unknown. This complication is likely to be less frequent than with intercostal nerve block because the pleural reflection is significantly more anterior to the exiting nerve root than to the intercostal nerves. Because the paravertebral space is contiguous from one level to the next and with the epidural space, injection at a small number of levels can result in more extensive analgesia than expected. Indeed, spread into the epidural space may produce bilateral sensory block. Subarachnoid injection is also possible when the needle is directed through the intervertebral foramen and penetrates the lateral dural cuff.

ILIOINGUINAL/ILIOHYPOGASTRIC NERVE BLOCK

Anatomy. The ilioinguinal, iliohypogastric, and genitofemoral nerves are the primary nerves supplying sensation to the groin region. The ilioinguinal and iliohypogastric nerves travel from the posterior abdominal wall anteriorly between the transversus abdominis and internal oblique muscles. The iliohypogastric nerve receives contributions from T12 and L1 and pierces the internal oblique muscle adjacent to the anterior superior iliac spine. The ilioinguinal nerve arises from L1 alone and pierces the internal oblique muscle somewhat medial to the anterior superior iliac spine where it enters the inguinal canal. The genitofemoral nerve receives contributions from L1 and L2 and divides very proximal in the retroperitoneum as it emerges from the psoas muscle. The genital branch courses inferiorly to enter the inguinal canal along with the spermatic cord and supplies sensation to the skin and fascia overlying the scrotum or labia majora. The femoral branch passes beneath the midportion of the inguinal ligament to sup-

ply sensation to the skin just inferior to the inguinal ligament over the anterior portion of the thigh. Blockade of the genitofemoral nerve is limited to treatment of chronic pain and will not be discussed further. Blockade of the ilioinguinal and iliohypogastric nerves takes advantage of the close anatomic proximity of the two nerves as they pass medial to the anterior superior iliac spine. Because of the variable depth of the nerves within the musculature of the abdominal wall, local anesthetic must be placed over a field that passes between various muscle layers.

Clinical uses. Combined block of the ilioinguinal and iliohypogastric nerves adjacent to the anterior superior iliac spine has been termed "hernia block" due to its usefulness in providing excellent postoperative analgesia during repair of simple direct and indirect inguinal hernias. This block can be combined with supplemental local anesthetic infiltration and light sedation for uncomplicated primary hernia repair. However, when there is a large hernia sac with extension of the peritoneum and bowel into the inguinal canal, the extensive dissection and peritoneal retraction required to repair the defect mandates the use of heavier sedation and extensive local infiltration. In many cases, general anesthesia with a hernia block for postoperative pain control is a more prudent approach. Likewise, the dissection required for repair of recurrent inguinal hernia or placement of mesh graft to repair an extensive abdominal wall defect is unlikely to proceed well with a hernia block alone. Finally, postherniorrhaphy pain is a common neuropathic pain problem and may involve the ilioinguinal, iliohypogastric, and/or genitofemoral nerves. Local anesthetic infiltration with or without a corticosteroid has been used for the diagnosis and management of postherniorrhaphy pain.

Block technique. The ilioinguinal and iliohypogastric nerves lie in close proximity to one another and adjacent to the anterior superior iliac spine. However, the ilioinguinal nerve pierces the internal oblique muscle at a variable location over the anterior abdominal wall; thus the two nerves may lie in separate fascial planes. To perform the block, a line is drawn between the anterior superior iliac spine and the umbilicus, and a skin wheal is raised at a point along this line approximately 1 cm medial and 1 cm cephalad to the anterior superior iliac spine (Fig. 7-8 on p. 82). A 25 gauge, $1\frac{1}{2}$ inch needle is advanced in an anterior to posterior plane to a depth of 2 to 4 cm and a total of 6 to 8 mL of local anesthetic (0.25% bupivacaine is often utilized) is injected while the needle is withdrawn. The needle is then angled 10 to 15° more medially, inserted to similar depth, and an additional 6 to 8 mL of local anesthetic is administered as the needle is withdrawn. This deposits a field of local anesthetic along the course of both nerves as they variably lie in different fascial planes.

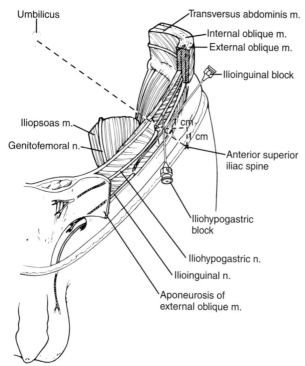

Figure 7-8 **Ilioinguinal and iliohypogastric nerve block.** The iliohypogastric and ilioinguinal nerves traverse from the lateral to anterior abdominal walls between muscle planes, and lie in close proximity adjacent to the anterior superior iliac spine. To perform the block, a single needle is inserted approximately 1 cm medial and 1 cm superior to the anterior superior iliac spine along a line connecting the anterior superior iliac spine and the umbilicus. The needle is initially passed directly posteriorly to a depth of 3 to 4 cm and local anesthetic is injected as the needle is withdrawn. A second pass of the needle is made in a more inferior direction to a similar depth, and local anesthetic again injected as the needle is withdrawn. (Redrawn from Brown DL: *Regional Anesthesia and Analgesia*, WB Saunders, Philadelphia, 1996, p. 569.)

Complications. Complications associated with ilioinguinal/iliohypogastric block are uncommon. When this block is combined with supplemental local anesthetic infiltration within the surgical field, fairly large volumes of local anesthetic may be required for bilateral blocks, and attention must be paid to the total dose administered to avoid systemic toxicity. Penetration of the bowel or the spermatic cord, and direct intravascular injection may also occur.

Case Study: Postherniorrhaphy Pain

A 32-year-old man returns to his surgeon 3 months after repair of an indirect inguinal hernia. The surgery was uncomplicated and completed without the need for mesh graft. He reports marked pain and sensitivity to light touch along the course of the incision and the lower abdominal wall. Examination reveals no evidence of a recurrent hernia.

Some degree of postherniorrhaphy pain persists at 3-month follow-up in 8 to 10% of patients who undergo primary repair of an inguinal hernia. This may involve the distribution of the ilioinguinal, iliohypogastric, and/or genitofemoral nerves. Persistent pain likely results from peripheral nerve injury caused by pressure exerted by the hernia or nerve stretch injury sustained in the process of repairing the hernia. In most cases, the pain gradually diminishes with time. Local anesthetic block of the peripheral nerves is often used to facilitate the diagnosis, and placement of local anesthetic and steroid may produce significant reduction in the persistent pain.

CONCLUSIONS

The widespread use of continuous epidural infusions to provide postoperative analgesia for major thoracic and abdominal surgeries has largely supplanted the use of single-shot peripheral nerve blocks of the trunk for hospitalized patients. Nonetheless, familiarity with these techniques can provide excellent anesthesia and postoperative analgesia for a variety of minor surgeries in ambulatory patients.

SUGGESTED READING

Brown DL: *Atlas of Regional Anesthesia*, Second Edition, WB Saunders, Philadelphia, 1999, pp. 217–251.

Kopacz DJ: Regional anesthesia of the trunk. In: *Regional Anesthesia and Analgesia*, WB Saunders, Philadelphia, 1996, pp. 292–318.

Neumann M, Raj PP: Thoracoabdominal pain. In: Raj PP (ed), *Practical Management of Pain*, Third Edition, Mosby, St. Louis, 2000, pp. 618–629.

CHAPTER 8

Lower Extremity Blocks

JOSEPH M. NEAL

CHRISTOPHER M. VISCOMI

INTRODUCTION

Lower extremity regional anesthesia is performed less frequently than upper extremity block. There are several reasons why anesthesiologists are less familiar with these techniques. In contrast to the relatively compact brachial plexus, the four major nerves to the lower extremity are widely spaced and reside deep within tissues that are identified by less familiar landmarks (Fig. 8-1 on p. 84). Despite its demand for time and patience, lower extremity block is beneficial in the practice of regional anesthesia, albeit contemporary use favors analgesic applications over the provision of surgical anesthesia. Lower extremity blockade offers the unique advantages of avoiding bilateral sympathectomy and side effects of neuraxial opioids, such as urinary retention, pruritus, and respiratory depression. This chapter reviews the anatomy pertinent to lower extremity regional anesthesia; describes commonly used approaches for blocking the two major plexi and/or individual nerves at the hip, popliteal fossa, and ankle; and discusses major complications.

BASIC ANATOMY

Four major nerves supply the lower extremity (Table 8-1). The femoral, obturator, and lateral femoral cutaneous nerves originate from the lumbar plexus and

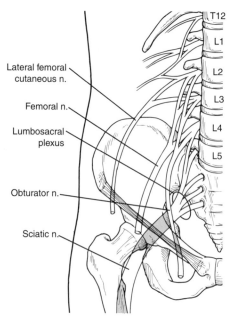

Figure 8-1   Anatomic layout of the lumbar and lumbosacral plexi. Note the widely spaced individual nerves. (Redrawn from Brown, DL: *Atlas of Regional Anesthesia*, Second Edition, WB Saunders, Philadelphia, 1999, p. 95, Fig. 11-1.)

primarily innervate the anterior leg. The posterior leg is innervated by the lumbosacral plexus, which forms the sciatic nerve (Fig. 8-2 on p. 85) (Box 8-1). An understanding of lower extremity neuroanatomy allows the anesthesiologist to select the appropriate approach for a specific surgery, identify which nerves require supple-

mental block, accurately assess the block prior to incision, and avoid complications.

Lower extremity cutaneous innervation consists of overlapping sensory fields from multiple nerve fibers (Fig. 8-3 on p. 86), thus making block assessment using loss of sensation imprecise. A simpler means of assessing lower extremity block – push, pull, pinch, punt – utilizes specific functions to evaluate individual terminal nerves (Fig. 8-4 on p. 86).

Clinical Caveat: Assessing Lower Extremity Block (Fig. 8-4)

PUSH – Patient plantar flexes the foot against resistance (sciatic nerve)
PULL – Patient adducts the thigh against resistance (obturator nerve)
PINCH – Anesthesiologist pinches the lateral buttock/upper thigh (lateral femoral cutaneous nerve)
PUNT – Patient punts an imaginary football against resistance (femoral nerve)

Lumbosacral Plexus

The lumbosacral plexus originates as the anterior rami of the fourth and fifth lumbar nerves (L4–L5) plus the first, second, and third sacral nerves (S1–S3), and wholly

---

Table 8-1   Major Nerves of the Lower Extremity

Nerve	Plexus of Origin	Roots of Origin	Motor Function	Sensory Function	Anatomic Relationships
Femoral	Lumbar	L2, L3, L4 posterior divisions	Quadriceps (knee extension) Sartorius (hip adduction)	Anterior thigh Medial lower leg - knee to great toe (saphenous n.) Articular branches to knee and hip	Groove between psoas and iliacus muscles Beneath inguinal ligament and lateral to femoral artery
Obturator	Lumbar	L2, L3, L4 anterior divisions	Thigh adduction	Lower medial thigh Articular branches to hip and knee	Deep in obturator canal Lateral to and below the pubic tubercle
Lateral Femoral Cutaneous	Lumbar	L2, L3 posterior divisions	None	Lateral thigh to mid thigh Anterolateral thigh from mid thigh to knee	Deep to inguinal ligament Medial and caudad to anterior superior iliac spine
Sciatic 1. Tibial n. 2. Common peroneal n.	Lumbosacral	Anterior rami of L4, L5; S1, S2, S3: 1. Ventral branches 2. Dorsal branches	Hamstrings (knee flexion) Muscles of the lower leg and foot (foot plantar or dorsi flexion)	Posterior femoral nerve Skin of lower leg and foot (except saphenous distribution) Articular branches to the knee	Exits pelvis at sacral notch Tibial and common peroneal nerves split at the popliteal fossa

entire lower leg and foot except for their medial portion (saphenous nerve). The sciatic nerve controls movement of the hamstrings and lower leg. The largest nerve in the body, the sciatic actually consists of two major trunks. The tibial nerve is the more medial and is comprised of the anterior branches of the lumbosacral plexus, while the posterior branches form the smaller and more lateral common peroneal nerve. The sciatic nerve exits the pelvis through the greater sciatic notch (sacrosciatic foramen), lies anterior to the piriformis muscle, and accompanies the posterior femoral cutaneous nerve. The sciatic nerve maintains a relationship to the femur throughout its proximal course. Initially it lies between the ischial tuberosity and greater trochanter, and then traverses distally along the posterior medial femur (Fig. 8-1 on p. 84). Near the cephalad border of the popliteal fossa, although occasionally more proximally, the tibial and common peroneal nerves split. At the knee, the tibial nerve maintains its relative medial position, while the common peroneal nerve courses farther laterally. Understanding and visualizing these anatomic relationships builds a basis for interpreting paresthesias or motor responses during sciatic nerve block (Table 8-2). For instance, foot plantar flexion indicates tibial nerve stimulation, and thus medial needle placement. Since the sciatic nerve consists of two distinct components, controversy exists as to whether multiple stimulation or injection techniques are more effective than a single injection.

Lumbar Plexus

The lumbar plexus originates as the anterior rami of the first through fourth lumbar nerves (L1–L4), with inconsistent contributions from the twelfth thoracic and fifth lumbar nerves. The rami further subdivide into posterior and anterior divisions. The femoral and lateral femoral cutaneous nerves originate from the posterior divisions, while the obturator nerve comprises the anterior division (Fig. 8-1 on p. 84). Superior and inferior branches of the L1 and T12 nerve roots become the iliohypogastric and ilioinguinal nerves, and the genitofemoral nerve, respectively (see Chapter 7). The lumbar plexus passes through the psoas compartment and courses within the psoas muscle as it divides into three distinct nerves (Table 8-1). The *femoral nerve* leaves the psoas muscle and is contained within a space between the psoas and iliacus muscles as it passes under the inguinal ligament, and gives off anterior and posterior branches. The key anatomic relationship of the femoral nerve is that it lies just lateral and partially posterior to the femoral artery. The anterior branch provides motor control to the sartorius and sensory innervation of the anterior thigh; the posterior branch controls the quadriceps muscles and sensory innervation to the majority of the knee joint, the hip joint, and the saphenous nerve. The *lateral femoral*

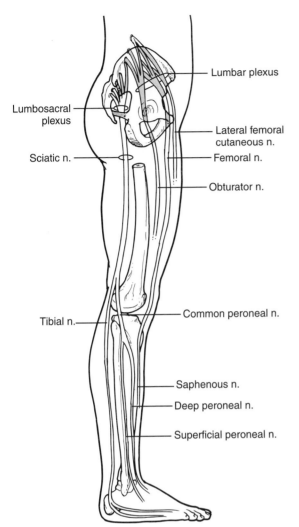

Figure 8-2 Lumbar and lumbosacral plexi. The lumbar plexus innervates the anterior thigh and medial lower leg, while the lumbosacral plexus innervates the posterior thigh and remainder of the lower leg. (Redrawn from Brown, DL: *Atlas of Regional Anesthesia*, WB Saunders, Philadelphia, 1992, p. 66, Fig. 8-2.)

constitutes the sciatic and posterior femoral cutaneous nerves (Fig. 8-1). The latter provides cutaneous innervation to the posterior thigh. The sciatic nerve provides sensory innervation to the posterior knee joint and the

Box 8-1 Components of the Lumbar and Lumbosacral Plexi

Lumbosacral plexus (sciatic nerve):
  Anterior rami of L4–5
  Anterior rami of S1–3
  Occasional contributions from S4
Lumbar plexus (femoral, obturator, lateral femoral cutaneous nerves):
  Anterior rami of L1–4
  Occasional contributions from T12 and L5

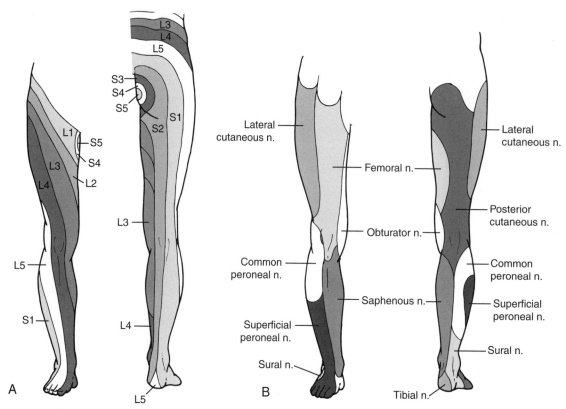

Figure 8-3 Dermatomes and sensory innervation of the lower extremity. (Redrawn from Wedel DJ: Nerve blocks. In: Miller RD (ed), *Anesthesia*, Fourth Edition, Churchill Livingstone, New York, 1994, p. 1547, Fig. 47-12.)

cutaneous nerve passes through the fascia lata to the abdominal wall, where it courses laterally and near the anterior superior iliac spine before dipping underneath the inguinal ligament. The only major nerve to the lower extremity that is purely sensory, it innervates skin of the

lateral hip and thigh down to the knee. The *obturator nerve* takes a medial course through the pelvis and exits via the obturator canal lateral to the pubic tubercle. Its anterior branch innervates the superficial thigh adductors, the hip joint, and has variable sensory innervation to

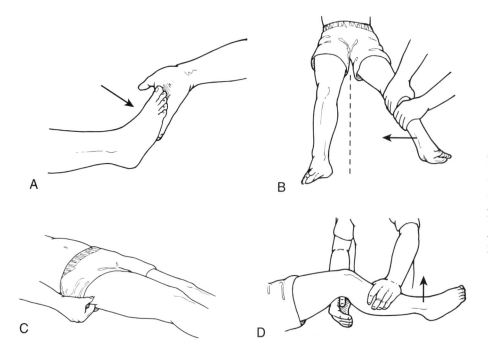

Figure 8-4 Assessment of lower extremity nerve block. **A**, Push (sciatic nerve) – **B**, pull (obturator nerve) – **C**, pinch (lateral femoral cutaneous nerve) – **D**, punt (femoral nerve). (Redrawn from Neal JM: Assessment of lower extremity nerve block: reprise of the Four Ps acronym, *Reg Anesth Pain Med* 27, 2002, pp. 618–620, Figs. 1-4.)

Table 8-2 Lumbar and Lumbosacral Plexi Stimulation: Expected Motor Response

Peripheral Nerve	Expected Motor Response
Femoral	Elevation of patellar tendon
Obturator	Contraction of thigh adductors
Mixed stimulation at the psoas compartment	Contraction of the quadriceps and/or thigh adductors
Lateral femoral cutaneous	None (purely sensory nerve)
Sciatic	
Tibial nerve	Foot plantar flexion
Common peroneal	Foot dorsiflexion or eversion
Mixed stimulation at the hip	Foot movement, typically inversion
Mixed stimulation at the popliteal fossa	Foot inversion

the medial thigh; the posterior branch innervates the deep adductors and supplies an articular branch to the knee. Understanding the anatomy of the lumbar plexus aids the anesthesiologist in block selection and evaluation (Table 8-2).

SCIATIC NERVE BLOCK

Proximal Approaches

Patient Selection

Patients undergoing lower leg amputation or surgery of the lower leg or foot benefit from sciatic nerve block, particularly if one wishes to limit the sympathetic perturbations that are occasionally associated with neuraxial block (Box 8-2). The sciatic nerve is rarely blocked in isolation; rather, supplemental femoral nerve block is required for surgery of the lower leg. All four major peripheral nerves must be blocked if a thigh tourniquet is to be used. Postoperatively, an isolated sciatic block provides analgesia after calcaneal surgery, but adds no further value to femoral nerve block after total knee arthroplasty. Because

Box 8-2 Indications for Sciatic Nerve Block

Below the knee amputation (with femoral nerve block)
Ankle and foot surgery (with saphenous nerve block, if indicated)
Analgesia following foot surgery
To avoid the hemodynamic consequences of bilateral lower extremity sympathectomy associated with neuraxial blockade

sciatic nerve block impairs leg strength and has a long duration, even with intermediate-acting local anesthetics, it may be inappropriate for ambulatory patients.

Block Techniques

Over half a dozen proximal approaches to the sciatic nerve have been described. Selection is based on personal preference or the ability to position the patient comfortably for block placement. Three approaches will be described – the classic approach of Labat and the recently described subgluteal posterior approaches, and the lateral approach. The latter is most useful when lateral or prone position increases patient discomfort, but it may spare the posterior femoral cutaneous nerve. Once mastered, either approach should be greater than 90% successful. Furthermore, both the classic and lateral approaches are efficacious in children. Other described approaches to the sciatic nerve include the anterior and lithotomy techniques. However, they are typically more painful to perform than those to be described, yet provide no unique benefit.

Classic (Labat) Approach

Labat's classic block approaches the sciatic nerve from the posterior direction. This block is executed in the lateral Sims position – on the side, leaning slightly forward, with the non-dependent heel (blocked leg) resting just below the knee of the dependent leg (Fig. 8-5). A line is drawn from the posterior superior iliac spine to the greater trochanter's cephalad prominence. A second perpendicular line that is extended caudally bisects this line. Needle placement is 3 to 5 cm down this perpendicular line. More exact measurement to adjust for patient height involves drawing a third line from the sacral hiatus to the same point on the greater trochanter, which will

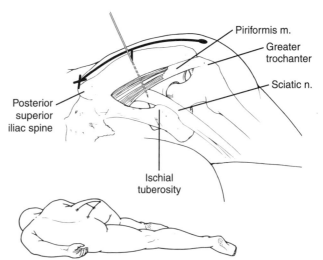

Figure 8-5 Classic (Labat) technique for sciatic nerve block. Note the first line drawn from the greater trochanter to the posterior superior iliac spine, which is then bisected by a second perpendicular line drawn caudally. (Redrawn from Brown, DL: *Atlas of Regional Anesthesia*, WB Saunders, Philadelphia, 1992, p. 84, Fig. 10-4.)

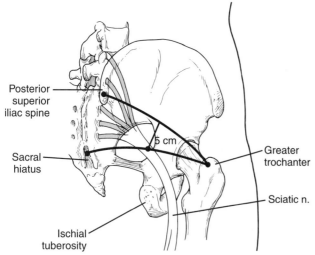

Figure 8-6   Classic sciatic nerve block. An additional line drawn from the sacral hiatus to the greater trochanter helps to adjust for patient height by determining how far caudad the anesthetizing needle should be placed. (Redrawn from Brown DL: *Atlas of Regional Anesthesia*, Second Edition, WB Saunders, Philadelphia, 1999, p. 99, Fig. 11-5.)

cross the perpendicular line at the site of needle entry (Fig. 8-6). A 22 gauge 6 inch needle or stimulating needle is aimed towards the symphysis pubis (perpendicular to all planes) and advanced until a paresthesia or motor response to the foot is elicited. Care should be taken not to misinterpret movement of the gluteal muscles as evidence of sciatic nerve stimulation. If one suspects entry into the sciatic notch, the needle should be redirected cephalad along the cephalad to caudad perpendicular line until bone is encountered, thus gauging the depth not to exceed if pelvic viscera are to be avoided. If bone is encountered prior to nerve stimulation, the needle is redirected back and forth along the sacral hiatus to greater trochanter line until an appropriate response is observed (typically at about 7 cm). After aspiration, a small amount of local anesthetic is slowly injected to rule out intraneural injection, followed by up to 30 mL of local anesthetic in divided doses. Seeking a second paresthesia or motor response reportedly improves block efficacy and reduces onset time. Sciatic nerve block may require up to 30 minutes to attain surgical anesthesia.

Clinical Caveat: Finding the Sciatic Nerve

When using the classic (Labat) approach, the sciatic nerve is best identified by systematically moving the block needle along the path defined by the sacral hiatus to greater trochanter line.

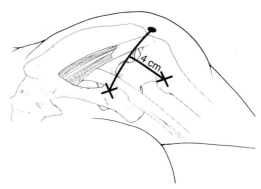

Figure 8-7   Subgluteus block landmarks. A line is drawn from the greater trochanter to the ischial tuberosity, and then bisected by a perpendicular line, which is extended caudally for 4 cm. (Redrawn from di Bendetto P, Casati A, Bertini L, et al.: Postoperative analgesia with continuous sciatic nerve block after foot surgery: a prospective, randomized comparison between the popliteal and subgluteal approaches, *Anesth Analg* 94:997, 2002, Fig. 1.)

Subgluteus Approach

An equally effective posterior method for sciatic nerve anesthesia is the subgluteus approach. Although it still requires the lateral Sims position, this approach has the added benefit of being more comfortable during the block and offers ease of placement of continuous catheter systems. A line is drawn from the ischial tuberosity to the greater trochanter, and is then bisected by a second perpendicular line that extends towards the foot. Needle entry occurs 4 cm along the perpendicular line (Fig. 8-7). Further confirmation of correct entry site is made by palpation of a skin depression formed by the biceps femoris and semitendinosus muscles. The needle is advanced perpendicular to the skin for 4–5 cm before stimulation is observed. Following test injection, 20 to 30 mL of local anesthetic is incrementally injected.

Lateral Approach

The lateral approach is useful when patients cannot lie comfortably in the lateral Sims position. The sciatic nerve is blocked in the subgluteal space as it passes posterior to the femur. With the patient supine, the greater trochanter is identified at its most lateral and posterior prominence, and a point is marked 3 cm distal (Fig. 8-8 on p. 89). A 22 gauge 5–6 inch needle or stimulating needle is advanced perpendicularly until the femur is contacted. The needle is then walked posteriorly and advanced underneath the femur until a paresthesia to or motor response of the foot is observed (Fig. 8-9 on p. 89). Since the peroneal component of the sciatic nerve is more lateral at this level, initial motor response is most often dorsiflexion and eversion of the foot (Table 8-2). Following test injection, 20 to 30 mL of local anesthetic is incrementally injected.

Complications

Complications following proximal sciatic nerve block include those common to peripheral nerve blocks in general – intravascular injection, hematoma, nerve injury, and

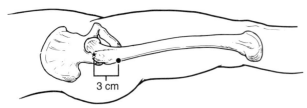

Figure 8-8   Surface landmarks for the lateral approach to the sciatic nerve. The lateral and posterior prominence of the greater trochanter is marked. A second mark is placed 3 cm distally. (Redrawn from Guardini R, Waldron BA, Wallace WA: Sciatic nerve block: a new lateral approach, *Acta Anaesthesiol Scand* 29:516, 1985, Fig. 4.)

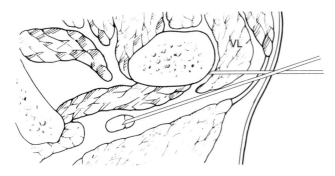

Posterior

Figure 8-9   Lateral approach to the sciatic nerve. Needle contacts periosteum and then is redirected posteriorly to slide beneath the femur. (Redrawn from Guardini R, Waldron BA, Wallace WA: Sciatic nerve block: a new lateral approach, *Acta Anaesthesiol Scand* 29:517, 1985, Fig. 6.)

infection. Delayed systemic local anesthetic toxicity is a particular concern with lower extremity regional techniques because they tend to block multiple nerves with relatively high volumes of local anesthetic. Minimal sympathectomy can occur in the blocked limb, but is rarely significant and may indeed be beneficial if increased blood flow is desirable. Unique to the classic approach is the theoretical risk of entering pelvic viscera, which is best avoided by limiting needle advancement beyond that depth identified by the bony rim of the sciatic notch (Box 8-3).

Popliteal Approaches

Patient Selection
Popliteal nerve blocks are ideally suited for patients undergoing foot or ankle surgery, and are especially use-

ful if postoperative analgesia is desirable. Because the thigh is not blocked, the anesthesiologist should ascertain that the surgery does not require a thigh tourniquet. Application of ankle tourniquets is generally well tolerated in patients anesthetized with popliteal approaches. If the surgical field includes the medial leg or foot, supplemental saphenous nerve anesthesia is required. Prior vascular surgery near the popliteal fossa is a relative contraindication to this approach.

Block Techniques
The sciatic nerve can be approached posteriorly via the popliteal fossa or from the lateral leg. The posterior approach, in particular, has been shown to be amenable for continuous techniques. It is also effective in small children. The lateral approach is ideal when the patient cannot tolerate the prone positioning required by the posterior approach.

The sciatic nerve typically branches into the tibial and common peroneal nerves 5-8 cm cephalad to the popliteal flexion crease, but the distance varies widely. Indeed, the two nerves may always be separate, or, conversely, not split until just above the popliteal crease. The nerves lie approximately half the distance between the skin and the femur, and are posterior and lateral to the popliteal vessels. Thus, aspiration of blood signifies needle tip placement that is too deep and likely too medial. As compared to a single injection, separately injecting local anesthetic onto motor responses corresponding to tibial and common peroneal nerve stimulation imparts higher success when the lateral, and perhaps the posterior, approach is used. The nature of the elicited motor response is important (Table 8-2). Inversion indicates needle placement near both nerves and reportedly leads to superior success when a high-volume (40 mL), single-injection posterior approach is used. Conversely, separate stimulation is more efficacious when a low-volume (20 mL), lateral approach is used (Box 8-4). Overall, both approaches result in equally good anesthetic conditions.

Box 8-3   Complications of Sciatic Block

Intravascular injection
Delayed systemic local anesthetic toxicity
Peripheral nerve injury
Classic approach - perforation of pelvic viscera
Popliteal approach - popliteal artery injury

Clinical Controversy: Single versus Double Injection for Popliteal Fossa Blocks

The ideal number of stimulations/injections for popliteal block is unclear. Success following the lateral approach is typically improved by a double-injection technique. When performing popliteal block from the posterior approach, the motor response of foot inversion leads to more complete anesthesia, but whether two stimulations are better remains unanswered.

Box 8-4 How to Interpret Foot Motor Responses Elicited at the Popliteal Fossa

Posterior approach:
  Inversion (mixed nerves) – ideal response for single-injection technique
  Plantar flexion (tibial nerve) – most common response, move needle laterally
  Dorsiflexion or eversion (common peroneal nerve) – move needle medially
Lateral approach:
  Dorsiflexion or eversion (common peroneal nerve) – most common response, inject then advance needle slightly farther to stimulate tibial nerve
  Plantar flexion (tibial nerve) – inject, then withdraw needle slightly to stimulate common peroneal nerve

Posterior Approach

The patient is placed prone, with the foot supported on a pillow to maintain slight flexion of the knee. Surface landmarks are drawn to match the superior dimensions of the popliteal fossa. A line is drawn across the popliteal crease, forming the base of a triangle whose lateral wall is the border of the biceps femoris muscle and medial wall is the border of the semitendinosus muscle (Fig. 8-10). The leg is returned to full extension after marking. A 50 mm stimulating needle is placed 7 cm above the popliteal crease, in the midline, at or near the triangle apex formed by the two muscles. The needle is advanced cephalad at a

20–30° angle to the skin. Inversion of the foot is sought, indicating stimulation of both the tibial and common peroneal nerves. If plantar flexion occurs, this signifies tibial nerve stimulation (the most common first response) and should prompt slight lateral redirection of the needle to seek foot inversion. After a slow test injection, 30–40 mL of local anesthetic is incrementally deposited as a single injection. Alternatively, if one chooses to seek two separate motor responses, 20 mL of local anesthetic can be injected near each nerve.

Lateral Approach

Asking the supine patient to flex slightly their knee accentuates landmarks for the lateral popliteal fossa block. The groove between the posterior border of the vastus lateralis muscle and the anterior border of the biceps femoris tendon is identified. The patient then relaxes the knee, extends the leg, and maintains the foot at a 90° angle to the leg. A second line is then drawn downward and laterally from the top of the patella, crossing the first line. At the resulting intersection, a 50 mm stimulating needle is directed slightly distal and posterior at a 20–30° angle. Care is taken not to misinterpret biceps femoris movement as an endpoint. The common peroneal nerve is typically stimulated first (dorsiflexion or foot eversion), followed by a tibial nerve motor response (plantar flexion) (Fig. 8-11). The double-injection technique deposits 20 mL of local anesthetic near each nerve. An alternative to the above technique is to direct the needle in a flatter plane, contact the femur, and then redirect it beneath the femur.

Saphenous Nerve Block

If the popliteal approach is chosen, surgery involving the medial leg or foot will require supplemental saphenous nerve block. The saphenous nerve (a component of the

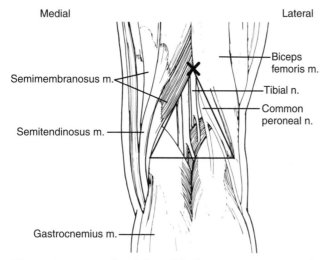

Figure 8-10 Popliteal fossa block, posterior approach. Note the triangle formed by the popliteal crease, the semitendinosus, and the biceps femoris. Needle entry is at the apex of the triangle, ~7 cm above the crease. (Redrawn from Brown DL: *Atlas of Regional Anesthesia*, Second Edition, WB Saunders, Philadelphia, 1999, p. 125, Fig. 15-1.)

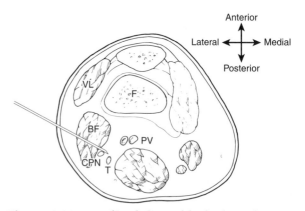

Figure 8-11 Popliteal fossa block, lateral approach. Needle entry is in the groove of the biceps femoris (BF) and vastus lateralis (VL), at the top of the patella. The needle is directed at a 20–30° posterior angle, contacting the common peroneal nerve (CPN) first. The tibial nerve (T) is medial, and lies posterior to the popliteal vessels (PV). (Redrawn from Zetlaoui PJ, Bouaziz H: Lateral approach to the sciatic nerve in the popliteal fossa, *Anesth Analg* 87:80, 1998, Fig. 1.)

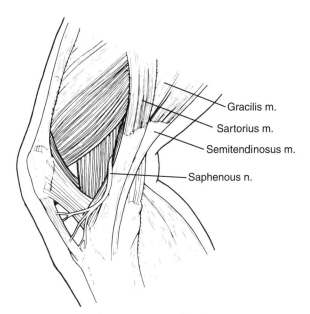

Gracilis m.
Sartorius m.
Semitendinosus m.
Saphenous n.

Figure 8-12   Saphenous nerve block. Note the superficial position of the nerve as it courses over the pes anserinus (insertion of the gracilis, semitendinosus, and sartorius tendons). (Redrawn from Brown DL: *Atlas of Regional Anesthesia*, Second Edition, WB Saunders, Philadelphia, 1999, p. 127, Fig. 15-4.)

lumbar plexus) is quite superficial just distal to the medial surface of the tibial condyle. The area can be further defined by palpating the pes anserinus, which consists of the insertion points of the sartorius, semitendinosus, and gracilis tendons (Fig. 8-12). Local anesthetic (5–10 mL) is fanned subcutaneously into this region. Sensory block requires 15 to 25 minutes to completion.

Complications

Complications related to popliteal fossa block are the same as for proximal sciatic blocks. The proximity of the popliteal artery and saphenous vein leads to the rare possibility of intravascular injection, hematoma, or direct vascular trauma.

ANKLE BLOCK

The ankle block is a staple of peripheral nerve block practice. It can be precisely performed with relatively small amounts of local anesthetic placed near individual nerves.

Innervation of the Foot

Five terminal nerves originate from the lumbar and lumbosacral plexi to eventually innervate the foot (Box 8-5). The *posterior tibial nerve* provides sensation to the plantar surface of the foot. It lies within a neurovascular bundle containing the posterior tibial artery and veins. The *saphenous nerve* accompanies the greater

Box 8-5   Innervation of the Foot

Lumbar plexus
　Saphenous nerve
Lumbosacral plexus
　Posterior tibial nerve
　Deep peroneal nerve
　Superficial peroneal nerve
　　Medial cutaneous branch
　　Intermediate cutaneous branch
　Sural nerve (lateral cutaneous nerve)

saphenous vein and lies below fascia in a groove between the medial (tibial) malleolus and the tibialis anterior tendon. It innervates the medial foot and medial great toe. The *deep peroneal nerve* shares a neurovascular bundle with the dorsalis pedis artery and supplies the interspace between the great and second toes. The *superficial peroneal nerve* divides into two branches as it crosses the anterior ankle. The medial dorsal cutaneous nerve is 1–2 cm medial to the intermediate branch, supplying sensation to second toe and adjacent skin of the great and third toes. The more lateral component (intermediate dorsal cutaneous nerve) crosses just medial to the fibular malleolus. It supplies sensation to the middorsum of the foot and the fourth plus part of the third and fifth toes. Finally, the *sural nerve* (lateral dorsal cutaneous nerve) courses behind the lateral (fibular) malleolus, innervating the lateral foot and lateral fifth toe. The neuroanatomy of the foot is detailed in Fig. 8-13 and Fig. 8-14 on p. 92.

Patient Selection

Ankle block is appropriate for any patient undergoing foot surgery distal to the ankle. Use of an ankle tourniquet is generally well tolerated in these patients.

Block Techniques

Precise identification of individual nerves to the foot facilitates ankle block being performed with as little as 8–10 mL of local anesthetic. Adjuvant epinephrine 1:400,000 is acceptable for application around the ankle if the patient has no vascular compromise. Selective nerve block can be tailored to specific surgical needs. To anesthetize the entire foot, begin with the two branches of the *superficial peroneal nerve*. The intermediate cutaneous branch is easily identified as it bowstrings beneath the examiner's finger when the foot is plantar flexed and slightly inverted. A 27 gauge needle is advanced alongside the nerve and 0.5 mL of local anesthetic injected superficially. The medial branch lies

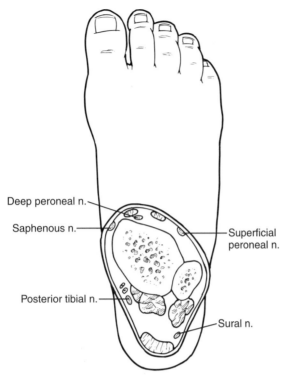

Figure 8-13   Ankle block. Cross-section demonstrating the five terminal nerves to the foot. (Redrawn from Brown DL: *Atlas of Regional Anesthesia*, Second Edition, WB Saunders, Philadelphia, 1999, p. 133, Fig. 16-2.)

about 1–2 cm further medial and is identified and anesthetized just as its associate branch was. The *sural nerve* is sought behind the lateral malleolus by dorsiflexion and slight adduction of the foot. It lies deep and is thus indirectly identified by its association with the lesser saphenous vein. Local anesthetic (1 or 2 mL)

injected subcutaneously in this vicinity will anesthetize the sural nerve. The *saphenous nerve* is then anesthetized by depositing 1 mL of local anesthetic next to the saphenous vein, in front of the medial malleolus and deep to the overlying fascia. Anesthesia of the *posterior tibial nerve* requires needle placement deep and posterior to the neurovascular bundle as it courses behind the tibial malleolus. With the foot abducted, the posterior tibial artery pulse is felt and the nerve appreciated as a cord-like structure inferior to it. After skin wheal, the needle is advanced posterior to the nerve and through the ligament before injecting 1–2 mL of local anesthetic after careful aspiration. Finally, the dorsalis pedis pulse is identified on the dorsum of the foot. A needle is advanced alongside the pulse until periosteum is encountered, whereby the *deep peroneal nerve* is anesthetized with 1–2 mL of local anesthetic.

Complications

Complications associated with ankle block are rare. Rarely, paresthesias may persist into the postoperative period, but typically for less than six weeks. Intravascular injection or infection is possible, especially in diabetic patients with vascular insufficiency.

FEMORAL NERVE BLOCK

Patient Selection

Femoral nerve block (FNB) is by far the most useful lower extremity regional anesthetic technique for the anesthesiologist. It can be used alone for quadriceps biopsy, or

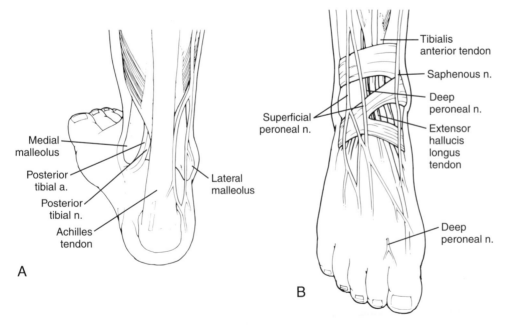

Figure 8-14   Ankle block. Surface anatomy relationships to the five terminal nerves. (Redrawn from Miller RD: *Anesthesia*, Fifth Edition, Churchill Livingstone, Philadelphia, 2000, p. 1537, Figs. 43-17 and 43-18.)

in combination with sciatic nerve block for lower leg and foot surgery. The block is most effective as an analgesic adjunct following total knee arthroplasty (where it has been shown superior to intrathecal morphine), anterior cruciate ligament repair, or midshaft femur fracture repair. For pain control, FNB is particularly amenable to continuous techniques, which have been shown to improve analgesia and rehabilitation following knee replacement and reconstruction (Box 8-6). Because FNB does not affect hamstring and lower leg motor function, it is well tolerated by ambulatory patients who have been properly instructed in the use of crutches.

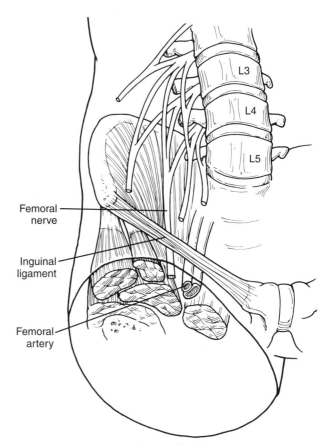

Figure 8-15   Femoral nerve block. The needle is placed just lateral to the femoral artery, in the inguinal crease. (Redrawn from Brown DL: *Atlas of Regional Anesthesia*, Second Edition, WB Saunders, Philadelphia, 1999, p. 109, Fig. 12-5.)

Block Techniques

The femoral nerve can be anesthetized using either a peripheral nerve stimulator (PNS) or a field block technique. There is no clinical data to recommend one technique over the other, but both have theoretical advantages. The PNS technique helps define needle-to-nerve proximity, but takes more time and does not deposit anesthetic solution across tissue planes. The field block technique has the advantages of being exceedingly easy to learn, rapid to implement, and deposits local anesthetic across multiple tissue planes. While this technique would seem to increase the risk of needle-to-nerve contact, femoral nerve injury is rarely reported. Either technique typically requires 20–30 mL of local anesthetic injected incrementally. For ambulatory patients undergoing knee reconstruction, bupivacaine 0.25% is as effective as 0.5%. For knee replacement patients, there is no value added by combining FNB with sciatic nerve block in terms of analgesia, patient satisfaction, or opioid sparing.

Peripheral Nerve Stimulator Technique

With the patient lying supine, the femoral artery is palpated. Cadaver studies suggest that placing the stimulating needle just lateral to the artery at the inguinal crease will optimize nerve localization (Fig. 8-15). This level is chosen in part because the femoral nerve branches substantially once it crosses under the ligament. The needle is advanced directly posterior until an acceptable motor response (elevation of the patella, quadriceps contraction) is observed at ≤0.5 mA. A sartorius motor response

is less desirable because it indicates stimulation of the anterior branch of the femoral nerve, which does not provide innervation to the knee. After negative aspiration, a small amount of local anesthetic is injected to rule out intraneuronal needle placement, followed by a total volume of 20–30 mL. Depositing smaller volumes of local anesthetic (4 mL) by redirecting the needle medial to lateral in response to stimulation of the vastus medialis, vastus intermedius, and vastus lateralis results in faster block onset and improved quality as compared with a single 12 mL injection. However, there is no evidence that this multi-stimulation, low-volume technique is superior to the more typical large-volume (20–30 mL) single injection.

When placing a continuous catheter (Fig. 8-16 on p. 94), the femoral nerve is located with a PNS in the same manner that was used for a single-shot block. Depending on the needle/catheter system selected, the catheter is placed alongside the nerve in one of two ways. If a non-stimulating catheter is used, 5–10 mL of local anesthetic is often injected through the stimulating needle with the (unproven) aim of dilating the perineural space. The catheter is then threaded 5–10 cm

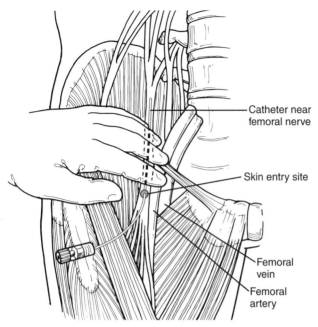

Figure 8-16 Continuous femoral nerve block. Note catheter alongside femoral nerve. (Redrawn from Brown DL: *Atlas of Regional Anesthesia*, Second Edition, WB Saunders, Philadelphia, 1999, p. 110, Fig. 12-6.)

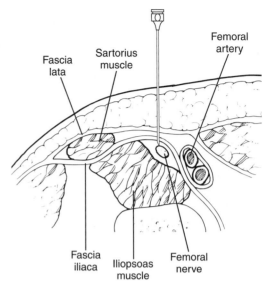

Figure 8-17 Femoral nerve block. Note that most of the femoral nerve lies deep to the fascia lata and fascia iliaca. (Redrawn from Wedel DJ: Nerve blocks. In: Miller RD (ed), *Anesthesia*, Fourth Edition, Churchill Livingstone, New York, 1994, Plate 19B.)

beyond the needle tip and secured. The hope is that the catheter will thread adjacent to the nerve in a retrograde fashion towards the psoas compartment; however, dye studies have shown this trajectory is not the rule. A stimulating catheter allows ongoing nerve stimulation as the catheter is threaded, ensuring that the catheter tip remains in close proximity to the nerve. This may allow more precise perineural placement, but there are no outcome studies to confirm its superiority to non-stimulating varieties. After localizing the nerve with the stimulating needle, the PNS is attached to the stimulating catheter and, through a series of twisting manipulations, threaded ~5 cm alongside the nerve while maintaining maximal motor response.

Field Block Technique

The same landmarks are used for the field block technique (Fig. 8-15 on p. 93). Local anesthetic (20 mL) is continuously injected during advancement and withdrawal of a 22 gauge regional block needle as it is fanned laterally away from the artery in three or four passes. On the first pass, the needle should be aspirated intermittently to assure it is not intravascular. As the needle is advanced posteriorly, the anesthesiologist should appreciate two distinct pops representing the fascia lata and fascia iliaca. Although the femoral nerve primarily resides deep to the fasciae lata and iliaca (Fig. 8-17), it undergoes significant branching underneath and proximal to the inguinal ligament. Because the field block technique deposits local anesthetic above, below, and between fascial compart-

ments, it theoretically increases the likelihood that all branches of the femoral nerve are exposed to local anesthetic.

Clinical Caveat: Ideal Motor Response for Knee Surgery

When performing a femoral nerve block with the aid of a peripheral nerve stimulator, a quadriceps motor response (elevation of the patella) is preferable to sartorius movement (hip adduction, or isolated twitch just medial and superior to the knee). This is ideal for analgesia after knee surgery because the former motor response indicates stimulation of the posterior branch of the femoral nerve, which supplies articular branches to the knee.

Complications

Proximity to the femoral artery predicts that FNBs may lead to local anesthetic toxicity or hematoma formation. Indeed, this anatomic relationship makes them relatively contraindicated in patients with previous peri-inguinal vascular surgery. For reasons unclear, nerve injury following femoral nerve block appears to be rare, with lower frequency compared with brachial plexus blocks. Also, the relatively contaminated groin area does not appear to increase infection risk for single-shot techniques, although there is some evidence that femoral catheters are prone to bacterial colonization without significant infection.

Clinical Controversy: Femoral Nerve Block in the Patient With Residual Neuraxial Block

The timing of femoral nerve block in patients undergoing knee surgery is controversial. Because there is no evidence that preoperative block placement provides substantial pre-emptive analgesia, many anesthesiologists elect to place the block after surgery to maximize analgesic duration. However, postoperative placement frequently involves patients who have residual neuraxial block. Most experts agree that placing a femoral nerve block soon after a neuraxial block is problematic, because patients are unlikely to feel a paresthesia or intraneural injection. A reasonable alternative is to wait for some return of neural function before placing the femoral block – recovery of motor function or occurrence of mild pain. In so doing, it is assumed (but not definitively known) that the patient will realize the intense pain generated by an intraneural injection. There is no clinical evidence that using a peripheral nerve stimulator in this setting is more or less safe than the field block approach.

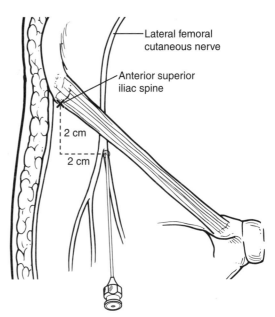

Figure 8-18   Lateral femoral cutaneous nerve block. The needle entry site is 2 cm medial and 2 cm caudad to the anterior superior iliac spine. (Redrawn from Brown DL: *Atlas of Regional Anesthesia*, Second Edition, WB Saunders, Philadelphia, 1999, p. 114, Fig. 13-2.)

LATERAL FEMORAL CUTANEOUS NERVE BLOCK

Patient Selection

The primary indication for lateral femoral cutaneous nerve (LFCN) block is the diagnosis and treatment of meralgia paresthetica, when the LFCN becomes irritated as it passes under the inguinal ligament. This condition should be distinguished from decreased sensation of the lateral thigh that may follow childbirth, but resolves rapidly. The LFCN is also anesthetized, along with the femoral, obturator, and sciatic nerves, if total anesthesia of the thigh is required for surgery or tourniquet tolerance.

Block Technique

The LFCN is blocked after it passes under the inguinal ligament. A point is marked 2 cm medial and 2 cm caudal to the anterior superior iliac spine. As a regional block needle is advanced from this point, one can appreciate its passage through the fascia lata. Local anesthetic (10 mL) is deposited on either side of the fascia lata in a fanning motion lateral and medial from the point of entry (Fig. 8-18). There are no serious complications associated with LFCN block.

OBTURATOR NERVE BLOCK

Patient Selection

Isolated obturator nerve block is occasionally used to diagnose and treat adductor spasticity related to neurologic illness, assess sources of hip pain, or prevent thigh adduction in response to unwanted stimulation of the nerve during transurethral surgery. Its combination with femoral, lateral femoral cutaneous, and sciatic nerve blocks is required for complete anesthesia of the thigh and knee. Nonetheless, obturator nerve block is rarely performed for any of these indications because of the technical challenge of consistently anesthetizing it. This difficulty may in part reflect the nerve's widely branched configuration, which occurs in up to 40% of patients.

Block Technique

The obturator nerve lies deep within the obturator canal. With the patient supine, the needle entry site is located 1.5 cm lateral and 1.5 cm below the pubic tubercle. An 8 cm, 22 gauge needle is directed towards the pubis until the horizontal (superior) ramus is contacted, and then redirected laterally and advanced an additional depth of 2 cm (Fig. 8-19 on p. 96). Local anesthetic (10–15 mL) is injected without seeking paresthesia. Seeking a motor response is optional for obturator block, but if used, adduction of the thigh confirms nerve localization.

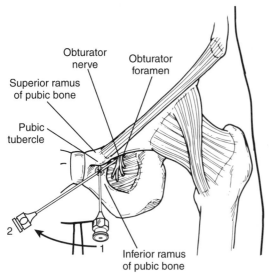

Figure 8-19   Obturator nerve block. Needle is placed 1.5 cm lateral and 1.5 cm below the pubic tubercle. The needle is advanced until it contacts the superior ramus, and is then redirected laterally in the horizontal plane and advanced an additional 2 cm. (Redrawn from Moore DC: *Regional Block*, Fourth Edition, Charles C. Thomas, Springfield, IL, 1965, p. 292, Fig. 200.)

Complications

Anesthetizing the obturator nerve is the most difficult of all lower extremity nerve blocks. The block is generally painful, and has the potential to enter vascular structures or the bladder, rectum, or vagina. Furthermore, the combined volume of local anesthetic required to anesthetize all four nerves to the lower extremity places the patient at substantial risk for local anesthetic systemic toxicity.

LUMBAR PLEXUS BLOCKS

Patient Selection

Continuous postoperative analgesia is desirable in select patients undergoing knee or hip surgery. In these cases, blocking the lumbar plexus at a more proximal location is preferred because it increases the likelihood of anesthetizing all three major nerves of the lumbar plexus with a single catheter system, and also eliminates the concerns inherent to using continuous neuraxial techniques in the setting of postoperative anticoagulation. Conversely, single-shot lumbar plexus blocks are less attractive for surgical anesthesia. For instance, the three-in-one block infrequently (~20% of blocks) anesthetizes the posterior component (knee articular branch) of the obturator nerve, as even large and potentially toxic volumes of local anesthetic tend to spread lateral, caudad (away from the lumbar plexus), and only slightly medial.

Box 8-7   Indications for Lumbar Plexus Block

Surgical
    Hip or knee surgery – but must be combined with a neuraxial or sciatic block
Continuous analgesia
    Total hip or knee arthroplasty
    Knee reconstruction
    Surgery of the thigh (may require additional sciatic catheter)

While the psoas compartment block is more effective for anesthetizing the obturator nerve than either the femoral or iliaca approach, and the fascia iliaca compartment block has been demonstrated to be more effective than the three-in-one block in children and adults, both are inadequate for most lower extremity surgery without a supplemental lumbosacral plexus or neuraxial block (Box 8-7).

Block Techniques

Psoas Compartment Block

The psoas compartment can be visualized as a space containing the lumbar plexus that lies anterior to the lumbar transverse processes, posterior to the psoas muscle, lateral to the vertebral body, and medial to the quadratus lumborum muscle (Fig. 8-20). Local anesthetic

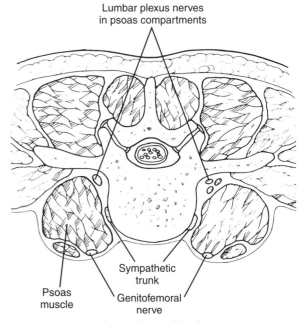

Figure 8-20   Lumbar plexus block – psoas compartment approach. The lumbar plexus lies within the psoas compartment. (Redrawn from Brown DL: *Atlas of Regional Anesthesia*, Second Edition, WB Saunders, Philadelphia, 1999, p. 88, Fig. 10.2.)

deposited within this compartment crest provides anesthesia throughout the lumbar plexus innervation and occasionally includes partial lumbosacral plexus distribution. This block is most useful as a continuous analgesic technique. With the patient in the lateral decubitus position (surgical side up), a line is drawn between iliac crests. A second line is drawn over the spinous processes; a third is drawn parallel to this line at the level of the posterior superior iliac spine (PSIS). The needle entry point is two-thirds of the distance from the vertebral to the PSIS line, and 1 cm cephalad from the intercrestal line (Fig. 8-21). A 5 inch stimulating needle is advanced perpendicular to the skin until the L4 transverse process is contacted, typically at ~7 cm in males and ~5 cm in females. The needle is then redirected caudad to walk off the transverse process (Fig. 8-22). Contact with the transverse process is desirable, as it confirms position and may prevent unintentionally deep needle placement. The lumbar plexus is typically contacted 18 mm into this advancement and is heralded by a quadriceps motor response. Following an initial bolus of 5 mL of local anesthetic, a catheter is threaded 5–8 cm laterally and caudally. Continuous infusion is commenced at 8–10 mL/hour. Using this technique, 83–88% of the patients will exhibit signs of ongoing analgesia at 24-hour follow-up.

Fascia Iliaca Compartment Block

The patient is placed supine and a line drawn along the inguinal crease from the anterior superior iliac spine to the pubic tubercle. The needle entry point is at the junction of the lateral and middle thirds of the inguinal line and 1 cm caudad. This block is classically described

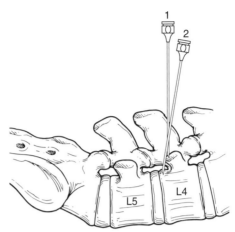

Figure 8-22   Psoas compartment block. Needle contacts the L4 transverse process and is then redirected to the lumbar plexus (~2 cm). (Redrawn from Brown DL: *Atlas of Regional Anesthesia*, Second Edition, WB Saunders, Philadelphia, 1999, p. 90, Fig. 10-4.)

as a loss-of-resistance technique. An 18 gauge Tuohy needle is angulated at 75° to the skin and aimed cephalad. After two distinct pops are felt, indicating loss-of-resistance to the fascia lata and fascia iliaca, the needle angle is decreased to 30° before advancing a final centimeter. After an incremental injection of 20 mL of local anesthetic, a catheter is threaded 5–8 cm into the fascia iliaca compartment (Fig. 8-23). Continuous infusion of a long-acting local anesthetic is commenced at 8–10 mL/hour. Higher volumes may be required to improve analgesia success rate, but even then, local anesthetic rarely reaches

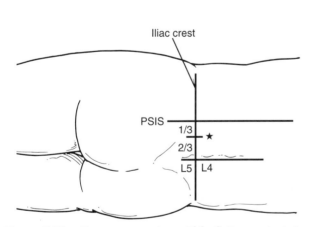

Figure 8-21   Psoas compartment block. Entry point is 1 cm cephalad to a line drawn between the superior portions of the iliac crests, and two-thirds of the distance from the vertebral spine to a parallel line drawn from the posterior superior iliac spine (PSIS). (Redrawn with permission from Capdevila X, Macaire P, Dadure C, et al.: Continuous psoas compartment block for postoperative analgesia after total hip arthroplasty: new landmarks, technical guides, and clinical evaluation, *Anesth Analg* 94:1608, 2002, Fig. 1.)

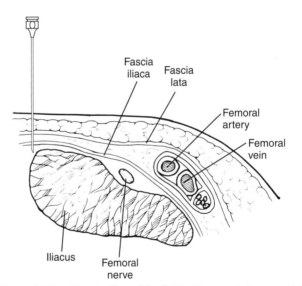

Figure 8-23   Fascia iliaca block. Needle entry is 1 cm caudal to the point where the lateral and middle third of a line connecting the anterior superior iliac spine to the pubic tubercle. (Redrawn from Liu SS, Salinas FV: Continuous plexus and peripheral nerve blocks for postoperative analgesia, *Anesth Analg* 96:267, 2003, Fig. 2.)

the lumbar plexus. Consequently, at 30 minutes, the femoral and LFC nerves are anesthetized in ~90% of patients, but the obturator is only affected in about 40% of patients.

Complications

Improper catheter position is relatively frequent following lumbar plexus blocks (3-5%). Both psoas compartment and fascia iliaca compartment blocks have the potential for intravascular injection or infection. A rare complication of psoas compartment block is bleeding into the psoas muscle, which has been reported with and without concomitant anticoagulation therapy. Unintended epidural spread of local anesthetic (bilateral segmental block) can happen in <5% of patients undergoing psoas compartment block. This occurs as a consequence of high volumes of local anesthetic entering the intervertebral foramen and spreading to the epidural space in a retrograde fashion. Nerve injury can present after either approach, but is particularly rare following the fascia iliaca compartment block because needle entry is significantly distant from the femoral nerve. As expected, the fascia iliaca approach has fewer side effects (hypotension, bradycardia, nausea and vomiting) as compared with epidural anesthesia and analgesia (Box 8-8).

> **Box 8-8 Complications of Lumbar Plexus Blocks**
>
> Improper catheter position (3-5%)
> Vascular puncture (including psoas hematoma)
> Infection
> Unintended epidural spread during psoas compartment block
> Lumbar plexus nerve injury

CONCLUSIONS

Lower extremity nerve blocks are a valuable part of the anesthesiologist's armamentarium. In the contemporary practice of regional anesthesia, these blocks are primarily used for postoperative analgesia. With practice, they are easy to perform, effective, and have a side effect profile that favorably compares with approaches to the upper extremity.

SUGGESTED READING

Brown DL: *Atlas of Regional Anesthesia*, Second Edition, WB Saunders, Philadelphia, 1999.

Capdevilla X, Biboulet P, Bouregba M, et al.: Comparison of the three-in-one and fascia iliaca compartment blocks in adults: clinical and radiographic analysis, *Anesth Analg* 86:1039-1044, 1998.

Capdevilla X, Macaire P, Dadure C, et al.: Continuous psoas compartment block for postoperative analgesia after hip arthroplasty: new landmarks, technical guidelines, and clinical evaluation, *Anesth Analg* 94:1606-1613, 2002.

di Benedetto P, Bertini L, Casati A, et al.: A new posterior approach to the sciatic nerve block: a prospective, randomized comparison with the classic posterior approach, *Anesth Analg* 93:1040-1044, 2001.

Guardini R, Waldron BA, Wallace WA: Sciatic nerve block: a new lateral approach, *Acta Anaesthesiol Scand* 29:515-519, 1985.

Hadzic A, Vloka JD: A comparison of the posterior versus lateral approaches to the block of the sciatic nerve in the popliteal fossa, *Anesthesiology* 88:1480-1486, 1998.

Hadzic A, Vloka JD, Singson R, et al.: A comparison of intertendinous and classical approaches to popliteal nerve block using magnetic resonance imaging simulation, *Anesth Analg* 94:1321-1324, 2002.

Vlodka JD, Hadzic A, Drobnik L, et al.: Anatomical landmarks for femoral nerve block: a comparison of four needle insertion sites, *Anesth Analg* 89:1467-1470, 1999.

Epidural Anesthesia

JOSEPH M. NEAL

Anesthesiologists perform more neuraxial blocks than any other regional technique. The various epidural approaches are especially relevant because they encompass all aspects of anesthetic management – from surgical and obstetric care to acute and cancer pain applications. The epidural space can be approached throughout its entirety, from the cervical to the caudal levels. Conduction blockade at each level offers unique physiologic advantage, but also requires specific technical modifications to enter the epidural space successfully. This chapter discusses in a comparative fashion the anatomy, physiology, pharmacology, and technical considerations pertinent to the four major approaches to the epidural space: cervical, thoracic, lumbar, and caudal.

EPIDURAL ANATOMY AND PHYSIOLOGY

Bony Anatomy

The structure of the vertebrae changes as one moves from cephalad to caudad. These differences in bony configuration have great relevance for the regional anesthetist. A typical vertebra consists of a spinous process that melds into bilateral laminae. The epidural space lies anterior to the laminae, and is bordered laterally by the pedicles and anteriorly by the vertebral body (Fig. 9-1 on p. 100). Access to the epidural space is through the interlaminar space. The superior and inferior articular processes define the facet joints, which provide the lateral articulating surfaces between adjacent vertebrae and play an important role in positioning for block placement. The sacral hiatus is the area where the fifth sacral vertebra (S5) lacks a spinous process and laminae posteriorly. The two sacral cornua lie on either side of the sacral hiatus and cephalad to the coccyx.

Individual vertebral components can affect epidural block technique. The *spinous processes* vary in their degree of angulation at the various vertebral levels (Fig. 9-2 on p. 100). At the cervical and lumbar regions the spinous process attaches to the lamina nearly horizontally, thus facilitating a midline perpendicular approach to the neuraxis (Fig. 9-3 on p. 101). Conversely, the midthoracic (T5–T9) spinous processes are acutely angulated to such an extent that paramedian approaches are

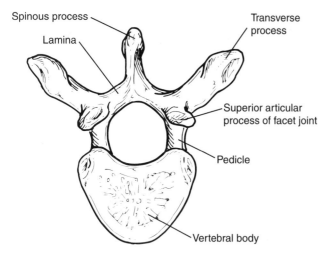

Figure 9-1   Major vertebral components (T9). (Redrawn from Stevens RA: Neuraxial blocks. In: Brown DL (ed), *Regional Anesthesia and Analgesia*, WB Saunders, Philadelphia, 1996, p. 324, Fig. 19-6.)

much easier than those performed in the midline. High (T1–T4) and low (T10–T12) thoracic spinous processes are intermediate in their orientation, and are thus amenable to either an acutely angulated midline or a paramedian approach. The *laminae* become more vertically oriented as one progresses caudally, therefore "walking off" the lamina is associated with progressively deeper needle placement from inferior to the superior in the cervical region; this also accounts for the more shallow lamina depth noted on entering the lumbar region from a paramedian approach. Positioning the patient for block placement is impacted by *facet* joint orientation. Since the lumbar facet joints are oriented in the sagittal plane and allow anterior–posterior movement, having a patient maximally flex their vertebral spine (the fetal position) serves to open the lumbar interlaminar spaces. Thoracic facet joints are primarily oriented in the coronal plane, allowing rotational movement of the spine. Therefore, exaggerated flexion serves no useful purpose during the performance of thoracic epidural blocks (Fig. 9-4 on p. 101) (Table 9-1).

Clinical Caveat: Positioning for Epidural Placement

For lumbar epidural placement, maximum flexion of the lumbar spine widens the interlaminar space
Because thoracic facet joints primarily allow axial rotation, exaggerated spinal flexion serves little benefit during performance of thoracic epidural block
Cervical facets allow some rotation, but primarily facilitate flexion and extension. Thus, neck flexion will improve access to the cervical epidural space

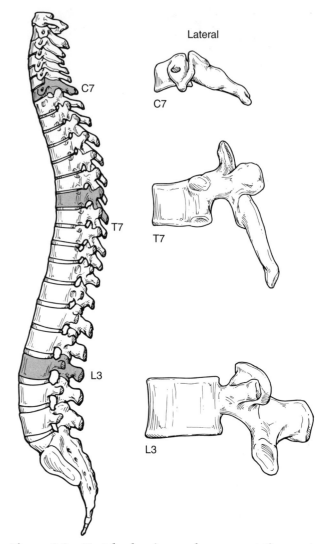

Figure 9-2   Vertebral spine and representative vertebrae from the cervical, thoracic, and lumbar regions. Note the varying angulation of the spinous processes, especially the extreme angulation in the mid thoracic region. (Redrawn from Brown DL: *Atlas of Regional Anesthesia*, Second Edition, WB Saunders, Philadelphia, 1999, p. 307, Fig. 41-3.)

Identification of a specific vertebral interspace based on palpation alone is notoriously inaccurate. Nevertheless, several surface landmarks (Fig. 9-5 on p. 102) assist in identifying vertebral levels more precisely (Box 9-1). In most humans, the C7 spinous process (the vertebrae prominens) is the most noticeable midline structure at the posterior neck base. A line drawn between the inferior angles of the scapulae identifies the T7 spinous process, while a line drawn between the iliac crests crosses the tip of the L4 spinous process or the L4-5 interspace. The spinal cord generally terminates at the L2 level; and the dural sac ends at S2 (the level of the posterior superior iliac spines). The tip of an equilateral triangle drawn between the posterior superior iliac spines and directed caudally overlies the sacral cornua and sacral hiatus.

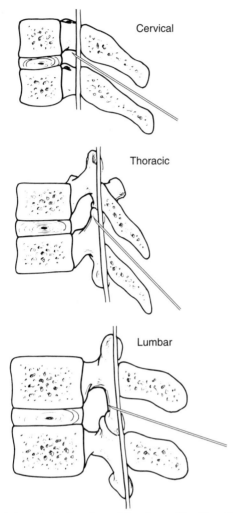

Figure 9-3   Variation in epidural needle direction as a function of spinous process angulation. (Redrawn from Cousins MJ, Veering BT: Epidural neural blockade. In: Cousins MJ, Bridenbaugh PO (eds), *Neural Blockade in Clinical Anesthesia and Pain Management*, Third Edition, Lippincott-Raven, Philadelphia, 1998, p. 255, Fig. 8-13.)

Epidural Space Anatomy

Just as the bony structure of the vertebral spine varies from the cervical to the sacral levels, so does the anatomy of the epidural space. The epidural space extends from the foramen magnum to the sacrococcygeal ligament. It is filled with epidural fat, a robust venous plexus, and loose areolar tissue (Fig. 9-6 on p. 103). These contents are not as prominent in the thoracic and cervical space as in the lumbar region, where epidural veins are at their largest diameter. The *ligamentum flavum* is a structure of variable thickness and completeness that defines the posterior-lateral soft tissue boundaries of the epidural space (Fig. 9-7 on p. 103). Because the ligamentum flavum's leather-like consistency resists active expulsion of fluid from a syringe, loss of this resistance is valuable in signaling entry into the epidural space. The ligament's structure is steeply arched and tent-like, so much so that the lateral reflection may be up to 1 cm deeper than at the midline (Fig. 9-7 on p. 103). In the cervical and thoracic epidural spaces, the ligamentum flavum is often not fused in the midline, which can become problematic during loss-of-resistance (LOR) techniques. When the dense ligamentum flavum is absent in the midline, it is possible to enter the epidural space without ever sensing significant resistance to injection (Fig. 9-8 on p. 104). The ligamentum flavum is thickest at the lumbar and thoracic levels, and thinnest at the cervical level. Its thickness also diminishes at the cephalad aspect of each interlaminar space, and as the ligamentum flavum tapers off laterally (Fig. 9-8 on p. 104). The *epidural space* itself progressively narrows in anterior–posterior dimension from the lumbar level (5–6 mm) to the thoracic level (3–5 mm), and is narrowest at the C3–6 levels (2 mm) (Table 9-1). Since the spinal cord typically terminates at the L2 level, unintentional needle puncture of the dura below this level encounters the free-floating nerve roots of the cauda equina, rather than a fixed spinal cord. Conversely, when the epidural space is entered at the thoracic and cervical levels, the narrow dimension of the cervical and thoracic epidural space results in close proximity of the spinal cord.

Figure 9-4   Articulation at the facet joints. The L2 facet joints are oriented in the sagittal plane, thus facilitating spine flexion and extension. The T6 facet joints are oriented in the coronal plane, thus facilitating axial rotation of the spine, but not flexion. (Redrawn from Netter FH: *Atlas of Human Anatomy*, Ciba-Geigy Corporation, Summit, NJ, 1989.)

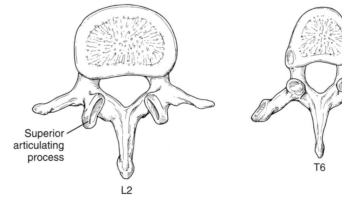

Table 9-1   Comparative Anatomy of Vertebral Spine Regions

	Cervical	Thoracic	Lumbar
Spinous processes	Horizontal	Steeply angulated (mid thoracic)	Horizontal
Facet joint orientation	Intermediate	Coronal	Sagittal
Primary movement	Intermediate	Axial rotation	Flexion/ extension
Ligamentum flavum			
Thickness (mm)	1.5–3.0	3.0–6.0	5.0–6.0
Midline fusion	Occasionally fails	Occasionally fails	Consistently fuses
Maximum epidural space antero- posterior dimen- sion (mm)	2	3–5	5–6

Box 9-1   Surface Landmarks Relevant to Epidural Anesthesia

Vertebral prominens at base of the neck = C7 spinous process

Line drawn between inferior angles of the scapulae = T7 spinous process

Line drawn between iliac crests = L4 spinous process or L4–5 interspace

Line drawn between the posterior superior iliac spines = S2, dural sac termination

Caudad tip of an equilateral triangle drawn between the posterior superior iliac spines = sacral hiatus

Above C7–T1 and at intermittent areas along the posterior spinal canal, the epidural space is best described as a potential space that is easily dilated by injection of anesthetic solutions. Distribution of solutions within the epidural space is not uniform, especially as distance from the injection site increases. Rather, solutions spread along various routes as determined by small, low-resistance channels that exist between the epidural fat and veins. Nevertheless, epidural anesthesia is generally successful, probably because anesthetic solutions flow preferentially along the spinal nerve root sheaths, and because the only significant barrier to epidural flow appears to be the posterior longitudinal ligaments, which serve to further direct anesthetic solutions towards the nerve roots (Fig. 9-9 on p. 104).

Sympathetic Nervous System

As opposed to single-shot spinal anesthesia, intermittent epidural anesthesia dosing regimens allow more control of anesthetic spread and sympathetic nervous system blockade, providing sufficient time elapses between small incremental doses of local anesthetic. These positive attributes are secondary to the segmental nature of epidural block resulting from the limited bi-directional spread of anesthetic agents from the point of injection. This phenomenon has implications for sympathetic nerve and motor function during epidural anesthesia.

Sympathetic nervous system control of the heart is modulated by the T1–T5 sympathetic nerve fibers (cardioaccelerator). Blocking these autonomic nerves results in diminished myocardial oxygen demand (bradycardia, decreased contractility) and increased supply (coronary vasodilation in patients with atherosclerotic disease). As a result, a segmental T1–T5 block will theoretically improve myocardial oxygen balance while avoiding hypotension. Indeed, segmental local anesthetic blockade of thoracic sympathetic fibers results in a lower heart rate, but higher blood pressure, than a

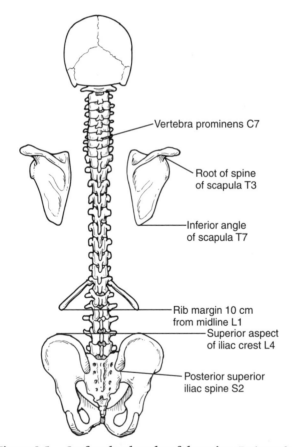

Vertebra prominens C7

Root of spine of scapula T3

Inferior angle of scapula T7

Rib margin 10 cm from midline L1

Superior aspect of iliac crest L4

Posterior superior iliac spine S2

Figure 9-5   Surface landmarks of the spine. (Redrawn from Cousins MJ, Veering BT: Epidural neural blockade. In: Cousins MJ, Bridenbaugh PO (eds), *Neural Blockade in Clinical Anesthesia and Pain Management*, Third Edition, Lippincott-Raven, Philadelphia, 1998, p. 250, Fig. 8-9.)

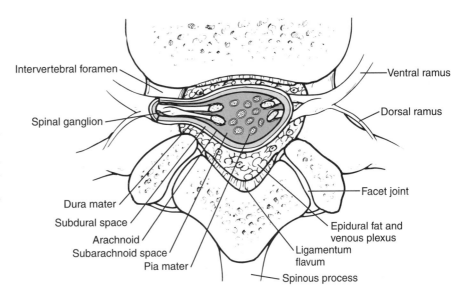

Figure 9-6   Epidural space anatomy. Fat and veins fill the epidural space. Spinal nerve roots, within dural cuffs, exit through the intervertebral foramina. (Redrawn from Miller RD: Atlas of regional anesthesia procedures. In: *Anesthesia*, Fifth Edition, Churchill Livingstone, Philadelphia, 2000, Plate 6.) (See colour inserts, Plate 4.)

block that extends from the high thoracic to the sacral levels (Fig. 9-10 on p. 105). Avoiding an extensive epidural block at the lumbar level reduces lumbar sympathetic nerve block, lowering the frequency of hypotension and improving a patient's ability to ambulate after surgery (less motor block). Sympathetic control of gut propulsion is derived from the T5–L2 spinal cord segments. Segmental blockade reduces postoperative ileus by allowing overriding parasympathetic tone from the unblocked vagus and sacral parasympathetic nerve fibers, which promote gut propulsion. The low thoracic/high lumbar sympathetic fibers (T9–L1) regulate vasomotor tone in the lower extremities. A segmental block above this level maintains diastolic perfusion pressure to the coronary arteries, because the unblocked caudad segments remain under central sympathetic con-

trol, thus maintaining normal systemic vascular resistance. Conversely, local anesthetic blockade of these same fibers improves vascular flow to the legs secondary to vasodilation (Box 9-2).

Motor Function

Epidural segmental block also has an impact on postoperative lower extremity motor function. Continuous thoracic epidural block with low-concentration local anesthetic avoids local anesthetic spread to the lumbar and lumbosacral plexi, thus preserving motor function and facilitating postoperative ambulation. Lumbar epidural analgesia is predictably associated with a higher incidence of motor block resulting in delayed ambulation and recovery.

Figure 9-7   Cryomicrotome of the T9 epidural space. Note steeply arched ligamentum flavum and the basivertebral vein (arrow). (Reproduced from Hogan QH: Epidural anatomy examined by cryomicrotome section. Influence of age, vertebral level, and disease, *Reg Anesth* 21:397, 1996, Fig. 2.)

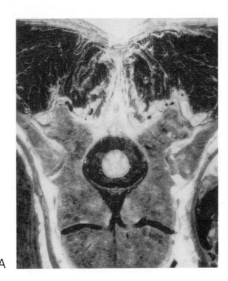

A

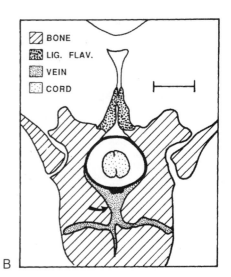

B

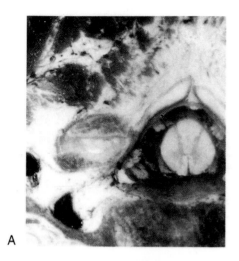

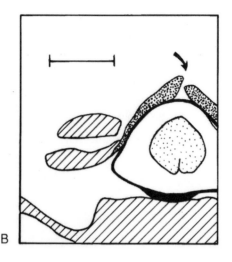

Figure 9-8 Cryomicrotome of the C7–T1 epidural space. Note failure of the ligamentum flavum to fuse at the midline. Nerve roots are seen gathering at the lateral margin of the dural sac. (Reproduced from Hogan QH: Epidural anatomy examined by cryomicrotome section. Influence of age, vertebral level, and disease, *Reg Anesth* 21:399, 1996, Fig. 5.)

EPIDURAL PHARMACOLOGY

Epidural Space Pharmacology

The pharmacodynamics and pharmacokinetics of drugs administered within the epidural space are complex and incompletely understood. Pharmacodynamic target sites of action differ between drug classes. For instance, local anesthetics most likely exert their initial effects on the spinal nerve roots and dorsal root ganglia as they exit the intervertebral foramina (Fig. 9-6 on p. 103 and Fig. 9-9). Neural blockade may also take place at the paravertebral levels, implying peripheral as well as central nervous system target sites. Individual nerve target sites are responsible for the segmental nature of epidural block when local anesthetics are employed. Conversely,

epidural opioids diffuse from the epidural space to the cerebrospinal fluid (CSF) and exert their primary pharmacodynamic effect on the spinal cord. Epidural opioids may also stimulate receptors on the dorsal root ganglia. Despite older teachings, epidural drugs do not reach the spinal cord by diffusion into the dural cuffs or transfer via the radicular arteries. Instead, opioids and local anesthetics diffuse across the meninges, where the arachnoid layer is the primary limiting membrane. Small amounts of epinephrine that diffuse into the CSF supplement anesthesia by exerting a direct agonist effect on spinal cord α_2-adrenergic receptors.

Drugs are cleared from the epidural space by two mechanisms. Some enzymatic degradation of epinephrine occurs from epidural and meningeal catechol-O-methyl transferase (COMT). However, most epidural

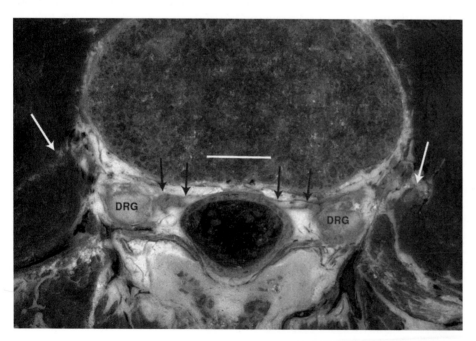

Figure 9-9 Cryomicrotome at the L3–4 interspace. Ink accumulates around the dura and extends to the intervertebral foramina, where it tracks along the segmental nerves and dorsal root ganglia (DRG). Flow is impeded by the posterior longitudinal ligament (black arrows) and directed out the foramina. White arrows indicate peripheral nerves within the psoas muscle. (Reproduced from Hogan Q: Distribution of solution in the epidural space: examination by cryomicrotome section, *Reg Anesth Pain Med* 27:152, 2002, Fig. 1.)

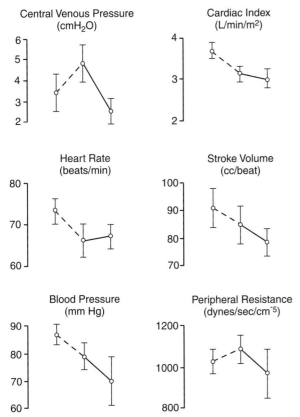

Figure 9-10   Hemodynamic consequences of segmental epidural block. Control (left) versus T1–4 block (center) versus T1–S5 block (right). (Redrawn from Cousins MJ, Veering BT: Epidural neural blockade. In: Cousins MJ, Bridenbaugh PO (eds), *Neural Blockade in Clinical Anesthesia and Pain Management*, Third Edition, Lippincott-Raven, Philadelphia, 1998, p. 264, Fig. 8-19.)

drugs are cleared by diffusion into epidural fat, areolar tissues, and especially the dural vascular plexus. After systemic uptake, drugs are metabolized in the liver and kidneys. Epidural drug clearance is especially relevant to the use of epinephrine admixed with local anesthetics. Epinephrine appears to prolong the duration of epidural local anesthetic action by reducing dural blood flow (but not spinal cord blood flow), thereby slowing drug clearance and prolonging exposure of neural elements to higher drug concentrations.

Box 9-2   Segmental Sympathetic Innervation

Cardioaccelerator fibers = T1–T5
Gastrointestinal propulsion = T5–L2
Lower extremity vasomotor tone = T9–L1

Local Anesthetics

The volume and total milligram dose (mass) of local anesthetic deposited within the epidural space is determined according to vertebral level. Typical volumes of local anesthetics placed in the lumbar epidural space range between 15 and 25 mL, depending on drug mass and patient age. Doses are reduced by 50 to 75% for thoracic and cervical techniques because the epidural space and nerve roots are smaller as compared to the lumbar region. Dosing should be more conservative in the elderly, as spinal deformity further reduces epidural space volume and egress through narrowed foramina is diminished. The total mass of local anesthetic is more significant than either volume or concentration for determining intensity, duration, and spread of epidural block. Solutions injected in the lumbar region tend to spread cephalad to a greater extent than caudad. Conversely, solutions injected into the high and mid-thoracic epidural spaces tend to spread more caudad than cephalad, and are equivalent in bi-directional longitudinal spread when placed in the low thoracic regions. Thus, the puncture site is the primary determinant of the cranial and caudal borders of thoracic sensory block, but local anesthetic doses are similar regardless of which thoracic level is entered (Fig. 9-11 on p. 106). Careful attention must be paid to local anesthetic selection, because even intermediate-acting agents such as lidocaine or mepivacaine can result in recovery times that far exceed surgical anesthetic requirements (Fig. 9-12 on p. 106) (Table 9-2).

Re-dosing regimens vary with the local anesthetic used and the clinical situation. A re-dose volume is typically one-third to one-half of that used for the initial loading dose. Re-dosing based on a fixed time interval may lead to relative over- or underdosing. Instead, hemodynamic signs such as tachycardia or hypertension can objectively guide therapy when the block is beginning to dissipate (Table 9-2).

Opioids

Epidural opioids may provide additive or synergistic analgesia when combined with local anesthetics. For instance, epidural morphine enhances spread and analgesia when combined with low-dose bupivacaine infusions. Similar to local anesthetics, epidural opioid dosing may require adjustment based on the vertebral level where they are deposited. It has long been stated that lipophilic opioids such as fentanyl or sufentanil exhibit little rostral movement within the CSF because they are rapidly absorbed by epidural fat and cleared. However, recent evidence suggests that bolus lipophilic opioids spread rapidly and extensively within the CSF, resulting in signi-

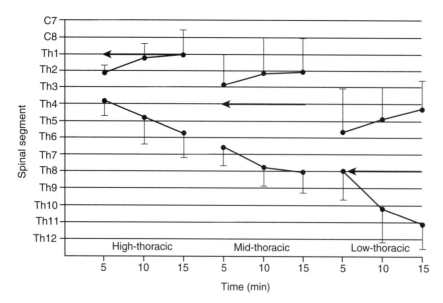

Figure 9-11   Segmental anesthesia after 6 mL of lidocaine 1%. Note the similarity of total dermatomal spread. Injection site (arrow) ultimately determines the level of the segmental band of anesthesia. (Redrawn from Visser WA, Liem TH, van Egmond J, Gielen MJM: *Anesth Analg* 86:334, 1998, Fig. 1.)

ficant CSF concentrations within the rostral CSF within minutes of administration. Early respiratory depression can potentially be a significant risk with the lumbar intrathecal administration of more lipophilic opioids. Conversely, when lipophilic opioids like fentanyl and sufentanil are administered via continuous infusion, most of the drug is found in epidural fat with lesser amounts detectable in the spinal cord white matter. This is likely to account for the wider band of analgesia afforded when hydrophilic opioids such as morphine and to a lesser extent hydromorphone are utilized to provide analgesia using continuous epidural infusion (Fig. 9-13 on p. 107). Because of this significant spread within the CSF, when opioids and/or local anesthetics are delivered by either bolus or continuous infusion, the drug dose and rate of infusion must be adjusted downward for thoracic catheters and in elderly patients.

APPROACHES TO THE EPIDURAL SPACE

The appropriate spinal level for epidural needle and catheter insertion is determined by anesthetic and physiologic goals. For optimal anesthesia and analgesia, epidural drugs are ideally delivered to that spinal level corresponding to the dermatomal midpoint of the incision. Although accurately identifying a specific spinal interspace is imprecise using only surface landmarks, the injected volume of epidural solution typically provides sufficient cephalad and caudad spread. It is also important to place the anesthetic solution at a level appropriate to optimize physiologic effects. For example, efforts to decrease ileus require blocking of the T5–L2 sympathetic nerve fibers. Thoracic epidural placement is therefore most appropriate for abdominal surgery, while lumbar placement is ideally

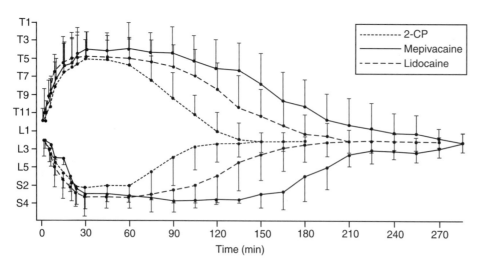

Figure 9-12   Duration of three epidural local anesthetics without epinephrine. (Redrawn from Kopacz DJ, Mulroy MF: Chloroprocaine and lidocaine reduce hospital stay and admission rate after outpatient epidural anesthesia, *Reg Anesth* 15:21, 1990, Fig. 1.)

Table 9-2	Approximate Duration of Initial Anesthesia and Interval to Re-dose: Epidural Local Anesthetics With Epinephrine		

Drug	Approximate Anesthetic Duration (min)	Interval to Re-dose (min)
2-Chloroprocaine, 3%	60	45
Lidocaine, 2%	100	60
Mepivacaine, 2%	110	60
Bupivacaine, 0.5%	180	120
Ropivacaine, 0.75%	180	120

Box 9-3	Matching Epidural Placement to Surgical Requirement

Thoracotomy = T4–T6
Upper abdominal = T6–T8
Lower abdominal = T10–T12
Lower extremity = L2–L4
Labor and delivery = L2–L4
   First stage of labor (T10–L1)
   Second stage of labor through delivery (S2–S4)

suited for lower extremity surgery, particularly when lumbar sympathectomy is desirable (Box 9-3).

Cervical Epidural Block

Clinical Uses

Cervical epidural block is the least frequently utilized epidural approach. The relative lack of familiarity with this

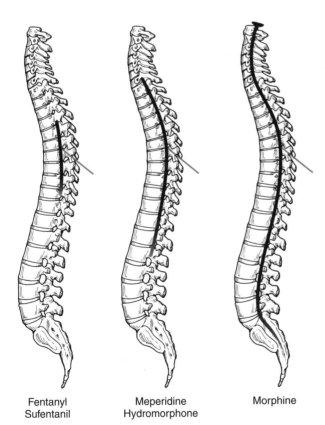

Fentanyl
Sufentanil
      Meperidine
      Hydromorphone
           Morphine

Figure 9-13 **Intraspinal opioid spread**. Note the more extensive and rostral spread of hydrophilic opioids such as morphine. (Redrawn from Love W, Rathmell JP, Tarver JM: Regional anesthesia for acute pain management, *Problems in Anesthesia* 12:3, 2000.)

block, combined with the proximity of the cervical spinal cord, suggests that those who undertake it should be well trained and experienced in the technique. Cervical epidural injection is most frequently used to place steroid solutions for treatment of inflammatory radiculopathy. Continuous techniques are applicable for managing chronic and cancer pain of the neck, upper extremities, or upper thorax. While less frequently used as an anesthetic technique, cervical epidural can be used for surgeries involving these same anatomic distributions. Cervical epidural local anesthetic blockade reduces phrenic nerve function and is associated with a slight increase in $PaCO_2$, but to a clinically insignificant extent. Hemodynamic consequences of cervical epidural block are similar to those associated with high thoracic segmental block (bradycardia, hypotension from decreased contractility).

Block Technique

Cervical epidural block is most commonly performed in the midline in sitting patients. Appropriate assistance is required to monitor these patients, as vasovagal syncope can occur and compromise patient safety. The paramedian approach is most efficacious for patients positioned in lateral decubitus. The C7–T1 interspace is commonly chosen for its wide interspinous space. Following local anesthesia of the skin, the epidural needle is placed low in the interspace and advanced horizontally into the interspinous ligament. The ligamentum flavum is typically 4 to 6 cm from the skin, may be unfused in the midline, and is only 1.5 to 3 mm thick. Once entered, the epidural space is typically only 2 mm in anterior–posterior dimension and the spinal cord is directly underneath the dura. For surgical anesthesia, 8 to 10 mL of local anesthetic is deposited and should be expected to cause upper extremity weakness. For continuous techniques, low-concentration local anesthetic solutions (e.g. bupivacaine 0.025–0.1%) are infused at 4 mL/hour.

Identification of the cervical epidural space can be accomplished with a loss-of-resistance technique. Alternatively, pressure within the cervical epidural space in sitting patients is negative with respect to atmospheric pressure and this fact makes identification of the epidural space using the hanging drop technique particularly useful. Negative pressure within the thoracic epidural space is due to transmission of negative intrapleural pressures to the epidural space, and like intrapleural pressure, the pressure within the epidural space fluctuates with respiration. In the lower cervical and lumbar epidural spaces, this negative pressure is postulated to be due to a combination of transmitted thoracic negative pressure and dural tenting. The hanging drop technique begins by seating a midline epidural needle into interspinous ligament. A small drop of saline is placed within the needle's hub; surface tension will allow a drop of sufficient size to bulge above the needle's hub and be easily seen. The needle is then advanced with careful observation of the saline drop. When the epidural space is entered, negative pressure pulls the drop inward and it is seen to retract into the hub of the epidural needle (Fig. 9-14).

Clinical Controversy: Identification of the Epidural Space

The epidural space is most commonly identified using a loss-of-resistance to air or saline technique. While both mediums have their proponents, there is little evidence to suggest that one is superior to the other. When unintentional dural puncture occurs using an air-filled syringe, intrathecal injection of the air may lead to pneumocephalus and significant headache that begins almost immediately. This headache is less likely to be postural than is a postdural puncture headache and typically resolves within a few hours after injection. The hanging drop technique is less frequently used because its endpoint can be less obvious. Hanging drop is most appropriate for thoracic and low cervical approaches, where negative epidural space pressure is maximal.

Thoracic Epidural Block

Clinical Uses

Patients undergoing thoracic or abdominal operations that involve large surgical incisions are optimally suited for thoracic epidural anesthesia and analgesia. Surgical incision determines the level of placement along the thoracic spine (Box 9-3). Segmental thoracic block offers several advantages in these patients. First, anesthetizing the sympathetic nerve fibers to the gut will decrease the incidence of ileus, while blocking the cardioaccelerator fibers benefits myocardial oxygen balance and may theoretically improve cardiac outcome. Second, avoiding lumbar nerve root anesthesia will greatly diminish the frequency of postural hypotension and lower extremity motor block, thus facilitating postoperative ambulation. There are no specific contraindications unique to thoracic epidural placement that would not also apply to other approaches.

Block Technique

Since high and mid-thoracic epidural blocks are easiest to perform with a paramedian approach, this technique will be described for thoracic block. Description of the midline technique will be discussed as it relates to lumbar epidural anesthesia. The midline and paramedian approaches can be used at all vertebral levels, and there are many advocates for each method. For thoracic placement, patients are comfortably placed in the lateral decubitus position with the spine parallel to the bed. The sitting position is a useful alternative for obese patients with poorly defined surface landmarks. The patient is sedated to a level of comfort that still allows communication with the anesthesiologist. At a minimum, a pulse oximeter monitors the patient, providing audible indication of both the heart rate and oxygen saturation. (See Chapter 4 for a complete discussion of monitoring during block placement.) After selecting the appropriate spinal interspace, the inferior portion of the spinous process is identified. This corresponds to the mid-portion of the underlying vertebral lamina. The needle entry point is marked just enough off midline to avoid the spinous process.

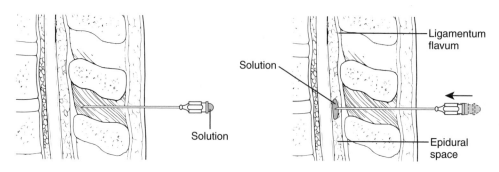

Figure 9-14 Hanging drop technique. Note how negative pressure draws the saline drop into the epidural needle hub as the epidural space is entered. (Redrawn from Miller RD: Atlas of regional anesthesia procedures. In: *Anesthesia*, Fifth Edition, Churchill Livingstone, Philadelphia, 2000, Plate 7B.)

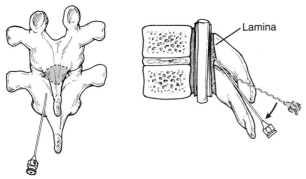

Lamina

Figure 9-15   Paramedian approach to the thoracic epidural space. Note how the needle is placed just off the midline at the inferior pole of the spinous process and then incrementally "walked" along the lamina and into the interlaminar space. (Redrawn from Stevens RA: Neuraxial blocks. In: Brown DL (ed), *Regional Anesthesia and Analgesia*, WB Saunders, Philadelphia, 1996, p. 325, Fig. 19-7.)

A small-gauge 1.5 inch needle is then used to anesthetize the skin and underlying tissues, including the laminar periosteum. This needle also acts as a "finder" to identify preliminarily underlying structures. An epidural needle with the bevel facing cephalad is advanced perpendicular to the skin until it comes in contact with the lamina. Because the epidural needle is placed just off midline, subsequent movement is primarily in the cephalad direction, with only minimal (≤10°) angulation towards the midline. The epidural needle is then methodically "walked along the lamina" in small (1 mm) increments until it is felt to just slip off of the cephalad aspect of the lamina and engage ligamentum flavum (Fig. 9-15). A saline-filled syringe with a small air bubble is then attached to the epidural needle. Pressure on the syringe barrel should meet resistance with consequent compression of the bubble. Next, the epidural needle is incrementally advanced a millimeter at a time, checking resistance after every advancement, until loss of resistance occurs and the saline and air bubble are easily injected into the epidural space (Fig. 9-16). An epidural catheter is advanced through the needle and 2 to 5 cm into the epidural space (4 to 5 cm in obese patients). Catheters positioned more than 5 cm in the epidural space are associated with a higher incidence of unilateral block, most likely because the catheter migrates laterally within the epidural space, at times even exiting via an intervertebral foramen (Fig. 9-6 on p. 103).

Figure 9-16   Loss-of-resistance technique. Note compressed bubble in saline that releases once the epidural space is entered. (Redrawn from Miller RD: Atlas of regional anesthesia procedures. In: *Anesthesia*, Fifth Edition, Churchill Livingstone, Philadelphia, 2000, Plate 7A.)

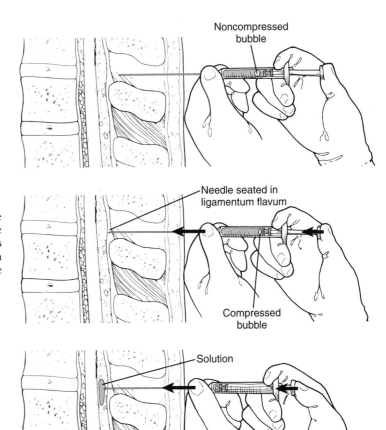

Noncompressed bubble

Needle seated in ligamentum flavum

Compressed bubble

Solution

Clinical Caveat: Unilateral Epidural Anesthesia

Unilateral epidural anesthesia is most likely due to a malpositioned catheter that has been advanced an excessive length (>3–5 cm) into the epidural space and has come to rest in a far lateral position or exited through an intervertebral foramen. The proposed existence of septae within the epidural space that are capable of impeding local anesthetic flow has been largely discredited.

Testing epidural catheter placement is essential to rule out intrathecal or intravascular placement. Although needle aspiration should be routinely performed, it is associated with a high false negative rate, especially for identifying intravenous needle or catheter placement. Aspiration through the catheter may apply a sudden and marked negative pressure at the catheter's tip. This collapses the vein and no blood appears within the catheter despite the intravascular placement. False negative aspiration is significantly less frequent with the use of multiorifice catheters. The standard epidural test dose consists of 3 mL of lidocaine 1.5% with 5 µg/mL epinephrine. If the needle or catheter is intravascular, the patient will manifest a 10–15% increase in heart rate within one minute of injection. Intravascular test doses are unreliable in patients taking β-adrenergic blocking agents, who are in the midst of uterine contractions, or who are sedated; they are variably reliable in elderly and anesthetized patients. Pulse oximetry is most convenient for monitoring intravenous test doses. This same test dose contains enough local anesthetic to rule out subarachnoid catheter or needle placement; sacral anesthesia should develop within 3 to 5 minutes of test dose injection, and can be tested by pin-prick within the sacral dermatomes.

When performing epidural anesthesia, it is possible to observe a false loss of resistance (Fig. 9-17). Such a scenario will occur if a space exists between a highly calcified interspinous ligament and the ligamentum flavum, or if the epidural needle crosses the midline while engaged in the interspinous ligament or ligamentum flavum. False loss of resistance is also possible if the needle tip enters a facet joint.

Lumbar Epidural Block

Clinical Uses

Lumbar epidural block is ideal for patients requiring labor analgesia or undergoing lower extremity surgery. Abdominal surgery, especially below the umbilicus, can also be accomplished with the lumbar approach; how-

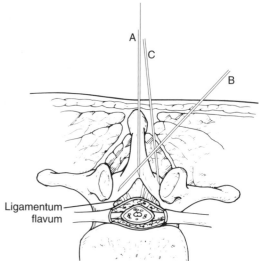

Figure 9-17   Potential areas to experience a false loss of resistance. A, Midline needle can enter a small space between a calcified interspinous ligament and the ligamentum flavum. **B,** A needle can cross the midline at the interspinous ligament or ligamentum flavum. **C,** Far lateral needles can enter a facet joint. (Redrawn from Brown DL: *Atlas of Regional Anesthesia*, Second Edition, WB Saunders, Philadelphia, 1999, p. 334, Fig. 43-3.)

ever, subsequent postoperative analgesia will be less than optimal because of the motor block that accompanies anesthesia of the lumbar nerve roots. Other disadvantages of the lumbar approach include lumbar sympathectomy leading to postural hypotension. Conversely, lumbar sympathetic block is desirable for improving vaso-occlusive disease or thromboembolic outcomes following peripheral vascular and hip surgery. The relative lack of sacral anesthesia secondary to sacral nerve root thickness limits the usefulness of lumbar anesthesia for perineal and below the knee anesthesia and analgesia.

Block Technique

Lumbar epidural block is typically performed via a midline approach, although paramedian techniques are useful in some patients, particularly those with calcified vertebral interspaces or parturients with accentuated lumbar lordosis. The sitting position may enhance surface landmark identification in obese patients, but lumbar epidural anesthesia is routinely performed in the lateral decubitus position. Extreme flexion of the spine (fetal position) serves to widen the interlaminar space and facilitate needle entry. Needle placement at the cephalad aspect of the interspace provides the most direct path to the epidural space (Fig. 9-3 on p. 101). A small-gauge needle is used to provide anesthesia within the skin and subcutaneous tissues and serves as a "finder" to identify the location of bony elements. Subsequently, the epidural needle will pass through the skin and subcutaneous tissue, the supraspinous ligament, and the interspinous ligament before encountering the ligamentum flavum's increased resistance. Once engaged in the ligamentum flavum, a syringe with saline and a small air bubble is attached to the epidural needle. Pressure on the syringe barrel should reveal firm resistance. The needle is slowly advanced, with constant pressure applied to the syringe barrel, until resistance is lost, signaling entry into the epidural space (Fig. 9-16 on p. 109). The depth from skin to lumbar epidural space is between 4 and 6 cm in the majority of patients (range 2 to >8 cm). An epidural catheter is advanced and tested as described for thoracic placement. Single-shot techniques involve a 3 mL test dose injected through the epidural needle, followed by incremental delivery of the anesthetic solution in 5 mL aliquots to observe for signs of intravascular or subarachnoid injection.

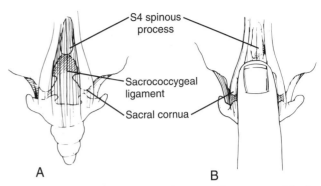

Figure 9-19   Palpation of the sacral cornua aids in localizing the sacral hiatus, particularly in children. (Redrawn from Stevens RA: Neuraxial blocks. In: Brown DL (ed), *Regional Anesthesia and Analgesia*, WB Saunders, Philadelphia, 1996, p. 347, Fig. 19-28.)

Caudal Block

Clinical Uses

The caudal approach, once the mainstay of obstetric analgesia, has largely been supplanted by the lumbar and thoracic epidural approaches. There are a number of reasons for this shift, including anatomic variability, the relative technical difficulty of the approach, and modern absence of extensive training in the technique. Contemporary indications for caudal anesthesia are essentially limited to postoperative analgesia in children, access to the epidural space for epidural steroids when the lumbar approach is compromised, and rarely as an anesthetic for anorectal, perineal, or lower extremity procedures.

Block Technique

For caudal block, adults are placed in the lateral decubitus position or prone (with hips slightly elevated and heels rotated laterally). Caudal block in children is typically performed under general anesthesia in the lateral decubitus position. The caudal canal is entered through the sacral hiatus. The sacral hiatus has a frequent anatomic variation in which the laminae and spinous

process may be partially present, making the caudal space inaccessible in up to 7% of adults. The sacral hiatus lies cephalad to the coccyx near the superior extent of the gluteal cleft. The apex of an equilateral triangle whose base spans the posterior iliac spines will lie over the sacral hiatus with the palpable sacral cornua on either side of midline (Fig. 9-18). In children the cornua are easily palpated (Fig. 9-19). Once the sacral hiatus is identified, a 22 gauge needle is directed at a 45° angle to the skin with the bevel facing anterior. When the sacrococcygeal membrane has been pierced, often with a notable "pop," the needle angle is flattened and advanced about 2 cm in adults or 1 cm in children (Fig. 9-20). Prior to local anesthetic injection the needle is aspirated to ensure it has not entered the dural sac, which typically terminates at the

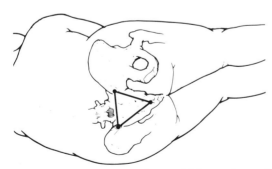

Figure 9-18   Localization of sacral hiatus. An equilateral triangle drawn between the posterior superior iliac spines, with the apex pointing caudally, will overlie the sacral hiatus. (Redrawn from Miller RD: Atlas of regional anesthesia procedures. In: *Anesthesia*, Fifth Edition, Churchill Livingstone, Philadelphia, 2000, Plate 17B.)

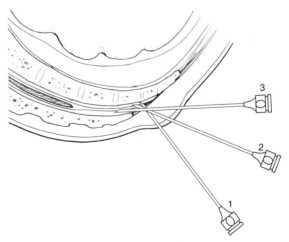

Figure 9-20   Caudal puncture technique. After penetration of the sacrococcygeal ligament, the needle is flattened and directed 1 to 2 cm into the caudal canal. (Redrawn from Miller RD: Atlas of regional anesthesia procedures. In: *Anesthesia*, Fifth Edition, Churchill Livingstone, Philadelphia, 2000, Plate 17C.)

Box 9-4   Pediatric Caudal Dosing: Bupivacaine 0.25%

Total bupivacaine dose should not exceed 3 mg/kg
Sacral block – 0.5 mL/kg
Low thoracic block – 0.75 mL/kg
Upper thoracic block – 1.25 mL/kg

S2 level in adults and even more caudad in children. A test dose will further rule out subarachnoid or intravenous injection. Continuous techniques are described with the caudal approach; in neonates, epidural catheters can be reliably advanced from the caudal canal to the lumbar or thoracic levels to provide analgesia after various types of surgery. In older children and adults, epidural catheters tend to curl in the caudal canal and cannot reliably be advanced more cephalad without x-ray guidance. In adults, 10–15 mL of local anesthetic will provide perineal anesthesia, while up to 35 mL is necessary to anesthetize the legs. Various dosage regimens in children exist (Box 9-4).

Complications of Epidural Anesthesia

Most complications of epidural anesthesia are not limited to a specific approach along the vertebral column (Box 9-5). The approximate incidences of complications are given in those cases where frequency has been examined. Block-specific complications are most likely to follow caudal anesthesia. Caudal needle punctures that pass lateral to the sacrum or penetrate the ventral sacral plate can contact vital structures, most notably the rectum or fetal parts during obstetric applications.

Cardiovascular Complications

Cardiovascular complications related to epidural anesthesia can occur from direct intravascular injection, delayed systemic uptake of local anesthetic, or indirectly from local anesthetic effects on sympathetic nerve fibers. Intravascular injection can lead to systemic local anesthetic toxicity that ranges from mild symptoms such as tinnitus or circumoral numbness, to convulsions, to cardiac collapse associated with potent long-acting agents such as bupivacaine (see Chapter 2 for an in-depth discussion of local anesthetic toxicity). These complications are best avoided through the routine use of epidural test dosing and incremental injection. Epidural and caudal anesthesia are associated with high local anesthetic plasma levels from delayed tissue uptake. While data are conflicting, epidural and caudal local anesthetic peak plasma levels are probably second in magnitude only to those observed after peripheral nerve blocks (especially intercostal blocks) and mucosal application of local anes-

---

Box 9-5   Complications and Side Effects of Epidural Anesthesia

Cardiovascular
  Intravascular injection (2–5%) – local anesthetic systemic toxicity
  Sympathectomy (common) – hypotension and bradycardia
Unintentional dural penetration
  High spinal anesthesia (<1%)
  Postdural puncture headache (2–5%)
Neurologic
  Epidural hematoma (<1:150,000, incidence is higher when coagulation disorder is present or anticoagulants are in use at the time of epidural placement or removal)
  Nerve root injury (0.001–0.6%)
  Infection – epidural abscess or meningitis (<1:10,000)
  Urinary bladder atony (common, manifests as urinary retention persisting after resolution of sensory and motor block)
  Cauda equina syndrome (<1:100,000, as a result of neural compression associated with either spinal epidural hematoma or abscess; or maldistribution of supernormal local anesthetic concentrations or doses)
  Paraplegia/quadriplegia (<1:250,000, as a result of neural compression associated with either epidural hematoma or abscess)
Needle-induced injury
  Pelvic organs or fetus (seen rarely with caudal anesthesia)

---

thetics. Anesthesia of the cardioaccelerator nerves is linked to bradycardia and hypotension, although the frequency of this side effect is less than that seen with spinal anesthesia. Appropriate early treatment with atropine, volume, and vasopressors is indicated. Hypotension from lumbar sympathetic nerve blockade is treated in a similar fashion, but is less frequently associated with concurrent bradycardia. Even though controversial, most studies report little benefit from prophylactic ephedrine or volume loading for preventing these side effects. However, volume loading (≥500 mL) is still frequently utilized prior to epidural analgesia for labor.

Unintended Dural Penetration

Unintentionally penetrating the dura with an epidural needle can lead to two significant complications. When unrecognized by aspiration of CSF or the subarachnoid test dose, injection of large volumes of local anesthetic into the subarachnoid space can result in rapid development of high spinal anesthesia. If this occurs, preparations should be in place to support the patient's respiratory and cardiovascular systems until the local anesthetic effect dissipates. The large dural rent made by the epidural needle also places the patient at ~70% risk of developing a postdural puncture headache (see Chapter 12 for a detailed discussion, including treatment of this entity).

Neurologic Complications

Permanent neurologic complications following epidural block are extremely rare, but are often debilitating. Epidural hematoma may occur spontaneously or be associated with epidural needle placement or catheter removal in a coagulopathic patient. (Specific guidelines for the management of the anticoagulated patient are detailed in Chapter 13.) If epidural hematoma occurs, prompt diagnosis and neurosurgical intervention are crucial, because significant neurologic recovery is infrequent if more than eight hours have elapsed since the onset of any neurologic deficit. Direct needle trauma to individual nerves is rare, but possible if the needle penetrates nerve roots and especially if anesthetic solution is subsequently injected into the nerve. Similar risk exists for intraspinal cord injection. Both of these complications are best avoided by not performing epidural anesthesia in heavily sedated or anesthetized patients. Because they cannot cooperate, young children are an exception to this rule when the potential benefits of epidural placement are substantial. Infection following epidural placement is also rare and may present as meningitis or epidural abscess. Meningitis typically presents with fever, headache, and photophobia. Epidural abscess, like epidural hematoma, typically begins with severe back pain and progresses to neurologic deficit within hours to days, depending on the location and rate at which the epidural mass expands. As with epidural hematoma, a high index of suspicion followed by rapid diagnosis and treatment is the only means of averting potentially devastating neurologic sequelae. A common neurologic side effect of caudal and lumbar epidural anesthesia is urinary bladder atony, which may require a postoperative indwelling catheter. The exact incidence of this condition is difficult to ascertain, but is reduced by the use of segmental thoracic approaches.

Relative Risk of Epidural Approaches

Because of the close proximity of the spinal cord itself, logic and emotion lead us to believe that cervical and thoracic epidural anesthesia carry a higher risk of complication than does the lumbar approach (Box 9-6). There are no data available for cervical epidurals, but reports of catastrophic outcomes are rare. Studies demonstrate equivalent complication profiles for upper and mid-thoracic versus low thoracic and lumbar approaches. The incidence of opioid-induced respiratory depression, and for neurologic and infectious complications, is equivalent. Indeed, postdural puncture headache, postural hypotension, and motor block occur less frequently when thoracic epidural anesthesia and analgesia is used. Lumbar and thoracic

---

Box 9-6   Clinical Controversy: Why Are Thoracic and Cervical Epidural Techniques Intimidating?

There is inconsistent midline fusion and a thinner ligamentum flavum that may lead to problems detecting a convincing loss-of-resistance during epidural placement.

There is a narrower epidural space as compared to the lumbar region.

The spinal cord lies directly anterior to the needle as it enters the epidural space and is relatively fixed in position beneath the dura, while the cauda equina floats freely within the dural sac in the lumbar region

Nevertheless, thoracic epidural placement carries no more risk than lumbar epidural placement; and is less likely to cause significant postural hypotension and motor block

---

epidural analgesia can be safely maintained on hospital wards and do not require intensive monitoring.

SUGGESTED READING

Brown DL: *Atlas of Regional Anesthesia*, Second Edition, WB Saunders, Philadelphia, 1999.

Cousins MJ, Veering BT: Epidural neural blockade. In: Cousins MG, Bridenbaugh PO (eds), *Neural Blockade in Clinical Anesthesia and Management of Pain*, Third Edition, Lippincott-Raven, Philadelphia, 1998, pp. 243–321.

Giebler R, Scherer R, Peters J: Incidence of neurologic complications related to thoracic epidural catheterization, *Anesthesiology* 86:55–63, 1997.

Hogan QH: Epidural anatomy examined by cryomicrotome section. Influence of age, vertebral level, and disease, *Reg Anesth* 21:395–406, 1996.

Hogan Q: Distribution of solution in the epidural space: examination by cryomicrotome section. *Reg Anesth Pain Med* 27:150–156, 2002.

Liu S, Allen H, Olsson G: Patient controlled epidural analgesia with bupivacaine and fentanyl on hospital wards. Prospective experience with 1,030 surgical patients, *Anesthesiology* 88:688–695, 1998.

Neal JM: Thoracic epidural analgesia, American Society of Anesthesiologists On-Line Pain Management Workshop, 2001, www.asahg.org/continuinged.htm (Nov 2002).

Tanaka K, Watanabe R, Harado T, Dan K: Extensive application of epidural anesthesia and analgesia in a university hospital: incidence of complications related to technique, *Reg Anesth* 18:34–38, 1993.

Visser WA, Liem TH, van Egmond J, Gielen MJM: Extension of sensory blockade after thoracic epidural administration of a test dose of lidocaine at three different levels, *Anesth Analg* 86:332–335, 1998.

CHAPTER 10

Spinal Anesthesia

CHRISTOPHER M. VISCOMI

INTRODUCTION

Spinal anesthesia is among the most commonly employed regional anesthetic techniques in contemporary anesthetic practice. It combines many favorable attributes of an ideal regional anesthetic, including technical ease, reliability, low complication rate, and ability to provide postoperative pain control.

Spinal anesthesia was pioneered by several German physicians. In 1884, Dr. Carl Koller first applied cocaine to the cornea and conjunctiva to produce topical anesthesia. In 1897, German surgeon Dr. August Bier utilized a spinal needle developed by a fellow University of Berlin physician, Dr. Iraneus Quincke, to inject cocaine into the subarachnoid space. In the course of the initial experiments, Bier and an assistant performed spinal anesthetics on each other. After recovering from the characteristic sensory and motor block, each of the investigators reported a severe postdural puncture headache.

Early spinal anesthesia was plagued by severe headaches, hypotension, limited pharmacologic options, and infectious complications. Each of these limitations has been largely overcome in contemporary practice. Pencil point spinal needles have lowered postdural puncture headache rates to less than 2.5%, and blood patch therapy has been developed as an effective treatment. Intravenous hydration and judicious use of vasoconstrictors allow simple and effective treatment of spinal anesthesia-induced hypotension. Many pharmacologic options now exist to tailor the block level and duration to that required by a particular surgical procedure. Finally, aseptic technique and disposable sterile spinal anesthesia kits have all but eliminated infectious complications.

ANATOMY

The spinal subarachnoid space begins at the foramen magnum and is continuous with the intracranial subarachnoid space (Fig. 10-1 on p. 115). The spinal subarachnoid space extends to approximately the second sacral level. The vertebral column shields the spinal cord and proximal nerve roots in a protective bony encasement, and

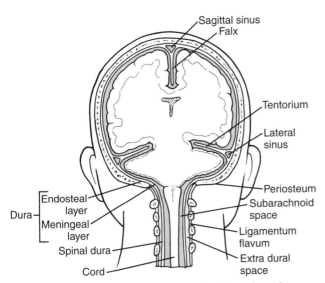

Figure 10-1   Intracranial and spinal subarachnoid spaces are continuous. (Redrawn from Cousins MJ, Bridenbaugh PO: *Neural Blockade*, Third Edition, Lippincott-Raven, Philadelphia, 1998, Fig. 7-4.)

is divided into seven cervical, twelve thoracic, and five lumbar vertebrae (Fig. 10-2 on p. 116). Caudad to the fifth lumbar vertebra are the sacrum and coccyx. Between the sacrum and coccyx is a posterior opening termed the sacral hiatus, used clinically to perform caudal epidural blocks.

The vertebral column has several clinically relevant curves. The highest (most anterior) points of the spinal column in the supine patient lie at C_5 and L_{4-5}, and the most posterior lie at T_5 and S_2. This anatomy, together with the baricity of the anesthetic injected, can be used to control the dermatomal level of anesthesia.

The individual vertebrae are connected by a series of ligaments (Fig. 10-3 on p. 116) that provide stability while allowing for movement. Anterior to the spinal canal, the vertebral bodies are connected by the anterior and posterior longitudinal ligaments. Posterior to the spinal canal, a series of three ligaments connect the laminae and spinous processes of adjacent vertebrae. The ligament flavum is the strongest of these ligaments, and extends from the articular processes to the midline spinous processes. The interspinous ligament connects anteriorly to the ligamentum flavum, posteriorly to the supraspinous ligament, and to the spinous processes superiorly and inferiorly. Finally, the supraspinous ligament runs from C_7 to S_1, and connects the apices of the spinous processes posteriorly.

Within the spinal canal are neural elements (spinal cord and cauda equina), cerebrospinal fluid (CSF), and blood vessels supplying the spinal cord. An important anatomical consideration is the inferior terminus of the

spinal cord, the conus medullaris (Fig. 10-4 on p. 117). The spinal cord extends as low as the third lumbar vertebral body (L_3) in children and L_{1-2} in adults. Inferior to this point, the neural elements contained within the spinal canal are nerve roots bathed in CSF which are termed the cauda equina (Latin for "horse's tail," describing the tail-like appearance of the nerve roots within the thecal sac below the conus medullaris). Spinal anesthetic injections are usually performed caudad to L_2 to avoid the potential for spinal cord trauma. Here, the nerve roots of the cauda equina are relatively mobile and are unlikely to be impaled by an advancing spinal needle.

The spinal cord is enveloped by three connective tissue layers termed meninges (Fig. 10-5 on p. 117). Enclosing the CSF are the closely approximated arachnoid meninges and dura mater. The space immediately outside the dura is termed the epidural space, while internal to the arachnoid is the subarachnoid space. Local anesthetic injection just external to the dura is termed epidural anesthesia. The subarachnoid space is also termed the "intrathecal space." Local anesthetics injected into the subarachnoid space produce sensory anesthesia termed "spinal anesthesia." The pia mater is the third meningeal covering, and is a highly vascular tissue layer closely adherent to the neural elements. Between the arachnoid and the pia are numerous delicate connections termed arachnoid trabeculae.

The neural elements of the spinal column are bathed in CSF, which is an ultrafiltrate of blood which is produced and secreted by the choroid plexus within the lateral, third, and fourth ventricles of the brain. The rate of production of CSF is relatively uniform at about 500 mL/day. CSF absorption is equal to production, and total CSF volume is typically 130–150 mL. CSF contains both proteins and electrolytes (principally sodium and chloride) and has a specific gravity of 1.003–1.009 at 37° C (Box 10-1).

PHYSIOLOGY

The injection of local anesthetics into the subarachnoid space produces a spectrum of physiologic responses. Knowledge of these effects is critical to optimizing the safety of spinal anesthesia.

Box 10-1   Physical Characteristics of CSF

pH: 7.3
Total volume (adult): 150 mL
Specific gravity: 1.003–1.009
CSF pressure (lateral decubitus): 60–80 mmHg
Protein: 30 mg/dL

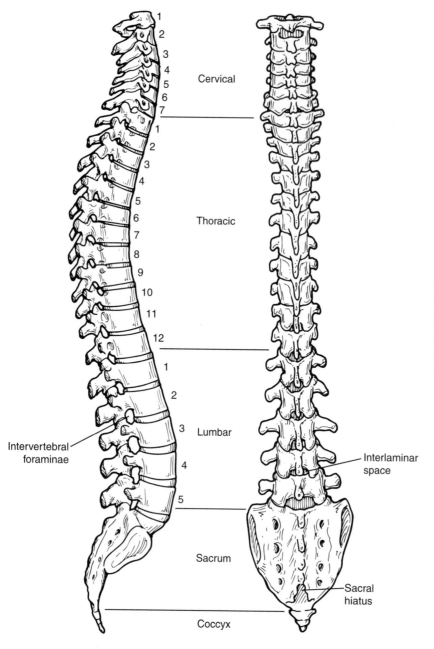

Cervical

Thoracic

Lumbar

Intervertebral foraminae

Sacrum

Coccyx

Interlaminar space

Sacral hiatus

Figure 10-2   Vertebral elements. The vertebral elements of the spinal column are divided into cervical, thoracic, and lumbar vertebrae; the fused vertebral elements into the sacrum and the coccyx. (Redrawn from Stoelting RK, Miller RD: *Basics of Anesthesia*, Churchill Livingstone, New York, 1989, Fig. 13-1.)

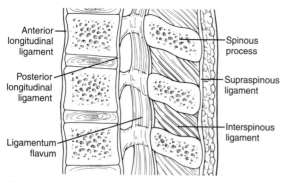

Anterior longitudinal ligament

Posterior longitudinal ligament

Ligamentum flavum

Spinous process

Supraspinous ligament

Interspinous ligament

Figure 10-3   Ligaments of the spine. Three ligamentous attachments connect and stabilize adjacent vertebrae. (Redrawn from Cousins MJ, Bridenbaugh PO: *Neural Blockade*, Third Edition, Lippincott-Raven, Philadelphia, 1998.)

Cardiovascular Effects

The cardiovascular response to spinal anesthesia is due to sympathetic nerve blockade induced by intrathecal local anesthetics. Sympathetic impulses are carried via Aδ and C nerve fibers, which are easily blocked by local anesthetics. Thus, sympathetic blockade typically extends several dermatomes higher than sensory blockade during spinal anesthesia. The sympathetic nerve fibers emerge from the spinal cord from T_1 to L_2, thus total sympathetic blockade is quite possible with thoracic levels of sensory block.

Sympathetic blockade produces arteriolar vasodilation, typically causing a 15–20% decrease in systemic vascular

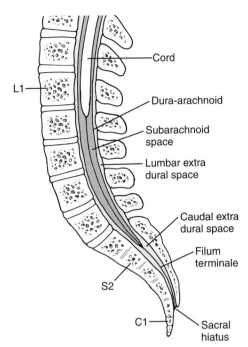

Figure 10-4   The inferior terminus of the spinal cord. (Redrawn from Cousins MJ, Bridenbaugh PO: *Neural Blockade,* Third Edition, Lippincott-Raven, Philadelphia, 1998.)

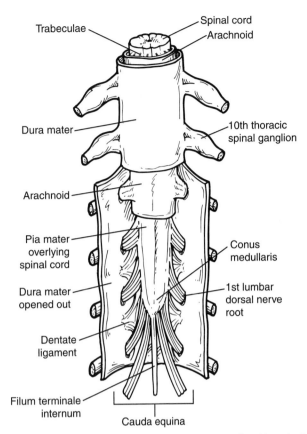

Figure 10-5   The meninges. Dura mater, arachnoid, and pia mater are the three connective tissue layers enveloping the brain and spinal cord. (Redrawn from Cousins MJ, Bridenbaugh PO: *Neural Blockade,* Third Edition, Lippincott-Raven, Philadelphia, 1998, Fig. 7-8.)

resistance. Of note, the arteriolar smooth muscle retains localized autoregulation under these circumstances, such that vasomotor tone can still be modulated by local metabolic demands. In contrast, venous tone is completely abolished by sympathetic blockade. Thus, venous pooling is pronounced during spinal anesthesia, and venous return becomes dependent upon gravity and negative intrathoracic pressure during spontaneous ventilation. Reverse Trendelenburg positioning can have dramatic effects on cardiac preload with high spinal anesthesia. Because systemic vascular resistance (afterload) is reduced during spinal anesthesia and preload becomes the major determinant of cardiac output, intravenous fluid administration and patient positioning are the primary means of preventing hypotension during spinal anesthesia.

Heart rate may decrease in conjunction with spinal anesthesia, particularly with high thoracic block levels. Bradycardia is principally due to blockade of sympathetic preganglionic cardioaccelerator fibers (T_1–T_4). An additional mechanism of bradycardia during high spinal anesthesia is right atrial chronotropic stretch receptors. When stretched, these receptors cause increase in heart rate but, with spinal anesthesia-induced venodilation, activation of atrial stretch receptors is absent and heart rate declines (Box 10-2).

Although heart rate typically falls by only 10–20%, athletic patients with a low resting heart rate have experienced asystole during spinal anesthesia. This extreme case may be partially mediated by the Bezold–Jarisch reflex, a reflex leading to bradycardia and hypotension that

is mediated through both afferent and efferent pathways within the vagus nerve and originates from unidentified chemoreceptors within the heart. The role of the Bezold–Jarisch reflex in mediating bradycardia and hypotension following spinal anesthesia remains in question.

The cardiac effects of spinal anesthesia are dependent upon the maintenance of cardiac preload; spinal anesthesia should not be performed on hypovolemic patients who already have decreased cardiac preload and active vasoconstriction maintaining blood pressure. Spinal anesthesia can lead to profound hypotension under these circumstances.

Myocardial oxygen supply and demand are both significantly influenced by spinal anesthesia. Myocardial oxygen supply is directly proportional to coronary blood flow. Coronary blood flow is, in turn, controlled by coronary perfusion pressure (CPP) and heart rate. Because approximately 80% of coronary blood flow is during diastole, then

Coronary Perfusion Pressure (CPP)	=	Diastolic Blood Pressure (DBP)	−	Left Ventricular End-Diastolic Pressure (LVEDP)

Box 10-2   Mechanism of Bradycardia during High Spinal Anesthesia

Blockade of sympathetic cardiac accelerator fibers (T1–T4) leading to unopposed vagal stimulation

Decreased preload following venodilation leading to decreased activation of right atrial stretch receptors

---

Spinal anesthesia changes each of these parameters. DBP typically falls 15–20%, which tends to reduce coronary perfusion. However, decreased preload and afterload both decrease LVEDP, which reduces myocardial oxygen demand, thereby offsetting the decrease in DBP, and resulting in only a modest (5–10%) fall in coronary perfusion pressure. Heart rate is important also, as diastolic time is disproportionately shortened (compared to systolic time) with elevated heart rates. Heart rate tends to be stable or to decrease with spinal anesthesia.

Myocardial oxygen demand is also influenced by heart rate, ventricular wall tension, and inotropic state. Cardiac sympathetic denervation lowers heart rate and inotropy by about 15–20%. Decreased afterload and preload both reduce the size of the left ventricle, thereby lowering wall tension. Overall, myocardial oxygen demand falls by about the same amount as myocardial oxygen supply. Thus, although both supply and demand change, overall metabolic balance is typically maintained.

Cerebral blood flow also merits discussion. Cerebral autoregulation typically controls cerebral blood flow at a constant level between mean arterial pressures of 50–150 mmHg. This is accomplished by locally mediated changes in cerebral vascular resistance that compensate for increased or decreased perfusion pressures. Two patient subsets warrant special consideration. In patients with chronic hypertension, the cerebral autoregulatory pressure range is shifted higher, typically in the 80–180 mmHg range. Thus, less hypotension should be permitted with spinal anesthesia in those with chronic hypertension. Patients with significant cerebrovascular atherosclerosis may be highly sensitive to decreases in mean arterial pressure. Because of significant fixed obstructive vascular lesions, cerebral vasodilation in response to hypotension is unlikely to maintain cerebral blood flow. These patients should have MAP maintained within 20% of baseline (Box 10-3).

Respiratory Changes

Resting tidal volume, minute ventilation, and arterial blood gases are unaltered by high thoracic spinal anesthesia. This is likely because inspiration is controlled by diaphragm function (phrenic nerve), which is unaffected. Normal exhalation is controlled by passive elastic recoil of the lungs. However, respiratory maneuvers which require active exhalation are impeded by spinal anesthesia that extends to the thoracic dermatomes. Maximum breathing capacity, maximum expiratory volume, and maximum exhalation pressure generated by coughing involve accessory muscles of respiration, including the anterior abdominal muscles and intercostal muscles. Spinal anesthesia that extends to the thoracic dermatomes will block the motor function of these muscles and may exacerbate symptoms of dyspnea in patients needing active exhalation (asthma) or pulmonary toilet (chronic bronchitis). It is uncommon for this to progress to respiratory failure (Box 10-4).

Box 10-3   Treatment of Spinal Anesthesia-Induced Hypotension

In healthy patients, blood pressure decreases of up to 30% are typically well tolerated

Keep blood pressure within 20% of baseline in patients with known or suspected coronary artery or cerebrovascular disease

Maintain or augment preload with IV fluids and slight (5–10°) Trendelenburg position

Use vasopressors such as ephedrine 5–10 mg or phenylephrine 50–100 μg if preload augmentation is ineffective

Consider spinal anesthesia using low doses of local anesthetic combined with a lipophilic opioid (such as 10–25 μg fentanyl). This produces significantly less hypotension compared to higher doses of local anesthetic used alone

---

Box 10-4   Respiratory Changes of High Thoracic Spinal Anesthesia

NO CHANGE

PaO_2
$PaCO_2$
pH
Tidal volume
Respiratory rate
Minute ventilation
Maximal inhalation

DECREASED

Maximal exhalation
Maximal minute ventilation
Maximal expiratory flow (cough)

In the setting of high (cervical) spinal anesthesia, phrenic nerve (C_{3-5}) function may be impaired. However, concentrations of local anesthetic necessary to block phrenic nerve motor function are higher than those typically found even under total spinal anesthesia. More likely, severe hypotension with high or total spinal anesthesia causes under perfusion of the medullary respiratory centers, leading to apnea. Restoration of blood pressure and cardiac output typically leads to prompt return of spontaneous ventilation.

Hepatic and Renal Blood Flow

Hepatic blood flow decreases with spinal anesthesia in direct proportion to decreases in mean arterial pressure. Hepatic venous oxygenation decreases, reflecting increased oxygen extraction by the liver. Similar changes are seen during general anesthesia. There are no human studies to suggest that either spinal or general anesthesia is preferable in patients with pre-existing hepatic disease. Surgical manipulation alone in the upper abdomen causes a greater decrease in hepatic blood flow than do general or regional anesthesia.

Renal blood flow is autoregulated in the range of 50–150 mmHg MAP. MAP below 50 mmHg results in decreased renal blood flow and urine output. In the absence of hypovolemia, renal function is usually well preserved, even with significant reduction in blood pressure.

Other Physiological Effects of Spinal Anesthesia

The hormonal and metabolic stress responses induced by surgical stimulation are more effectively blunted by spinal anesthesia than by general anesthesia. However, after resolution of spinal block, postoperative stress responses are similar in patients receiving either spinal or general anesthesia.

Gastric motility is typically augmented by spinal anesthesia. Sympathetic innervation to the large and small intestines is via the T_5–L_1 spinal nerve roots. With sympathetic blockade, unopposed vagal innervation leads to active peristalsis.

CLINICAL USES

Spinal anesthesia is suitable for most lower extremity and genitourinary procedures. Lower abdominal procedures, such as cesarean delivery, post-partum tubal ligation, and uncomplicated hysterectomy, are also amenable to spinal anesthesia. Most procedures involving upper abdominal surgery are better performed with general

---

Box 10-5 Advantages of Spinal Anesthesia

Fewer postoperative deep venous thromboses after hip repair and hip replacement
Improved postoperative analgesia when neuraxial opioids are administered
Less nausea and vomiting

---

anesthesia. While an adequate sensory level can be established with spinal anesthesia, peritoneal traction and surgical retraction often cause discomfort.

Duration of surgery influences the choice between spinal or general anesthesia. Nearly unlimited duration of anesthesia can be achieved by performing either combined spinal–epidural anesthesia or continuous spinal anesthesia. However, patient selection and judicious use of sedation are important, as many patients will become uncomfortable lying in the same position for many hours.

Most studies report less nausea and vomiting following spinal anesthesia compared to general anesthesia. Addition of neuraxial opioids can often improve pain control after surgery (Box 10-5). There do not appear to be any significant clinical differences in major cardiac outcomes comparing general versus spinal anesthesia, even in high-risk patients. Significant improvements in pulmonary outcome (lower rates of postoperative atelectasis, oxygen desaturation, and pneumonia) have been found when patients at high risk (e.g. obese patients receiving upper abdominal incisions) receive pain control after surgery with continuous epidural infusions of local anesthetic. However, there are no demonstrable improvements in outcome in patients who receive spinal anesthesia for surgery. This likely reflects the need for ongoing analgesia in the days following surgery to improve pulmonary toilet and the fact that most spinal anesthetics are carried out for low-risk pulmonary procedures involving the lower extremities.

Contraindications to neuraxial regional anesthesia are discussed in detail in Chapters 9, 13, and 16. Spinal anesthesia should not be used in the presence of coagulopathy due to the risk of epidural hematoma. Systemic or localized infection over the lumbar region may predispose to local abscess formation or meningitis. Significant hypovolemia may predispose patients to develop profound hypotension and the potential for cardiac arrest with spinal anesthesia. Finally, spinal anesthesia is often avoided in patients with specific intracardiac lesions where maintenance of preload and/or afterload are critical (Box 10-6).

Clincial Caveat: Why is Spinal Anesthesia Hazardous in Patients With Certain Cardiac Lesions?

Spinal anesthesia causes a significant decrease in both systemic vascular resistance (afterload) and venous return (preload). These physiologic effects combine to produce moderate hypotension in individuals with normal cardiac function. In those with reduced contractility (e.g. those with prior myocardial infarction), the reduction in afterload can actually reduce left ventricular wall tension and improve cardiac output. However, in those cardiac abnormalities where cardiac output is dependent on maintenance of elevated preload (e.g. Eisenmenger's syndrome) or where cardiac output is fixed by a restrictive lesion (e.g. aortic stenosis), spinal anesthesia can lead to profound hypotension and cardiac arrest. Use of spinal anesthesia in these individuals is controversial. When spinal anesthesia is used in patients with these critical cardiac lesions, strict attention must be paid to maintaining preload (intravenous hydration) and restoring systemic vascular resistance using vasoconstrictors.

Box 10-6   Contraindications to Spinal Anesthesia

Cutaneous infection at puncture site
Sepsis
Hypovolemia
Coagulopathy
Patient refusal
Cardiac lesions (spinal anesthesia is relatively contraindicated in patients with the following conditions; see further discussion in the Clinical Caveat box):
   Moderate-to-severe aortic stenosis
   Eisenmenger's syndrome
   Asymmetric septal hypertrophy
   Right-to-left intracardiac shunts

TECHNIQUE

Pre-block Preparations

Because induction of spinal anesthesia often results in marked hemodynamic changes, patients should be monitored continuously, and resuscitative drugs and equipment should be immediately available. It is helpful to have an assistant to position the patient and provide psychological support. Sedation (analgesics and anxiolytics) is frequently administered prior to performing spinal anesthesia to reduce discomfort and anxiety. These drugs may cause significant cardiorespiratory compromise, and may mask the pain or paresthesia of an intraneural injection. It is important to keep in mind that not every spinal anesthetic is successful, and that spinal anesthesia in itself can cause respiratory compromise. Thus, every spinal anesthetic has the potential to require rapid conversion to general anesthesia. Appropriate drugs and airway management equipment must be immediately available.

Patient Positioning

The lateral decubitus, sitting, and prone positions may all be used to perform spinal anesthesia. Each position has advantages and disadvantages. The lateral decubitus is the most common position used. Patients are typically comfortable in this position, and are less prone to movement compared to the sitting position. Syncope is less common than with the sitting position. The patient is positioned at the edge of the operating table (Fig. 10-6 on p. 121) with both the hips and shoulders vertically oriented. Slender males typically have a slightly up-sloping vertebral axis, reflecting slightly greater shoulder width compared to hip width. Slender females typically have a slightly down-sloping vertebral axis. Both the hips and the upper thorax should be flexed to provide a reverse lordotic position that maximizes the distance between lumbar vertebral spinous processes.

The sitting position is routinely chosen by some practitioners, and is often chosen when caring for obese patients. In the obese population, palpation of midline spinous processes is often difficult or impossible. In these cases, position of the midline can be estimated by connecting an imaginary line between the most prominent cervical vertebra (C7, the vetrebra prominens) and the intergluteal cleft and this is easier to do with the patient sitting. An assistant is required to maintain a stable position, particularly if the patient has been sedated. Patients are asked to slump their shoulders forward, and attempt to flex their spine (Fig. 10-7 on p. 121). A common mistake is having the patient merely bend forward at the waist. The sitting position also allows for spinal anesthesia restricted to the pelvis. This produces a "saddle block," or sensory block limited to the perineal surfaces typically in contact with the saddle or seat when riding horseback (Fig. 10-8 on p. 121). The injection of hyperbaric local anesthetic into the CSF in a sitting patient causes the local anesthetic to pool in the most dependent regions of the subarachnoid space (the sacrum). This technique is useful for instrumental vaginal deliveries, as well as certain urologic and gynecologic surgeries.

The prone position is occasionally chosen to provide spinal anesthesia to a patient having anal surgery in the

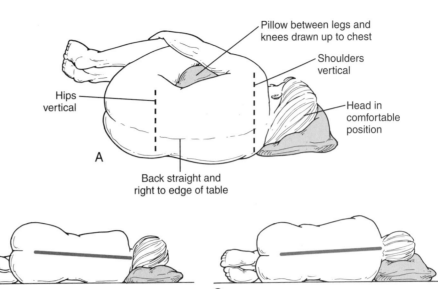

Figure 10-6   Lateral position for dural puncture. (A) Note slope of vertebral axis differs between slender females (B) and males (C). (Redrawn from Cousins MJ, Bridenbaugh PO: *Neural Blockade*, Third Edition, Lippincott-Raven, Philadelphia, 1998, Fig. 7-17.)

jack-knife position (Fig. 10-9 on p. 122). The patient is placed in the surgical position, and lumbar puncture is made. Hypobaric local anesthetic injections are used to restrict the anesthetic effect to the sacral and low lumbar dermatomes.

Puncture Site

Dural puncture is typically attempted below L_2 to avoid the spinal cord which ends at L_1–L_2. Although there is variation from individual to individual, a line drawn between the iliac crests typically passes through the L_{4-5} interspace (Fig. 10-7). Careful aseptic technique is important. This includes widely prepping the lumbar region with an iodine and/or alcohol solution, and utilizing sterile drapes.

Midline or Paramedian Approach

Two approaches to the subarachnoid space are commonly used: midline and paramedian (Fig. 10-10 on p. 122). Both are simple and effective. Practitioners should have familiarity with both approaches so that they can employ an alternative technique in those cases where the first approach fails. For the midline approach, the spinous processes are palpated in the lumbar region. After cleansing the region and raising a skin wheel between spinous processes, a spinal needle is advanced in the sagittal plane with a 10° cephalad needle orientation. This orientation is necessary as the interlaminar space is slightly cephalad to the palpable interspinous space.

The paramedian approach is often chosen in patients with excessive lumbar lordosis, and pregnant patients

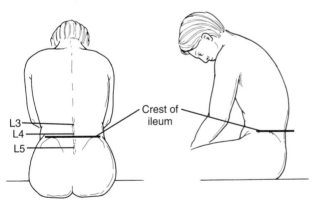

Figure 10-7   The seated position for dural puncture. Curling forward reverses the lumbar lordosis and increases the distance between adjacent spinous processes, thereby facilitating spinal needle placement. (Redrawn from Cousins MJ, Bridenbaugh PO: *Neural Blockade*, Third Edition, Lippincott-Raven, Philadelphia, 1998, Fig. 7-18.)

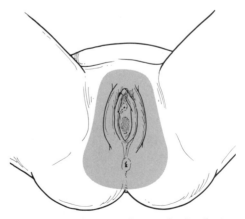

Figure 10-8   Distribution of anesthesia during saddle block. A hyperbaric local anesthetic injected in the sitting position will result in a dense sacral block (shaded area, "saddle block").

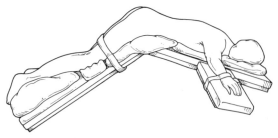

Figure 10-9   The jack-knife position for anal surgery. Hypobaric spinal anesthesia is performed with the patient already in this position. (Redrawn from Brown DL: *Atlas of Regional Anesthesia*, Second Edition, WB Saunders, Philadelphia, 1999, Fig. 42-4.)

who cannot flex their vertebral column. With excessive lordosis, the spinous processes are close together in the midline, and may prevent passage of the spinal needle to the spinal canal. The paramedian approach is less affected by suboptimal flexion of the spine. The paramedian approach is also chosen in elderly patients with calcified interspinous ligaments. With the paramedian approach, a skin wheel is raised with local anesthetic approximately 1-1.5 cm inferior and lateral to the desired vertebral interspace. The spinal needle is advanced with a 15° cephalad and medial orientation.

The Taylor approach is a variant of the paramedian approach used to enter the L_5-S_1 interspace. This interspace is the largest lumbar vertebral interspace and can often be entered using this approach even when entry at higher interspaces is difficult. The inferior aspect of the posterior superior iliac spine (PSIS) is palpated. Needle puncture is made 1 cm medial and 1 cm inferior to the PSIS inferior border (Fig. 10-10). The spinal needle is advanced with a needle angulation toward midline

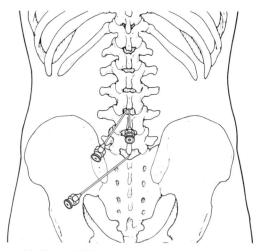

Figure 10-10   Midline and paramedian approaches to dural puncture. The Taylor approach is shown with the lowest needle, and is a paramedian approach to the L5-S1 interspace. (Redrawn from Hahn MB, McQuillan PM, Sheplock GJ: *Regional Anesthesia*, Mosby, St. Louis, 1996, Fig. 32-3.)

(45-55°) and steeply cephalad (45-55°). In obese patients, the needle direction should be in a 30-45° cephalad and medial orientation to account for tissue depth. If bone is contacted, the needle is angled more cephalad to walk off of the bony lamina into the interspace.

Continuous Spinal Anesthesia

To provide continuous spinal anesthesia, a catheter is placed into the subarachnoid space. Typically an 18 gauge Tuohy epidural needle is placed into the subarachnoid space via either a midline or paramedian approach. After dural puncture, a catheter is threaded 2-5 cm into the lumbar cistern (the most common method is to use the same catheter that is used to provide epidural anesthesia). This allows rapid and reliable titration of a spinal block (small repeated doses can be given) and duration is unlimited (the catheter allows for repeat dosing as the block recedes).

Clinical Controversy: Spinal Microcatheters

Small-diameter spinal "microcatheters" were approved for use in the USA during the 1980s. Thereafter, multiple reports of cauda equina syndrome appeared with large doses of intrathecal lidocaine and tetracaine administered via spinal microcatheters (24-32 g), leading the FDA to remove spinal microcatheters from the US market.

The small internal diameter of the microcatheters causes the local anesthetic solution to exit the catheter at a low velocity. This prevents adequate mixing of the local anesthetic with CSF. Toxicity results from localized pooling of lidocaine in the lumbar cistern, allowing neurotoxic concentrations of lidocaine to build up directly around the cauda equina. With appreciation of the mechanism leading to neurotoxicity and the use of appropriate doses of less toxic local anesthetics, microcatheters are being re-evaluated.

Patient Positioning and Desired Block

By choosing patient position together with the mass and baricity of the local anesthetic solution, block height can be relatively controlled, and a degree of unilateral block can be achieved. However, it can take as much as 15-20 minutes in the lateral position to establish a unilateral block. More commonly, the patient is kept on their side for just a few minutes and then turned supine. This leads to a nearly equal bilateral block after a few minutes. As an example of using baricity and patient position, the term "saddle block" refers to injecting a small dose of hyperbaric lidocaine (e.g. 25 mg of 5%

lidocaine in 7.5% dextrose) into the lumbar cistern of a patient in the sitting position. The patient is kept in a sitting position for 5-10 minutes after injection, allowing the local anesthetic solution to pool over the sacral nerve roots. Dense perineal anesthesia occurs (Fig. 10-8 on p. 121), and minimal hypotension ensues (since block height is well below the L_2 terminal of the sympathetic nerve fibers).

PHARMACOLOGIC CHOICES

Nearly all spinal anesthetics involve the injection of local anesthetics, either alone or in combination with adjuvant drugs. The pharmacology of these agents has been reviewed in earlier chapters. This chapter focuses on the specific subarachnoid use of these drugs (Table 10-1).

Local Anesthetics

Lidocaine, bupivacaine, and tetracaine are all commonly used local anesthetics for spinal anesthesia.

Lidocaine

Lidocaine (short-to-intermediate duration spinal anesthesia) in doses of 20-100 mg is frequently chosen for cases estimated to take 75 minutes or less. Lidocaine is most commonly used as a 5% solution in 7.5% dextrose; however, 1.5 and 2% lidocaine are also useful. The addition of epinephrine 0.2 mg prolongs anesthesia by 15-40 minutes, depending on the dose of local anesthetic used, but is associated with significantly prolonged motor block and delayed micturition. Fentanyl 15-25 µg is another useful additive. It allows a substantial reduction in lidocaine dose (to permit rapid recovery, and lower incidence of transient neurologic symptoms) and effectively blocks lower extremity tourniquet pain.

Bupivacaine

Bupivacaine (intermediate-duration spinal anesthesia) in doses of 5-15 mg is suitable for surgeries lasting 90-150 minutes, although duration of bupivacaine block tends to have a wider standard deviation as compared with lidocaine. Spinal anesthesia is commonly carried out with 0.75% bupivacaine in 8.25% dextrose. Bupivacaine 0.5% solution without dextrose is isobaric or slightly hypobaric, and is commonly used for lower extremity surgery. Epinephrine prolongs motor and sensory blockade by approximately 30-45 minutes when added to small-dose (7.5 mg) bupivacaine. Fentanyl is also used as an adjuvant to permit lower bupivacaine doses (with less hypotension) and enhanced analgesia (Box 10-7).

Table 10-1	Clinical Applications: Recommendations for Spinal Anesthesia			
Inpatient/ Outpatient	Expected Surgical Duration	Upper Extent of Desired Block	Examples	Spinal Recommendation
Outpatient	<1 hour	<T_{10}	Knee arthroscopy, vein stripping	Isobaric (2%) or hypobaric (0.5%) lidocaine 30-40 mg + fentanyl 20 µg
Outpatient	<1 hour	≥T_7	Inguinal or umbilical hernia repair	Hyperbaric lidocaine (5% in dextrose) 50 mg + fentanyl 20 µg
Outpatient	>1 hour	<T_{10}	ACL reconstruction	Isobaric bupivacaine (0.5%) 7 mg + fentanyl 20 µg
Inpatient	<1 hour	<T_{10}	TURP, bladder tumor, laser surgery	Hyperbaric lidocaine (5% in dextrose) 30 mg + fentanyl 20 µg
Inpatient	1-2 hours	<T_{10}	Primary knee or hip arthroplasty, hip fracture	Isobaric bupivacaine (0.5%) 5-7 mg + fentanyl 20 µg
Inpatient	>3 hours	<T_{10}	Femoral-popliteal vascular surgery	Hyperbaric (1% + dextrose) or isobaric (1% without dextrose) tetracaine 12 mg + epinephrine 0.2 mg

---

Box 10-7 Spinal Anesthesia in the Elderly: Low-Dose Bupivacaine Plus Fentanyl (versus Higher-Dose Bupivacaine Alone)

Less hypotension
Less vasopressor use
Lower fluid requirements

Tetracaine

Tetracaine (long-duration spinal anesthesia) in doses of 4–12 mg provides surgical anesthesia for 3 to 4 hours. Tetracaine is one of the oldest spinal anesthetics. It is available commercially as either niphanoid crystals (20 mg) or a 1% solution. Tetracaine is less stable in liquid solution than lidocaine or bupivacaine and has resulted in low-potency tetracaine ampules where some of the drug had degraded during storage. Tetracaine is unique among spinal anesthetics in that the successful blockade seems highly dependent on co-administration of epinephrine. Block failure rates of up to 35% occur with plain tetracaine. Tetracaine with epinephrine is the longest acting spinal anesthetic, resulting in lower abdominal anesthesia of approximately 4 hours, and lower extremity anesthesia of 5–6 hours.

Spinal Anesthesia Additives

Vasoconstrictors

Vasoconstrictors are often added to intrathecal local anesthetics in order to inhibit vascular uptake and thereby prolong blockade. Epinephrine and, less commonly, phenylephrine are agents used for this purpose. In addition to vasoconstriction, epinephrine may promote analgesia by α_2 receptor stimulation. Indeed, clonidine, an α_2 agonist, prolongs motor and sensory block with tetracaine spinal anesthesia to a greater degree than epinephrine.

In addition to prolonging sensory blockade, adding epinephrine to spinal local anesthetics substantially prolongs motor blockade and delays micturition. These two factors delay recovery from spinal anesthesia. For outpatient surgery, most centers avoid intrathecal epinephrine. Instead, intrathecal lipophilic opioids are used to augment and prolong anesthesia without impeding recovery.

Opioids

Opioid analgesics can be added to spinal anesthetics. Opioids appear to produce supra-additive (synergistic) anesthesia when added to intrathecal local anesthetics. This synergy appears particularly pronounced with visceral pain. Spinal opioids block pain pathways with minimal additional blockade of motor or sympathetic fibers. Two discrete classes of opioids are used in spinal anesthesia and analgesia.

Hydrophilic opioids are typically added to prolong postoperative analgesia. Morphine sulfate 0.1–0.3 mg is commonly chosen. This agent has analgesic effects within 45 minutes of lumbar administration, and lowers the need for additional analgesia postoperatively for 12–24 hours. Morphine slowly ascends the spinal column, and reaches the brainstem by rostral CSF circulation approximately 8 hours after lumbar administration. This corresponds to the delayed respiratory depression that has been reported with intrathecal morphine: peak effects are seen 8–10 hours after administration.

Spinal morphine has a number of other undesirable side effects. Nausea and vomiting rates appear higher than with systemic opioids. Pruritus is common (60–80%) and can be severe (20%). Micturition is substantially impaired, probably by inhibition of the detrusor mechanism. Because of the small risk of delayed respiratory depression and impaired ability to void, this drug is inappropriate for outpatient surgery (Box 10-8).

Lipophilic opioids (fentanyl and sufentanil) are gaining popularity in spinal anesthesia (Box 10-9). Fentanyl 10–25 μg or sufentanil 2.5–10 μg can be added to spinal anesthetics to achieve a number of goals. These agents have rapid onset of anesthetic synergy, and improve intraoperative anesthesia. This has been particularly well demonstrated with reduced tourniquet pain during lower extremity orthopedic procedures, as well as decreased pain and vomiting during cesarean deliveries.

Lipophilic opioids also allow reduction of the dose of co-administered local anesthetic, permitting more rapid motor recovery from spinal anesthesia in outpatients. For instance, lidocaine 30 mg (0.5%) combined with fentanyl 20 μg provides good anesthesia for knee arthroscopy with lower incidence of nausea and improved postoperative pain control when compared with standard doses of hyperbaric lidocaine. Likewise, 3.75 mg bupivacaine (0.75% hyperbaric in 8.25% dextrose) combined with fentanyl 25 μg results in excellent anesthesia for outpatient oocyte retrieval during

---

Box 10-8 Intrathecal Morphine

ADVANTAGES

Excellent analgesia for moderate pain
10–20 hour duration

DISADVANTAGES

Delayed (8–10 hours postinjection) respiratory depression
Pruritus: 70% mild, 20% severe
Nausea and vomiting increased
Delayed micturition
Inappropriate for outpatients

Box 10-9 Intrathecal Lipophilic Opioids

The most common lipophilic opioid used to supplement spinal anesthesia is fentanyl 10–25 μg. Addition of fentanyl to spinal local anesthetic:
Increases tourniquet tolerance
Allows reduced local anesthetic dose: less motor block, less hypotension, faster recovery
Has not been associated with the delayed respiratory depression observed following intrathecal morphine
Does not inhibit micturition
Typically leads to 2–4 hours of postinjection analgesia
Is ideal for outpatient surgery

Box 10-10 Clinical Applications: Hyperbaric Spinal Anesthesia

Selective anesthesia of perineum ("saddle block"). In obstetric, urologic, gynecologic, and rectal surgery, the perineum can be anesthetized without causing widespread sensory and sympathetic blockade. The lumbar puncture is made with the patient in a sitting position. With lateral aperture spinal needles, the hyperbaric injection is made with the needle aperture directed caudad. The patient is kept in the sitting position for 5–10 minutes to allow the block to "set-up."

Selectively anesthetizing one limb. The patient is positioned in a lateral decubitus position with the surgical site on the dependent side. Lumbar puncture is performed with the needle aperture aimed toward the dependent side during injection. The patient stays in the lateral position for 15–20 minutes. Producing a truly unilateral block using this technique rarely warrants the time necessary; most patients are rolled to the supine position early after spinal placement and attain similar bilateral block.

Abdominal anesthesia (e.g. cesarean delivery). In a supine person, the most dependent regions of the neuraxis will be the sacrum and approximately T_4 (Fig. 10-11). If a hyperbaric intrathecal injection is made in the mid-lumbar region, and the patient is quickly turned supine, the local anesthetic will tend to spread quickly to the dependent regions of the neuraxis. This will result in an approximately T_4 spinal block.

the course of in vitro fertilization. Respiratory depression is uncommon with intrathecal lipophilic opioids. Unlike morphine, micturition is not inhibited beyond the spinal local anesthetic effect.

Physicochemical Properties

Injectate baricity

Three definitions are important to understanding baricity and local anesthetic injections.

Density: The density of a solution is the mass in grams of 1 mL of the solution at standard temperature.

Specific gravity: A ratio that compares the density of a solution to the density of water.

Baricity: A ratio comparing the specific gravity of one solution to that of another solution. If the second solution is water, then baricity will be the same as specific gravity.

Intrathecal injections are usually described as "hypobaric" (lower specific gravity than CSF), "isobaric" (equivalent specific gravity to CSF), and "hyperbaric" (higher specific gravity compared to CSF). The specific gravity of CSF ranges from 1.003 to 1.009.

By varying patient position and spinal injectate baricity in concert, the location and level of spinal anesthetic block can be controlled to a significant degree. In clinical practice, hyperbaric injections are most common. These solutions are made hyperbaric by adding dextrose to local anesthetic. The addition of dextrose to the solution increases the solution density, which increases the specific gravity to a level greater than the specific gravity of CSF. Because these solutions are more dense compared to CSF, they tend to "sink" to dependent areas of the intrathecal space (Box 10-10).

Isobaric local anesthetic injections are also gaining in popularity. The patient position does not influence block spread with isobaric injections. Thus, it is unnecessary to keep a patient in a certain position to allow the block to "set-up" in the supine position. Isobaric solutions tend to remain

more localized near the injection site. Clinically useful isobaric solutions include 0.5 or 0.75% bupivacaine, and 2% lidocaine. It should be noted that 0.5% bupivacaine and 2% lidocaine have specific gravities near the lower end of the range of normal CSF specific gravity. Thus, these solutions may act somewhat hypobaric in clinical use (i.e. the nondependent region attains a denser block). Also, warming solutions to 37° C lowers the density of the solution, and makes 0.5% bupivacaine and 2% lidocaine clinically hypobaric.

Because of their limited block spread, isobaric solutions are ideally suited for lower extremity and extraperitoneal

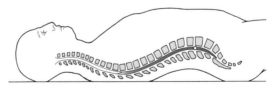

Figure 10-11 Curvature of the normal spine in the supine position. In supine patients, T_4 and S_5 are the most dependent regions of the neuraxis. Hyperbaric spinal anesthesia will typically yield a T_4 block if the patient is placed supine immediately after injection. (Redrawn from Barash PG, Cullen BF, Stoelting RK: *Clinical Anesthesia,* Fourth Edition, Lippincott, Williams & Wilkins, Philadelphia, 2001, Fig. 26-11.)

Box 10-11   Clinical Cases: Hypobaric Spinal Anesthesia

Repair of hip fracture. Patients with a fractured hip are often more comfortable with the fractured hip nondependent. Patients may be placed in a lateral decubitus position with the fractured hip nondependent. With a pencil-point needle, the aperture should be directed toward the nondependent side. Isobaric bupivacaine 0.25% (6 mg) + 20 µg fentanyl is used.

Hemorrhoidectomy. A patient is scheduled for hemorrhoidectomy in the jack-knife position (Fig. 10-9 on p. 122). The patient desires spinal anesthesia. The patient is positioned in the jack-knife position. A lumbar puncture is performed with the Whitacre needle aperture directed caudad. Hypobaric lidocaine 0.5% (40 mg) and fentanyl 20 µg are injected.

pelvic surgery. Intra-abdominal surgery is usually not performed with isobaric spinal anesthesia.

Hypobaric solutions are also occasionally clinically utilized. Bupivacaine 0.25–0.5%, and lidocaine 1–1.5% are hypobaric when warmed to body temperature. Hypobaric solutions will "float" to nondependent regions of the intrathecal space (Box 10-11).

Factors Affecting Block Spread

Many factors have been examined to help predict block height. Certain procedural variables will clearly have an impact on block spread: mass of drug, baricity of

Table 10-2   Factors Affecting Spinal Anesthetic Block Height

Major Factors	Minor Factors	Not Significant
Volume of the intrathecal space	Age	Gender
Patient position/ drug baricity	Height	Valsalva maneuver
Mass of drug	Temperature of drug	Barbotage (attempts to mix local anesthetic with CSF by repeated injection and withdrawal of CSF into a syringe attached to the spinal needle)
Direction of needle aperture	Rate of injection (with hypobaric drug)	Vasoconstrictor

drug, position of patient, and direction of needle aperture (with pencil point needles). Age has an impact on block height, with the elderly typically achieving 2–3 dermatome higher blocks compared to young adults. With hyperbaric spinal anesthesia, patient height is a minor variable, as spinal anatomy determines block spread.

Unfortunately, the factor that best predicts block height cannot be measured clinically. Variability in lumbosacral CSF volume explains the vast majority (80%) of differences in block height seen with spinal anesthesia. Height, gender, and age do not closely predict lumbosacral CSF volume. Patient weight correlates with spinal volume, but the correlation is not close enough to be clinically useful. Finally, block height has been shown to correlate directly with CSF density (Table 10-2).

COMPLICATIONS

Complications of spinal anesthesia include headache, neurologic symptoms, hypotension, respiratory depression, and cardiac arrest. Postdural puncture headache and neurologic injury are discussed in Chapters 12 and 14.

Hypotension is a common accompaniment to spinal anesthesia. Depending on the patient population and spinal anesthetic utilized, hypotension (>20% drop in systolic blood pressure) occurs during 20–70% of spinal anesthetics. Although fluid boluses prior to spinal anesthesia are commonly given to prevent hypotension, the effectiveness of this practice is low. Cardiac output is better maintained with pre-hydration, but blood pressure is minimally affected. Volume administration simultaneously with spinal anesthetic block development and vasoconstrictors are more effective compared to pre-hydration.

An effective approach to minimizing hypotension is to alter the drugs utilized in spinal anesthesia. Lipophilic opioids are often added to spinal local anesthetics, and allow dramatic (50–70%) reductions of local anesthetic dose. This, in turn, causes significant reductions in the rate and severity of hypotension, vasopressor use, and fluid requirements.

An analysis of the American Society of Anesthesiologists Closed Claims Database revealed 14 cases of unexpected cardiac arrest during spinal anesthesia. Two patterns were identified. The first pattern occurred in patients who were receiving sufficient intravenous sedation to produce a sleep-like state in which there was no spontaneous verbalization. In these cases, cardiac arrest was often heralded by cyanosis, pointing toward respiratory insufficiency as contributing to the arrests. The second pattern occurred in a group of patients who developed high spinal blockade and profound hypotension prior to cardiac arrest. The analysts of these adverse outcomes emphasize the importance of prompt augmentation of central venous filling by position changes (Trendelenberg) and prompt and aggressive use of alpha-agonists (epi-nephrine) to restore cardiac output.

Numerous factors can cause cardiac arrest, which is associated with spinal anesthesia to a significantly greater extent than epidural anesthesia or peripheral nerve block. Severe hypotension can cause cardiac arrhythmias, central nervous system (CNS) underperfusion, and apnea. All of these factors can cause cardiac arrest. There is also a surprising group of patients that appear to be at high risk for cardiac arrest. Younger, athletic patients with low resting heart rates seem to be predisposed to severe bradycardia and asystole with spinal anesthetic. Further risk factors that have been identified for this "athletic heart syndrome" include prolonged P-R interval, and spinal block height above T4. This latter factor probably indicates sympathetic blockade of T_2–T_4 (cardiac accelerator fibers), yielding unopposed vagal input to the heart.

Respiratory depression is unusual with spinal anesthesia, with reported rates of 0.2–1.0%. There are several causes of respiratory depression, with individual cases often having multiple contributing factors. Intrathecal opioids may cause respiratory depression, particularly with higher doses of intrathecal morphine. This respiratory depression peaks 8–10 hours after spinal morphine. Respiratory depression can also occur from high spinal anesthesia. Loss of consciousness and apnea are probably secondary to hypotension and inadequate CNS perfusion. Probably the most common cause of respiratory depression is over-sedation. Monitoring the patient with voice contact, pulse oximetry, and capnography should help prevent over-sedation.

CONCLUSION

Spinal anesthesia remains the most commonly performed regional anesthetic. With expertise in the procedural, pharmacologic, and physiologic aspects of spinal anesthesia, this block can be safely, reliably, and efficiently performed.

SUGGESTED READING

Adriani J: *Labat's Regional Anesthesia*, Third Edition, WB Saunders, Philadelphia, 1967.

Barash PG, Cullen BF, Stoelting RK: *Clinical Anesthesia*, Fourth Edition, Lippincott, Williams & Wilkins, Philadelphia, 2001.

Brown DL: *Atlas of Regional Anesthesia*, Second Edition, WB Saunders, Philadelphia, 1999.

Caplan RA, Ward RJ, Posner K, Cheney FW: Unexpected cardiac arrest during spinal anesthesia: a closed claims analysis of predisposing factors, *Anesthesiol* 87:1008–1009, 1988.

Cousins MJ, Bridenbaugh PO: *Neural Blockade*, Third Edition, Lippincott-Raven, Philadelphia, 1998.

Greene NM, Brull SJ: *Physiology of Spinal Anesthesia*, Fourth Edition, Williams and Wilkins, Baltimore, 1993.

Hahn MB, McQuillan PM, Sheplock GJ: *Regional Anesthesia*, Mosby, St. Louis, 1996.

Ostheimer GW: *Manual of Obstetric Anesthesia*, Second Edition, Churchill Livingstone, New York, 1992.

Stoelting RK, Miller RD: *Basics of Anesthesia*, Second Edition, Churchill Livingstone, New York, 1989.

CHAPTER 11

Sympathetic Blocks

JAMES P. RATHMELL

INTRODUCTION

The autonomic nervous system is divided into sympathetic and parasympathetic divisions that control many of the homeostatic functions within the body. The two systems are largely opposite in their functions; balance between activity in the two divisions maintains the normal function of many organs. For instance, sympathetic innervation to the bowel reduces gastrointestinal motility while parasympathetic innervation increases peristalsis. The parasympathetic nerves arise from the brainstem and the sacral portion of the spinal cord and are termed the craniosacral division of the autonomic nervous system. The sympathetic nerves arise from the thoracic and lumbar portion of the spinal cord and are termed the thoracolumbar division of the autonomic nervous system.

To the regional anesthesiologist and pain specialist, the sympathetic nervous system is important as it not only supplies efferent impulses responsible for vascular tone, but because the sympathetic chain carries afferent nociceptive impulses toward the spinal cord. A number of acute, post-traumatic, and chronic neuropathic pain conditions are maintained through nociceptive impulses that travel through the sympathetic nervous system and these conditions often improve with sympathetic blockade.

ANATOMY AND PHYSIOLOGY OF THE SYMPATHETIC NERVOUS SYSTEM

The preganglionic sympathetic neurons have their cell bodies located in the intermediolateral column of the thoracic and lumbar spinal cord (Fig. 11-1 on p. 129). The sympathetic nerves leave the spinal cord with the ventral nerve roots to join the spinal nerve roots as they exit the bony vertebral canal. The axons branch from the spinal nerve to travel via the white communicating rami where they reach the paravertebral sympathetic ganglia to synapse on the postganglionic neuronal cells. Some postganglionic sympathetic fibers then travel back toward the spinal nerve roots via the gray communicating rami. These postganglionic sympathetic fibers rejoin the spinal nerves and travel to their peripheral sites of termination along with the sensory nerves. Other postganglionic sympathetic fibers travel directly from the paravertebral ganglia to their effector organs. The anatomy of the sympathetic chain is shown in Fig. 11-2 on p. 129.

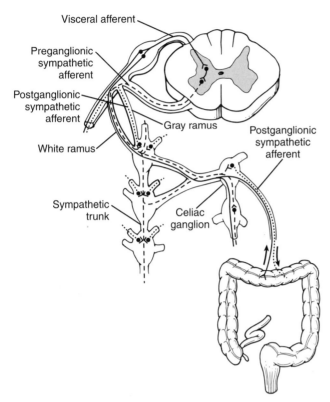

Figure 11-1 **Location and course of the sympathetic nerves and visceral afferent fibers.** (Redrawn from Brown DL: *Regional Anesthesia and Analgesia*, WB Saunders, Philadelphia, 1996, p. 358.)

The predominant functions of the sympathetic nervous system are detailed in (Box 11-1). Pain arising from the viscera and sympathetically maintained pain that arises after injury in the periphery can be effectively relieved in many instances by using local anesthetic or neurolytic blockade of the sympathetic nervous system at one of three main levels: the cervicothoracic ganglia (including the stellate ganglion); the celiac plexus; or the lumbar ganglia (Fig. 11-3 on p. 130). Pain that is relieved by sympathetic blockade is termed "sympathetically maintained pain" (see further explanation in Box 11-2). Sympathetically maintained pain is a subset of the larger category of neuropathic pain, or abnormal pain that occurs following injury to the nervous system. Neuropathic pain, including the subset of sympathetically maintained pain, carries a common set of clinical symptoms that distinguish it from the well-localized pain that typically follows tissue injury (see Clinical Caveat box).

STELLATE GANGLION BLOCK

Anatomy

The stellate ganglion is named for its fusiform appearance. The ganglion is comprised of the fused superior thoracic sympathetic ganglion and the inferior cervical

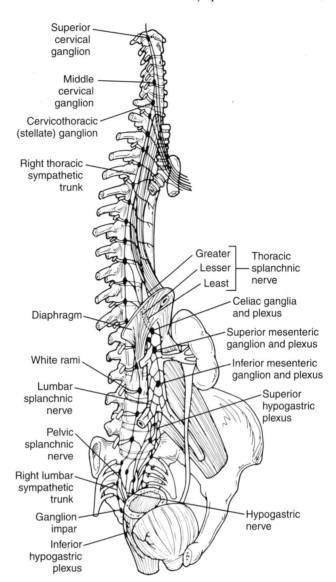

Figure 11-2 **Anatomy of the sympathetic chain.** (Redrawn from Brown DL: *Regional Anesthesia and Analgesia*, WB Saunders, Philadelphia, 1996, p. 359.)

ganglion and typically lies over the anterior surface of the first thoracic vertebral body adjacent to the articulation with the first rib. Cell bodies for the sympathetic nerves that supply the head and neck arise from the first and second thoracic segments while those supplying the upper extremities arise from T2–T8 and occasionally T9. Preganglionic fibers travel via the white communicating rami to the sympathetic chain where they travel cephalad to synapse in the inferior (stellate), middle, or superior cervical ganglia. Postganglionic fibers either follow in close apposition to the internal and external carotid arteries or travel along the gray communicating rami to join the cervical plexus or upper cervical nerve roots to supply the head, neck, and upper extremities. For successful sympathetic block of the head and neck, the stellate ganglion

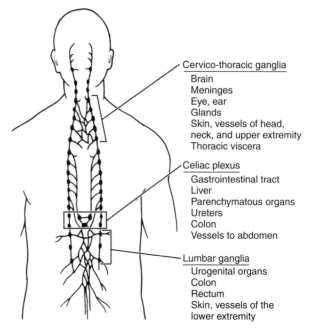

Figure 11-3   The three main levels of sympathetic blockade and the painful regions that may be effectively blocked. (Redrawn from Cousins MJ, Bridenbaugh PO (eds): *Neural Blockade in Clinical Anesthesia and Management of Pain,* Third Edition, Lippincott-Raven, Philadelphia, 1998, p. 413.)

should be blocked because all sympathetic fibers either synapse in this ganglion or their preganglionic fibers pass through this ganglion en route to the middle and upper cervical ganglia. Preganglionic fibers to the upper extremities arise within the second through ninth thoracic segments and travel via white communicating rami to the sympathetic chain where they ascend to synapse within the second and first thoracic ganglion and the inferior cervical ganglion (stellate). Postganglionic fibers enter the gray communicating rami to join the ventral spinal nerve roots that form the brachial plexus (C5–T1). Some postganglionic fibers join the subclavian artery to form the perivascular plexus within the upper extremity.

The stellate ganglion lies over the anterolateral surface of T1 just posterior to the subclavian artery where the vertebral artery arises. The cupola of the lung lies directly

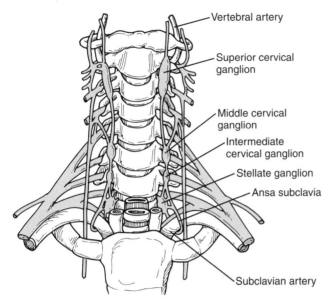

Figure 11-4   Detailed anatomy of the cervical sympathetic ganglia and stellate ganglia. Note the close apposition of the subclavian artery and the stellate ganglia at the level of T1. (Redrawn from Raj PP: *Practical Management of Pain*, Third Edition, Mosby, St. Louis, 2000, p. 656.)

lateral and just slightly superior to the ganglion in this location (Fig. 11-4). To reduce the incidence of pneumothorax and to avoid intravascular injection, the classic approach to blocking the stellate ganglion is carried out somewhat cephalad at the level of the anterior tubercle of the transverse process of C6 (Chassaignac's tubercle). A volume of local anesthetic is injected that ensures spread along the prevertebral fascia to bathe the ganglion at T1. The vertebral artery arises at the level of T1 and traverses posteriorly to enter the transverse vertebral foramen at the level of C6. This foramen is posterior to Chassaignac's tubercle and affords the artery some protection from direct penetration during stellate ganglion block at this level.

Clinical Uses

Stellate ganglion block has long been the standard approach to diagnosis and treatment of sympathetically maintained pain syndromes involving the upper extremity, such as complex regional pain syndrome. Other neuropathic pain syndromes, including ischemic neuropathies, herpes zoster (shingles), early postherpetic neuralgia, and postradiation neuritis, may also respond to stellate ganglion block. Blockade of the stellate ganglion has also proven successful in reducing pain and improving blood flow in vascular insufficiency conditions such as intractable angina pectoris, Raynaud's disease, frostbite, vasospasm, and occlusive and embolic vascular disease. Finally, the sympathetic fibers control sweating, and thus stellate ganglion block can be quite effective in controlling hyperhidrosis (recurrent and uncontrollable sweating of the hands).

Clinical Caveat: The Abnormal Sensations of Neuropathic Pain

Pain is a normal physiologic process and serves as a signal that tissue injury has occurred and that the injured region should be protected while healing ensues. As the tissue heals, the pain diminishes and usually resolves completely. Pain associated with tissue injury is usually well localized and associated with sensitivity in the region. Pain signals are carried toward the central nervous system via the peripheral sensory nerves. This type of pain is termed nociceptive pain.

In contrast, pain associated with many nerve injuries, termed neuropathic pain, including chronic pain states in which pain signals are carried through the sympathetic nervous system share a number of characteristics. The diagnosis of neuropathic pain is made largely on the basis of the patient's description of one or more of the following characteristics:

Spontaneous pain – pain that occurs without a specific sensory stimulus (e.g. the sudden lancinating pain described by those with postherpetic neuralgia)

Paresthesias/dysesthesias – abnormal pain distant from the site of actual tissue injury that may be spontaneous or evoked (e.g. the radiating pain associated with lumbar nerve root compression)

Hyperalgesia – an exaggerated painful response to a normally noxious stimulus (e.g. light pinprick leads to extreme and prolonged pain)

Allodynia – a painful response to a normally nonnoxious stimulus (e.g. light touch causes pain)

Block Technique

Stellate ganglion block can be a frightening experience for many patients, and it is essential that the procedure is carefully described well in advance. Mild sedation with an oral or intravenous anxiolytic can be used to facilitate patient comfort. However, the block is brief and relatively superficial, and many patients do well without sedation. Placing an intravenous line prior to stellate ganglion block is not considered mandatory in all pain clinics. When placed, the IV can be used for administration of sedative agents and resuscitative drugs in the rare event they are needed. In skilled hands, stellate ganglion block can be performed quickly and with relatively little discomfort. Whether or not an IV is placed prior to the block, it is imperative that IV supplies as well as full monitoring and resuscitative equipment are immediately available whenever this block is performed.

The most common technique for stellate ganglion block is the anterior approach at C6. The patient is asked to lie supine and a thin pillow is placed under the upper back to facilitate extension of the neck (Fig. 11-5 on p. 132). The

Patient position

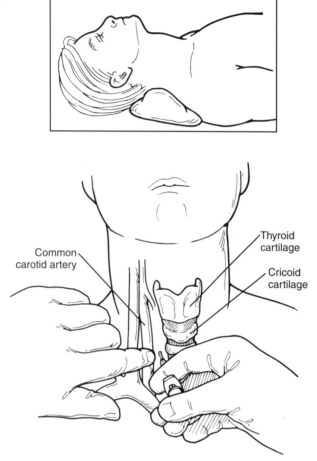

Figure 11-5   Stellate ganglion block. (Redrawn from Raj PP: *Practical Management of Pain*, Third Edition, Mosby, St. Louis, 2000, p. 656.)

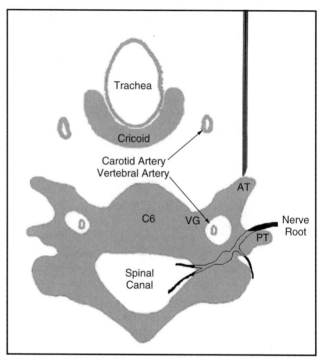

Figure 11-6   Chassaignac's tubercle and adjacent structures. Axial view of Chassaignac's tubercle (anterior tubercle, AT) and adjacent structures with needle shown in proper position. Note that angulation of the needle slightly medially will result in needle seating on the vertebral gutter (VG), an acceptable position that will lead to successful stellate ganglion block. However, more lateral angulation will result in needle placement on the posterior tubercle (PT) and will lead to somatic block of the exiting nerve root and adjacent brachial plexus. Note the close proximity of the carotid artery (shown in its usual anatomic location – the carotid artery is typically retracted laterally during stellate ganglion block). The vertebral artery lies within the transverse foramen in close proximity to the needle's final position.

operator stands to the side of the patient and locates the cricoid cartilage in the midline (which lies at approximately C6) using their nondominant hand. The syringe is held in the dominant hand. After placing one or two fingers on the cricoid cartilage, the fingers are gently pulled to the lateral margin of the trachea and into the paratracheal groove. The carotid artery will be palpable just beneath the fingertips. Firm pressure is applied with the fingertips to retract the carotid artery laterally and palpate the anterior tubercle of C6 (Chassaignac's tubercle). Once the tubercle is located, the skin is prepared with antiseptic solution and a 10 mL syringe containing local anesthetic (typically 0.25% bupivacaine) attached to a 21 or 23 gauge, $1\frac{1}{2}$ inch needle is assembled. The tubercle is again located with the nondominant hand, a small skin wheal of local anesthetic is placed directly over the tubercle, and the needle is advanced to contact the tubercle. The needle should be advanced perpendicular to all planes in a direct anterior to posterior direction (Fig. 11-6). If the needle is advanced more than several centimeters, it is likely that the tubercle

has been missed. The needle should be withdrawn, the tubercle again identified, and the needle advanced in a slightly more medial direction. Once seated on the tubercle, the nondominant hand releases pressure from the skin and steadies the base of the syringe while the injection is carried out with the dominant hand. Local anesthetic should be given only after meticulous aspiration to avoid intravascular injection. If the needle moves at all during injection, aspiration must be repeated.

Evidence of successful block often is apparent within minutes of the block, but may take as much as 20 minutes using longer-acting local anesthetics such as bupivacaine. Sympathetic block to the head can be documented by observing the presence of Horner's syndrome: miosis (pupillary constriction), ptosis (drooping of the eyelid), and enophthalmos (sinking of the eyeball). Associated findings include conjuctival injection, nasal congestion, and anhidrosis (reduced sweating on the side of blockade). Evidence of sympathetic block to the upper extremity includes venodilation and temperature rise within the hand (Box 11-3).

Horner's syndrome
    Miosis (pupillary constriction)
    Ptosis (drooping of the upper eyelid)
    Enophthalmos (recession of the globe within the orbit)
Anhidrosis (lack of sweating)
Nasal congestion
Venodilation in the hand and forearm
Increase in temperature of the blocked limb by at
    least 1° C

Box 11-4   Complications of Stellate Ganglion Block

Seizure (direct intravascular injection into the carotid or
    vertebral artery will result in onset of seizure within
    seconds and may occur after the injection of a very
    small volume of local anesthetic (e.g. <0.5 mL))
Hoarseness (block of the adjacent recurrent laryngeal
    nerve)
Cervical nerve root block
Brachial plexus block
Phrenic nerve block
High epidural or spinal block
Pneumothorax (unlikely when the block is carried out
    at the level of C6)

Complications

There are many structures within the immediate vicinity of the needle's tip once it is properly positioned over Chassaignac's tubercle for stellate ganglion block (Fig. 11-6 on p. 132). Commonly, diffusion of local anesthetic blocks the adjacent recurrent laryngeal nerve. This often leads to hoarseness, a feeling of having a lump in the throat, and a subjective feeling of shortness of breath and difficulty swallowing. Bilateral stellate ganglion block should not be performed as bilateral recurrent laryngeal nerve blocks may well lead to loss of laryngeal reflexes and respiratory compromise. The phrenic nerve is also commonly blocked by direct spread of local anesthetic and will lead to unilateral diaphragmatic paresis. Diffusion of local anesthetic as well as direct placement of local anesthetic adjacent to the posterior tubercle will result in somatic block of the upper extremity. This may take the form of a small area of sensory loss due to diffusion of local anesthetic or a complete brachial plexus block when the local anesthetic is placed within the nerve sheath. Patients with significant somatic block to the upper extremity should be sent home with a sling in place and counseled to guard their limb, just as one would instruct a patient who had received a brachial plexus block.

Major complications associated with stellate ganglion block include neuraxial block (spinal or epidural) and seizures. Extreme medial angulation of the needle from a relatively lateral skin entry point may lead to needle placement into the spinal canal through the anterolaterally oriented intervertebral foramen. In this manner, local anesthetic can be deposited in the epidural space or, if the needle is advanced far enough, it may penetrate the dural cuff surrounding the exiting nerve root and lie within the intrathecal space. More likely is placement of the needle tip on the posterior tubercle and spread of local anesthetic proximally along the nerve root to enter the epidural space. In this case, partial or profound neuraxial block, including high spinal or epidural block with loss of consciousness and apnea may ensue. Airway protection,

ventilation, and intravenous sedation should be promptly administered and continued until the patient regains airway reflexes and consciousness. Because the maximal effects of epidural local anesthetic may require 15-20 minutes to develop when using longer-acting local anesthetics, it is imperative that patients are monitored for at least 30 minutes after stellate ganglion block.

Intravascular injection during stellate ganglion block will likely result in immediate onset of generalized seizures. The carotid artery lies just anteromedial to Chassaignac's tubercle while the vertebral artery lies within the bony transverse foramen just posteromedial to the tubercle. If the carotid artery is not sufficiently retracted laterally, the needle's path may well pass directly through the carotid artery. Likewise, if the needle is directed medially and passes either superior or inferior to the transverse process, the vertebral artery can easily be penetrated. Because the local anesthetic injected enters the arterial supply traveling directly to the brain, generalized seizures typically begin rapidly and after only small amounts of local anesthetic (as little as 0.2 mL of 0.25% bupivacaine have led to seizure). However, because the local anesthetic rapidly redistributes, the seizures are typically brief and do not require treatment. In the event of a seizure, halt the injection, remove the needle, and begin supportive care (Box 11-4; see Chapter 2 for more detail).

CELIAC PLEXUS AND SPLANCHNIC NERVE BLOCK

Anatomy

The celiac plexus is comprised of a diffuse network of nerve fibers and individual ganglia that lie over the anterolateral surface of the aorta at the T12/L1 vertebral level. Sympathetic innervation to the abdominal viscera arises from the anterolateral horn of the spinal cord between the T5 and T12 levels. Nociceptive information from the abdominal viscera is carried by afferents that accompany the sympathetic nerves. Presynaptic sympathetic fibers travel from the thoracic sympathetic chain toward the ganglion, traversing over the anterolateral aspect of the inferior thoracic vertebrae as the greater (T5–T9), lesser (T10–T11), and least (T12) splanchnic nerves. Presynaptic fibers traveling via the splanchnic nerves synapse within the celiac ganglia, over the anterolateral surface of the aorta surrounding the origin of the celiac and superior mesenteric arteries at approximately the L1 vertebral level. Postsynaptic fibers from the celiac ganglia innervate all of the abdominal viscera with the exception of the descending colon, sigmoid colon, rectum, and pelvic viscera.

Celiac plexus block using a transcrural approach places the local anesthetic or neurolytic solution directly on the celiac ganglion anterolateral to the aorta (Fig. 11-7). Spread of the solution toward the posterior surface of the aorta may thus be limited, perhaps reducing the chances of nerve root or penetrating artery involvement. In contrast, splanchnic nerve block avoids the risk of penetrating the aorta, uses smaller volumes of solution, and the success is unlikely to be affected by anatomic distortion caused by extensive tumor or adenopathy within the pancreas. In most cases, the blocks can be used interchangeably to effect the same results. While there are those who strongly advocate one approach or the other, there is no evidence that either results in superior clinical outcomes.

Clinical Uses

Celiac plexus and splanchnic nerve block are used to control pain arising from intra-abdominal structures. These structures include the pancreas, liver, gall bladder, omentum, mesentery, and alimentary tract from the stomach to the transverse colon. The most common application is neurolytic celiac plexus block used to treat pain associated with intra-abdominal malignancy, particularly pain associated with pancreatic cancer. Neurolysis of the splanchnic nerves or celiac ganglion can produce dramatic pain relief, reduce or eliminate the need for supplemental analgesics, and improve quality of life in patients with pancreatic cancer and other intra-abdominal malignancies. The long-term benefit of neurolytic celiac plexus block in those with chronic nonmalignant pain, particularly those with chronic pancreatitis, is debatable.

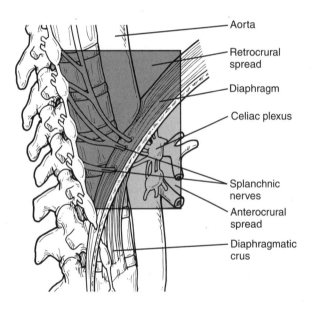

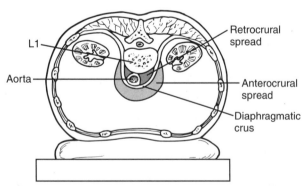

Figure 11-7   Celiac plexus block – retrocrural and anterocrural relationships. (Redrawn from Brown DL: *Atlas of Regional Anesthesia*, Second Edition, WB Saunders, Philadelphia, 1999, p. 288.) (See colour inserts, Plate 5.)

Case Study: Neurolytic Celiac Plexus Block

A 64-year-old man is hospitalized with jaundice and intractable abdominal pain. Evaluation reveals a mass in the head of the pancreas which proves to be adenocarcinoma. He describes his pain as a constant and severe boring pain just below the xiphoid process that worsens whenever he eats. Despite large doses of intravenous morphine, he continues to have pain and severe nausea. A diagnostic celiac plexus block is performed. During placement of a left-sided needle, blood can be freely aspirated as the needle is advanced anterior to the L1 vertebral body. The needle is advanced until blood can no longer be aspirated and injection of 2 mL of radiographic contrast confirms the needle is in position over the anterior surface of the aorta. Local anesthetic is given incrementally (30 mL of 25% bupivacaine). Over the next 20 minutes he develops abdominal cramping and sudden diarrhea and a decline in his blood pressure from 130/70 to 100/60. One hour later he reports complete resolution of his abdominal pain that lasts for nearly 4 hours after the block. The following day, neurolytic celiac plexus block is carried out using 30 mL of 12% phenol using the same block technique. Within 2 hours of the neurolytic block, he reports near complete resolution of his abdominal pain, but again has diarrhea and mild hypotension. The diarrhea and hypotension resolve over the following days and he is discharged from the hospital with only mild and intermittent abdominal pain and no further problems with nausea.

Block Technique

Several means of blocking the celiac ganglion and splanchnic nerves have been described. There is general agreement that radiographic guidance is useful to assure proper needle placement during celiac plexus block, and both plain x-ray (fluoroscopy) and computed tomography (CT) have been advocated. Blockade of the splanchnic nerves can be carried out by placing needles over the anterolateral surface of the L1 vertebral bodies. In this location, the needle tips lie posterior to the diaphragmatic crura and spread of solution will be retrocrural (Fig. 11-7 on p. 134). To ablate directly the celiac ganglion itself, the needles must be advanced through the diaphragm until they lie adjacent to the anterolateral surface of the aorta. This can be accomplished by advancing two separate needles adjacent to the anterolateral surface of the aorta (Fig. 11-8 (left panel)) or using a single needle advanced through the aorta (Fig. 11-8 (right panel)). Using transcrural needle placement in a transaortic or para-aortic location, the spread of solution will remain below the diaphragm in a plane anterior to the aorta (Fig. 11-7 on p. 134).

For either technique, the patient is placed prone in the CT scanner or fluoroscopy suite. Surface landmarks are identified, including the midline (spinous processes) and the inferior margin of the 12th rib. An entry mark is made 7–8 cm from midline at a point 1 cm below the inferior margin of the 12th rib. Radiographic guidance (using either CT or fluoroscopy) is then used to guide a 22 gauge 5 inch (thin to average build) to 8 inch (obese) needle toward the anterolateral margin of the T12-L1 interspace for splanchnic nerve block and to the anterolateral margin of L1 for celiac plexus block (Fig. 11-9 on p. 136). For splanchnic nerve block, the needle must be kept in close apposition to the lateral margin of the vertebral body, and on lateral radiography, the needle tip should lie over the anterior one-third of the vertebral body without extending beyond the anterior margin of the vertebral column. The same procedure is then repeated on the opposite side. For celiac plexus block, the left-sided needle is typically inserted first. This is the side of the aorta, and if radiographic contrast injected through the first needle spreads anterior to the aorta and across midline, the placement of a second needle is unnecessary. The first needle is passed slightly (about 0.5 cm) lateral to the anterolateral margin of L1. As the needle is advanced beyond the vertebral body, the position should be followed using lateral radiography and using continuous aspiration. The needle is advanced 2 to

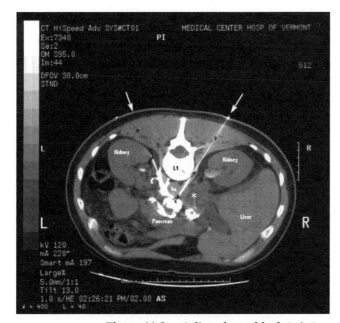 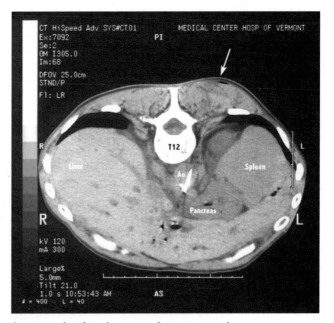

Figure 11-8   Celiac plexus block. Left: Computed tomography after placement of two transcrural needles for neurolytic celiac plexus block. The arrows indicate the approximate needle trajectory on each side. Radiocontrast extends over the left anterolateral surface of the aorta and anteriorly along the posterior surface of the pancreas. There is a large soft tissue mass adjacent to the right-sided needle (asterisk) consistent with either metastatic tumor or adenopathy. Neurolytic solution has not yet been placed through the right-sided needle. Right: Computed tomography after placement of a single transaortic needle. The arrow indicates the approximate trajectory of the needle. The medial pleural reflection can be seen passing in close proximity to the needle path. (From Rathmell JP, Gallant JM, Brown DL: Computed tomography and the anatomy of celiac plexus block, *Reg Anesth Pain Med* 25:411–416, 2000.)

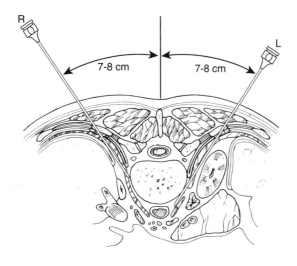

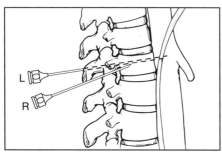

Figure 11-9   Retrocrural and transcrural needle placement for celiac plexus block. Inset: The left needle (R) is retrocrural and results in spread of solution to block the splanchnic nerves; the right needle (L) is transcrural and blocks the celiac plexus directly. (Redrawn from Raj PP: *Practical Management of Pain*, Third Edition, Mosby, St. Louis, 2000, p. 669.)

3 cm beyond the anterior margin of the vertebral column while continuously aspirating. If blood is encountered, the needle has likely entered the aorta, and aspiration and needle advancement should be continued just until blood can no longer be withdrawn, indicating needle passage through the anterior wall of the aorta.

Once the needles are in position using any of the techniques described, a small volume (2–3 mL) of radiocontrast (iohexol 180 mg/mL or the equivalent) is injected to confirm proper needle placement and assure that the needle tip does not lie within a blood vessel. In the case of splanchnic block, the contrast should spread tightly against the anterolateral margin of T12 on each side. During celiac block, the contrast should outline the anterior margin of the aorta, and the contrast typically appears pulsatile on fluoroscopy.

For splanchnic block, only 5–8 mL of local anesthetic or neurolytic solution are required on each side. For celiac block, 20 to 30 mL of solution may be required to achieve effective spread. For diagnostic or temporary

block, 0.25% bupivacaine is the typical anesthetic used. For neurolysis, either 50–100% ethanol or 10–12% phenol can be used. Phenol can be dissolved directly in radiographic contrast so that the spread of injectate can be monitored throughout the course of the injection.

Alcohol typically causes marked abdominal pain on injection while phenol has an immediate local anesthetic effect. Both neurolytic solutions appear to be effective, but there have been no studies comparing the two.

Complications

There are several physiologic side effects that are expected following celiac plexus block. These include diarrhea and orthostatic hypotension. Blockade of the sympathetic innervation to the abdominal viscera results in unopposed parasympathetic innervation of the alimentary tract, and may produce abdominal cramping and sudden diarrhea. Likewise, the vasodilation that ensues often results in orthostatic hypotension. These effects are invariably transient, but may persist for several days after neurolytic block. The hypotension seldom requires treatment other than intravenous hydration.

Complications of celiac plexus and splanchnic nerve block include hematuria, intravascular injection, and pneumothorax. Computed tomography allows visualization of the structures that lie adjacent to the celiac ganglion as the block is being performed (Fig. 11-8 on p. 135). The kidneys extend from between T12 and L3 with the left kidney slightly more cephalad than the right. The aorta lies over the left anterolateral border of the vertebral column. The celiac arterial trunk arises from the anterior surface of the aorta at the T12 level and divides into the hepatic, left gastric, and splenic arteries. Using the transaortic technique, caution must be used to avoid needle placement directly through the axis of the celiac trunk as it exits anteriorly. The inferior vena cava lies just to the right of the aorta over the anterolateral surface of the vertebral column. The medial pleural reflection extends inferomedially as low as the T12–L1 level.

Neurolytic celiac plexus block carries small, but significant additional risk. Intravascular injection of 30 mL of 100% ethanol will result in a blood ethanol level well above the legal limit for intoxication, but below danger of severe alcohol toxicity. Intravascular injection of phenol is associated with clinical manifestations similar to that of local anesthetic toxicity: CNS excitation, followed by seizures, and in extreme toxicity, cardiovascular collapse. The most devastating complication associated with neurolytic celiac plexus block using either alcohol or phenol is paraplegia. The theoretical mechanism is spread of the neurolytic solution toward the posterior surface of the aorta to surround the spinal penetrating arteries. At the level of T12 or L1, it is common to have a single, dominant penetrating artery, the

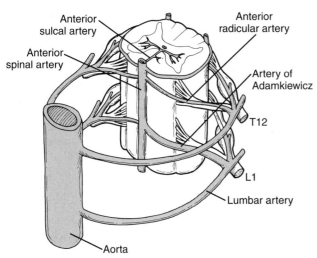

Figure 11-10   Anatomy of the arterial supply to the spinal cord adjacent to the celiac plexus. Spread of neurolytic solution posteriorly leading to spasm or necrosis of the artery of Adamkiewicz has been proposed as the mechanism for paraplegia that occurs rarely after neurolytic celiac plexus block. (From *Reg Anesth* 20:352–355, 1995.)

artery of Adamkiewicz. In some individuals, this artery is the dominant arterial supply to the anterior two thirds of the spinal cord in the low thoracic region (Fig. 11-10). Neurolytic solution may cause spasm or even necrosis and occlusion of the artery of Adamkiewicz leading to paralysis. The actual incidence of this complication is unknown, but appears to be less than 1:1,000 (Box 11-5).

Box 11-5   Complications of Celiac Plexus Block

Block with local anesthetic solution:
    Intravascular injection – direct needle placement into a blood vessel, including the aorta, inferior vena cava, or lesser vessels (the volume of local anesthetic used for celiac plexus block is enough to result in significant systemic toxicity)
    Hematuria – direct needle placement through the kidney, usually self-limited
    Pneumothorax – direct needle placement through the lung or pleural reflections
Additional complications unique to neurolytic celiac plexus block:
    Alcohol intoxication – intravascular injection of ethanol
    Phenol toxicity – intravascular injection of phenol (manifestations similar to local anesthetic toxicity with seizures and cardiovascular collapse)
    Paraplegia – posterior spread of neurolytic solution causing spasm or necrosis of the artery of Adamkiewicz

---

LUMBAR SYMPATHETIC BLOCK

Anatomy

The lumbar sympathetic chain consists of four to five paired ganglia that lie over the anterolateral surface of the second through fourth lumbar vertebrae. The cell bodies that supply the lumbar sympathetic ganglia lie in the anterolateral region of the spinal cord from T11 to L2, with variable contributions from T10 and L3. The preganglionic fibers leave the spinal canal with the corresponding spinal nerve root, join the sympathetic chain as white communicating rami, and then synapse within the appropriate ganglion. Postganglionic fibers exit the chain to join either the diffuse perivascular plexus around the iliac and femoral arteries or via the gray communicating rami to join the nerve roots that form the lumbar and lumbosacral plexi. Sympathetic fibers accompany all of the major nerves to the lower extremities. The majority of the sympathetic innervation to the lower extremities passes through the second and third lumbar sympathetic ganglia and blockade of these gangli results in near complete sympathetic denervation of the lower extremities.

Clinical Uses

Lumbar sympathetic blockade has been used extensively in the treatment of sympathetically maintained pain syndromes involving the lower extremities. The most common of these are the complex regional pain syndromes, type 1 (reflex sympathetic dystrophy) and type 2 (causalgia). The local anesthetic block can produce marked pain relief of long duration, and this block is used as part of a comprehensive treatment plan to provide analgesia and facilitate functional restoration.

Patients with peripheral vascular insufficiency due to small vessel occlusion may also be treated effectively with lumbar sympathetic blockade. Proximal fixed lesions are best treated with surgical intervention using bypass grafting or intra-arterial stent placement to restore blood flow. In those patients with diffuse, small vessel occlusion, lumbar sympathetic block can improve microvascular circulation and reduce ischemic pain. If local anesthetic block improves blood flow and reduces pain, these patients will often benefit from surgical or chemical sympathectomy.

Other patients with neuropathic pain involving the lower extremities have shown variable response to lumbar sympathetic block. In those with acute herpes zoster and early postherpetic neuralgia, sympathetic block may reduce pain. However, once postherpetic neuralgia is well established (beyond 3 to 6 months from onset), sympathetic blockade is rarely helpful. Likewise, deafferentation syndromes such as phantom limb pain and neuropathic lower extremity pain following spinal cord injury have shown variable and largely disappointing responses to sympathetic blockade.

Block Technique

Lumbar sympathetic blockade is typically carried out using a single-needle technique and using a large volume of local anesthetic to produce cephalad and caudad spread to adjacent ganglia. The ganglia of the lumbar sympathetic chain lie between L2 and L4 with the majority of ganglia over the inferior portion of L2 and the superior portion of L3. Thus a single needle placed over the anterolateral margin of the inferior portion of L2, the L2/3 interspace, or the superior margin of L3 is employed.

The patient is placed in the prone position with a pillow under the lower abdomen and iliac crest to reduce the lumbar lordosis (Fig. 11-11). A mark is made 10 cm from midline midway between the inferior margin of the 12th rib and the iliac crest. With the increasing availability of fluoroscopy in most pain clinics, lumbar sympathetic block is commonly carried out with radiographic guidance. For placement without radiographic guidance, a 22 gauge, 5 inch (7-8 inch for obese patients) needle is advanced toward the anterolateral surface of the vertebral body at an angle of 35-45° from the plane of the back. Once the vertebral body is contacted, the needle is withdrawn and the angle is increased slightly and the needle reinserted. During each needle pass, the depth at which the vertebral body is contacted is noted by placing a depth marker on the needle. This process is continued until the needle is walked off of the vertebral body. The needle is then advanced an additional 2 to 3 cm to lie over the anterolateral surface of the vertebral body.

Using fluoroscopy, a single needle entry and direct passage of the needle to the anterolateral surface of the vertebral body is possible, thus eliminating the discomfort of multiple needle passes and reducing the possibility of incorrect needle placement. Proper needle position is verified using anteroposterior (AP) and lateral radiographs. When the needle's tip is located in close apposition to the vertebral body, it will appear medial to the lateral vertebral margin in the AP view and just posterior to the anterior vertebral margin in the lateral view (Fig. 11-12 on p. 139).

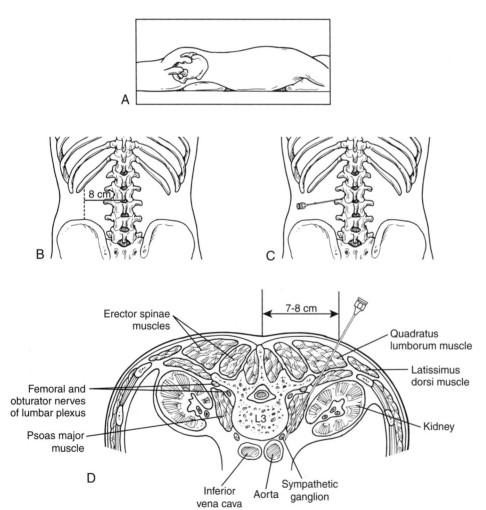

Figure 11-11 Lumbar sympathetic block. A, The patient is placed prone with a pillow under the lower abdomen and iliac crests to reduce the lumbar lordosis. **B, C,** The skin entry is made half way between the 12th rib margin and the iliac crest at a point 7 to 8 cm from the midline. **D,** Axial view of the lumbar sympathetic ganglion and adjacent structures with the needle in final position for lumbar sympathetic block. (Redrawn from Raj PP: *Practical Management of Pain,* Third Edition, Mosby, St. Louis, 2000, p. 674.)

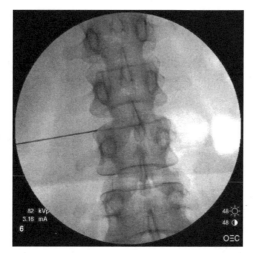 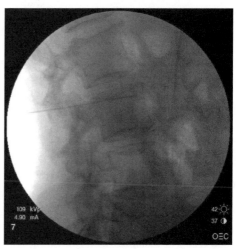

Figure 11-12   Lumber sympathetic block. Radiographs (left, anteroposterior view; right, lateral view) of needle tip in position over the anterolateral surface of the superior margin of L3 for left lumbar sympathetic block.

Clinical Caveat: Advantages of Radiographic Guidance for Lumbar Sympathetic Blockade

Patient comfort - using radiographic guidance, the needle can be passed through a single skin entry point to the anterolateral surface of the vertebral body without multiple redirections of the needle

Safety - final needle position can be confirmed and the small risk of advancing the needle into the spinal canal through the intervertebral foramen can be avoided

Box 11-6   Complications of Lumbar Sympathetic Block

Intravascular injection - direct needle placement into a blood vessel (the volume of local anesthetic used for lumbar sympathetic block is enough to result in significant systemic toxicity)

Hematuria - direct needle placement through the kidney, usually self-limited

Nerve root, epidural, or intrathecal injection - these complications arise when the needle is advanced through the intervertebral foramen and is avoided entirely through use of radiographic guidance

Once the needle is in position, aspiration to detect intravascular needle placement is carried out, followed by the incremental injection of local anesthetic (20 to 30 mL of 0.25% bupivacaine). The addition of epinephrine (1:200,000) will facilitate identifying intravascular injection and prolong the duration of the block. Signs of successful sympathetic blockade in the lower extremities include venodilation and temperature rise. The skin temperature should be monitored in both feet to assess for changes unrelated to the block. A rise in temperature of at least 1° C without a rise in the contralateral limb should occur with successful sympathetic block.

Complications

Complications of lumbar sympathetic block include intravascular injection and hematuria from needle passage through the kidney. When the technique is carried out without radiographic guidance, the needle can be advanced directly through an intervertebral foramen and produce nerve root, epidural, or spinal block (Box 11-6).

SUPERIOR HYPOGASTRIC PLEXUS BLOCK

Anatomy

The superior hypogastric plexus is composed of a flattened band of intercommunicating nerve fibers that descend over the aortic bifurcation. The plexus carries sympathetic afferents and postganglionic efferent fibers from the lumbar sympathetic chain as well as parasympathetic fibers that arise from S2-S4. The plexus is retroperitoneal in location and lies over the anterior surface of the fourth and fifth lumbar and the first sacral vertebrae. Sympathetic nerves passing through the plexus innervate the pelvic viscerae, including the bladder, uterus, rectum, vagina, and prostate.

Clinical Uses

Superior hypogastric plexus block is used in the treatment of pain arising from the pelvic viscerae. In patients with pain of nonmalignant origin, temporary block may be useful in better defining the source of the pain. More often, superior hypogastric neurolysis is used to treat intractable pelvic visceral pain associated with malignancy. Patients with locally invasive cancers involving the proximal vagina, uterus, ovaries, prostate, and rectum that are associated with pelvic pain often gain significant pain relief from this approach.

Block Technique

The use of fluoroscopic guidance is essential for performing superior hypogastric plexus block. The patient is placed prone with a pillow under the lower abdomen and iliac crests to facilitate posterior tilting of the pelvis which will improve access to the lumbosacral junction. The axis of the x-ray beam is directed 30–45° caudad and 25–35° oblique to midline into the pelvis to identify the L5–S1 intervertebral disc space. There is a small triangular window through which the needle must pass to reach the anterolateral margin of the lumbosacral junction. The triangle is bounded superiorly by the transverse process of L5, laterally by the iliac crest, and medially by the L5/S1 facet joint, structures that are readily identified using fluoroscopy

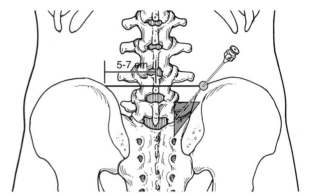

Figure 11-13   Superior   hypogastric   plexus   block. Posterior–anterior view showing the anatomic triangle through which the needle must pass for superior hypogastric plexus block. The triangle is bordered superiorly by the transverse process of L5, laterally by the iliac crest, and medially by the L5/S1 facet joint.

(Fig. 11-13). A skin entry point is made over the lowest point of this triangle, and typically overlies the iliac crest, 5 to 7 cm from midline at the level of the L4 spinous process. A 22 gauge, 5 inch needle (8 inch in obese patients) is advanced using fluoroscopic guidance to lie anterolateral to the L5–S1 interspace (Fig. 11-14). A small volume (2–3 mL)

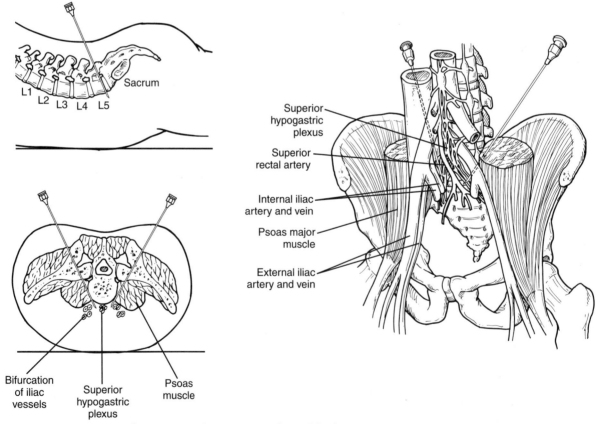

Figure 11-14   Superior hypogastric plexus block. (Redrawn from Cousins MJ, Bridenbaugh PO (eds): *Neural Blockade in Clinical Anesthesia and Management of Pain*, Third Edition, Lippincott-Raven, Philadelphia, 1998, p. 413.)

of radiographic contrast material will spread along the anterior surface of the lumbosacral junction confirming correct needle position. The same procedure is then carried out on the contralateral side. Temporary block is performed with 8-10 mL of local anesthetic (0.25% bupivacaine). In those patients considered candidates for neurolysis who report 50% or more pain reduction with local anesthetic block, neurolysis is carried out using the same procedure, injecting 8 mL of 10% phenol on each side.

Complications

There are only a limited number of reports detailing use of superior hypogastric plexus block and none have reported complications with this procedure. Due to the close proximity of the iliac vessels, intravascular injection can easily occur.

CONCLUSIONS

Sympathetic blocks are an important tool in treating chronic and cancer-related pain. Performing these techniques safely and effectively can be accomplished by most practitioners who have familiarity and technical facility with the regional anesthesia techniques used to provide surgical anesthesia.

SUGGESTED READING

de Leon-Cassasola OA: Sympathetic nerve block: pelvis. In: Raj PP (ed), *Practical Management of Pain*, Third Edition, Mosby, St. Louis, 2000, pp. 683-688.

Eisenberg E, Carr DB, Chalmers TC: Neurolytic celiac plexus block for treatment of cancer pain: a meta-analysis, *Anesth Analg* 80:290-295, 1995.

Ischia S, Polati E, Finco G, et al.: 1998 Labat Lecture: the role of the neurolytic celiac plexus block in pancreatic cancer pain management: do we have the answers?, *Reg Anesth Pain Med* 23:611-614, 1998.

Lamer TJ: Sympathetic nerve blocks. In: Brown DL (ed), *Regional Anesthesia and Analgesia*, WB Saunders, Philadelphia, 1996, pp. 357-384.

Plancarte R, de Leon-Cassasola OA, El-Helely M, et al.: Neurolytic superior hypogastric plexus block for chronic pelvic pain associated with cancer, *Reg Anesth* 22:562-568, 1997.

Rathmell JP, Gallant JM, Brown DL: Computed tomography and the anatomy of celiac plexus block, *Reg Anesth Pain Med* 25:411-416, 2000.

Rauck R: Sympathetic nerve blocks: head, neck, and trunk. In: Raj PP (ed), *Practical Management of Pain*, Third Edition, Mosby, St. Louis, 2000, pp. 651-682.

SAFETY, COMPLICATIONS, AND OUTCOMES

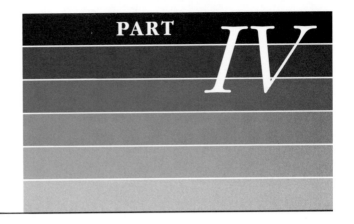

Postdural Puncture Headache

JOSEPH M. NEAL

INTRODUCTION

Postdural puncture headache (PDPH) remains one of the most common side effects in regional anesthesia practice and a frequent reason for consultation. While improvements in spinal needle design have markedly reduced the frequency of PDPH, there have been no major therapeutic breakthroughs in the past four decades. The pathophysiology of PDPH remains controversial and based on the observation of indirect physiologic consequences.

PATHOPHYSIOLOGY

Since August Bier and his assistant experienced postural headache the morning after their first successful experiment with spinal anesthesia, physicians have speculated that its cause is linked to intracranial hypotension. Recent studies have suggested that this explanation may be too simplistic. For decades, the pathophysiology of PDPH has been thought to involve a bimodal mechanism (Fig. 12-1 on p. 146). First, cerebrospinal fluid (CSF) leakage through a spinal needle-induced dural rent leads to low CSF pressure, which allows cranial contents to sag and place traction on pain-sensitive blood vessels and related structures that anchor the brain to the cranium. Second, these vascular structures reflexively vasodilate in response to traction, causing a migraine-like vascular component to PDPH pain. While never directly proven, this theory has indirect support from several observations. Intracranial hypotension is present in most, but not all, patients with PDPH. Evidence that sagging intracranial contents place traction on cranial and occipital nerves (the major referred pain pathways for PDPH) is indirectly seen with audiography. Patients with PDPH experience some degree of hearing loss (secondary to cranial nerve VIII stretching and endolymphatic fluid pressure changes) that reverts to baseline when the headache resolves (Fig. 12-2 and Fig. 12-3 on p. 146). Indeed, the magnitude of hearing loss directly correlates to the degree of CSF leakage. An alternative hypothesis to this long-held theory proposes that PDPH is purely a consequence of the potently painful stimulus of cerebral vasodilation. Proponents of this theory note that magnetic resonance scanning confirms sagging intracranial contents in some (but not all) patients with PDPH. Experiments in pigs have demonstrated that removal of small amounts of CSF are consistently linked to increased cerebral blood flow (CBF), which is presumably due to vasodilation. Conversely, epidural blood, as would be deposited with an epidural blood patch, causes vasoconstriction, normalization of CBF, and consequent pain relief. Ultimately, the pathophysiology of PDPH remains controversial and may involve altered cerebrovascular dynamics, physical stretching of pain-sensitive anchoring structures, or a combination of both.

Clinical Controversy: Pathophysiology of PDPH

The bimodal theory asserts that PDPH is a combination of intracranial hypotension, which allows the brain to sag and place traction on pain-sensitive anchoring structures and blood vessels. These same vessels also reflexively vasodilate, adding a migraine-like component to PDPH pain

An alternative theory suggests that PDPH is entirely the consequence of CSF loss, which causes cerebrovascular dilation (a potently painful stimulus)

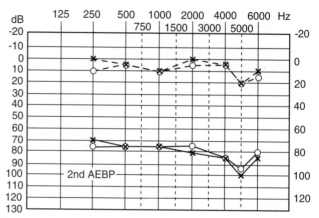

Figure 12-2 Audiogram before (bottom tracing) and after epidural blood patch. (Redrawn from Lybecker H, Andersen T: Repetitive hearing loss following dural puncture treated with autologous epidural blood patch, *Acta Anaesthesiol Scand* 39:389–394, 1995.)

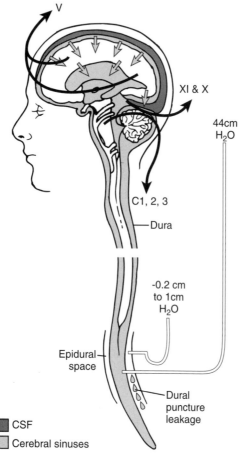

Figure 12-1 Pathophysiology of postdural puncture headache. (Redrawn from Brownridge P: The management of headache following accidental dural puncture in obstetric patients, *Anaesth Intens Care* 11:9, 1983.)

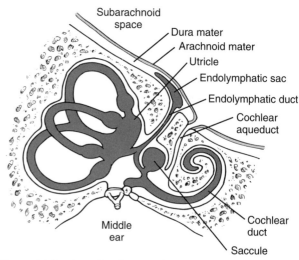

Figure 12-3 Hearing loss and intracranial hypotension. The relationship of inner ear pressure to subarachnoid pressure. (Redrawn from Lybecker H, Andersen T, Helbo-Hansen HS: The effect of epidural blood patch on hearing loss in patients with severe postdural puncture headache, *J Clin Anesth* 7:457–464, 1995.)

CLINICAL PRESENTATION

Signs and Symptoms

Postdural puncture headache classically presents as a postural headache that follows a known dural puncture. Symptoms are exacerbated by sitting or standing, and

improved by resuming the supine position. The headache is classically bilateral, and frontal, occipital, or both (Fig. 12-1). Neck pain and nausea are often present, and may be the only presenting symptom. Traction on cranial nerves may produce hearing loss or ocular muscle palsies (Box 12-1).

Postdural puncture headache is a diagnosis of exclusion. Meningitis, pregnancy-induced hypertension, intracranial pathology, and other maladies have all been misdiagnosed as PDPH. Any lateralizing neurologic sign (other than the aforementioned cranial nerve signs), fever, photophobia, or mental status changes are not compatible with the diagnosis of PDPH. Basic neurologic examination should be documented prior to diagnosing PDPH.

History compatible with dural puncture
Onset delayed 12 to 48 hours after dural puncture
Headache clearly improves in the supine position
Bilateral, throbbing headache; usually frontal, occipital,
or both
Associated symptoms – nausea, neck pain, tinnitus or
hearing loss, diplopia
Symptoms *not associated* with PDPH – fever, mental sta-
tus changes, photophobia, lateralizing neurologic
signs

In the absence of a compatible history, and especially if
initial treatment attempts fail, neurologic consultation
should be sought.

Clinical Course

Symptoms of PDPH classically present 12 to 48
hours after dural puncture, with ~70% presenting within
24 hours and ~90% within 48 hours (Fig. 12-4). Left
untreated, the vast majority of PDPH resolves spontaneously within 2 to 5 days of onset (Fig. 12-5). This latter
point is important when evaluating treatment efficacy,
as a large percentage of PDPH will resolve without
intervention.

Risk Factors

Postdural puncture headache is most common in
younger patients, reaching its peak incidence in the late

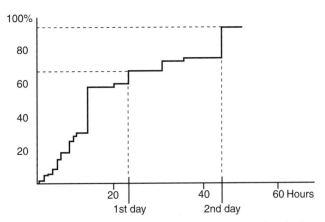

Figure 12-4   Onset of postdural puncture headache.
Cumulative onset of postdural puncture headache over time in 75
patients. (Redrawn from Lybecker H, Djernes M, Schmidt J:
Postdural puncture headache (PDPH): onset, duration, severity, and
associated symptoms. An analysis of 75 consecutive patients with
PDPH, *Acta Anaesthesiol Scand* 39:605–612, 1995.)

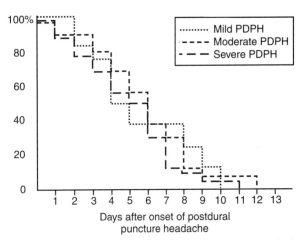

Figure 12-5   Recovery from postdural puncture headache.
Recovery from postdural puncture headache as a function of
headache severity. (Redrawn from Lybecker H, Djernes M, Schmidt
J: Postdural puncture headache (PDPH): onset, duration, severity,
and associated symptoms. An analysis of 75 consecutive patients
with PDPH, *Acta Anaesthesiol Scand* 39:605–612, 1995.)

teens and early 20s and then markedly declining over
age 40. Overall incidence is approximately 3.5% (ranging
from >5% in teenage patients to <1% in those >40
years). There is no gender difference. Previous suggestion
that young women are more prone to developing PDPH
is explainable by the higher incidence of neuraxial blockade performed during pregnancy. Repeated dural punctures increase the risk of PDPH, whereas early ambulation
does not. Besides age, the largest impact on PDPH frequency is spinal needle size and design. Smaller spinal
needles reduce the risk of PDPH by causing smaller dural
tears and, consequently, less CSF leakage. Headache is
clearly worse and more difficult to treat if it follows large
(<20 gauge) needle punctures. Spinal needle diameters
of 24 to 27 gauge are the optimal size to balance PDPH
risk with increased technical difficulty and block failure
rates. Perhaps more important than needle size is the
configuration of the needle tip. Non-cutting designs, such
as the pencil-point Whitacre or Sprotte needles, markedly
reduce the incidence of PDPH as compared to cutting tip
Quincke needles (see further discussion and illustrations
of needles in Chapter 4).

PREVENTION

Attention to certain principles significantly reduces
the incidence of PDPH (Box 12-2). When possible, avoid
spinal anesthesia in patients <25–30 years of age. Select
small (24 to 27 gauge) spinal needles with non-cutting
tips. If cutting tips or epidural needles are used, the needle
bevel should be parallel with the long axis of the spine
(see Fig. 4-2 on p. 38). Tangential needle passage through
the dura, as would occur with a paramedian approach,

Box 12-2 Prevention of Postdural Puncture Headache

Avoid spinal anesthesia in patients <25–30 years of age
Use 24 to 27 gauge diameter, non-cutting tip needles
   (Whitacre, Sprotte, Gertie Marx)
Insert epidural needles and cutting tip needles with the
   bevel parallel to the long axis of the spine

may also reduce the incidence of PDPH by creating a well-apposed dural flap. All of these concepts are supported by in vitro studies (Fig. 12-6). When continuous spinal catheters are utilized, there is some evidence to suggest that keeping them in place for ≥24 hours reduces the incidence of PDPH, particularly in parturients.

TREATMENT

Reassurance and oral analgesics are the mainstays of conservative therapy. Especially if secondary to a small-gauge spinal needle, most PDPH will resolve spontaneously within 24 to 48 hours; therefore conservative treatment is reasonable if the patient is able to remain supine during that time. Forced hydration, caffeinated beverages, abdominal binders, non-steroidal anti-inflammatory drugs, and steroids are without proven benefit.

Several minimally invasive and pharmacologic treatment options have been proposed to treat PDPH, but suffer from high recurrence rates or lack of rigorous scientific support. Epidural saline bolus and/or infusion is moderately successful (≤88%), but over half of patients will relapse when the infusion is discontinued. Epidural dextran 70 will remain in the epidural space for a longer period, but is associated with anaphylaxis. Caffeine therapy is moderately successful (75 to 90%) as an initial treatment, but 30% or more patients will relapse. Caffeine presumably works by reversing the vasodilation associated with PDPH. It is administered orally as a 300 mg single dose, or intravenously as caffeine sodium benzoate 500 mg every 4 hours. Other pharmacologic therapies, including sumatriptin, adrenocorticotropic hormone, and theophylline, have been proposed, but have not undergone randomized clinical trials. Similarly, preliminary reports of fibrin glue administered into the epidural space are intriguing but have not undergone rigorous study. If efficacious, fibrin glue would be a good alternative to epidural blood patching in patients with sepsis.

Epidural Blood Patch

Epidural blood patch (EBP) remains the treatment of choice for PDPH. It consistently provides at least partial relief in 90–95% of patients after the first attempt, and in ~97% after the second attempt. Failure is correlated with large spinal or epidural needle punctures, and incorrect diagnosis. The mechanism of EBP is not

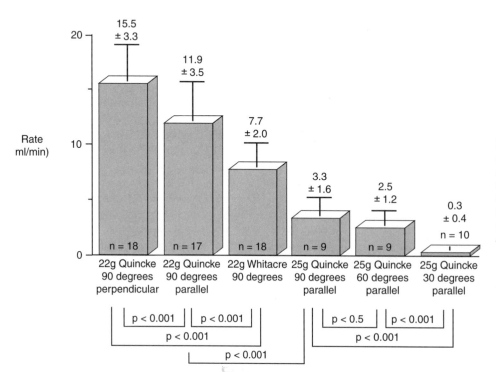

Figure 12-6 In vitro transdural fluid leak. Influence of needle type, bevel orientation, and needle angulation. (Redrawn from Ready L, Cuplin S, Haschke R, et al.: Spinal needle determinants of rate of transdural fluid leak, *Anesth Analg* 69:457–460, 1989.)

completely understood. Initial elevation of epidural space pressure and, by extension, subarachnoid space pressure, may temporarily provide relief from CSF hypotension. Epidural blood is observed in animal models to form a fibrin patch and plug over the area of dural rent, thereby preventing further CSF leakage. Rat studies suggest that both creation of a tamponade effect and sealing the dural rent are necessary for successful correction of CSF hypotension. The irritation of epidural blood on neural tissues has also been shown to cause vasoconstriction and decrease CBF. The timing of EBP placement is controversial. Although some studies suggest that effectiveness is improved by delaying EBP for several days after headache onset, this observation is most likely explainable by large dural rents causing more pain, thereby demanding earlier treatment, and then being more likely to fail as compared to small needle-induced PDPH. Because blood administered into the epidural space preferentially spreads rostrally, performing EBP at the level of the initial dural tap or an interspace below is recommended (Fig. 12-7). The ideal volume for injected epidural blood is believed to be in the 15 to 20 mL range, with injection stopping when symptoms of backache, neckache, or radicular pain occur.

Clinical Caveat: Ideal Volume of Blood for Epidural Blood Patch

The ideal volume of blood to use for an epidural blood patch is not precisely known. Success is improved with volumes over 10 mL, but may not be further enhanced by volumes over 20 mL. A reasonable approach is to stop blood administration after 20 mL has been injected, or when the patient notes back, neck, or radicular discomfort, whichever occurs first.

Side effects from EBP are common. Backache will occur in 75% of patients and leg discomfort in about half, some of whom will have radicular symptoms for several days afterwards. Transient cranial nerve palsies may occur following EBP. Transient bradycardia is common immediately following injection of epidural blood. Infectious complications are decidedly rare, including central nervous system spread of human immunodeficiency virus (HIV). Previous EBP does not affect the quality of subsequent epidural anesthetics.

Prophylactic EBP remains controversial. Suitable randomized clinical trials to support or refute this practice do not exist. Because the risk of PDPH following unintentional epidural needle dural penetration is so high

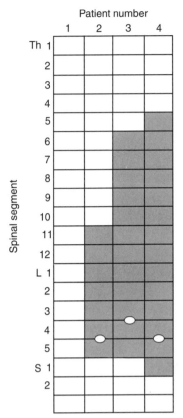

Figure 12-7   Spread of blood during epidural blood patch. Epidural blood preferentially spreads rostrally (open dots represent injection site). (Redrawn from Djurhuus H, Rasmussen M, Jensen EH: Epidural blood patch illustrated by CT-epidurography *Acta Anaesthesiol Scand* 39:613–617, 1995.)

(~70%), prophylaxis may be of reasonable benefit. The risk of prophylactic EBP is the development of the aforementioned side effects. Typically, sterile autologous blood is injected through the epidural catheter prior to its removal.

SUGGESTED READING

Boezaart AP: Effects of cerebrospinal fluid loss and epidural blood patch on cerebral blood flow in swine. *Reg Anesth Pain Med* 26:401–406, 2001.

Camann WR, Murray RS, Mushlin PS, Lambert DH: Effects of oral caffeine on postdural puncture headache. A double-blind, placebo controlled trial, *Anesth Analg* 70:181–184, 1990.

DiGiovanni AJ, Galbert MW, Wahle WM: Epidural injection of autologous blood for postlumbar-puncture headache. II. Additional clinical experiences and laboratory investigation, *Anesth Analg* 51:226–232, 1972.

Hatfalvi BI: Postulated mechanisms for postdural puncture headache and review of laboratory models, *Reg Anesth* 20: 329–336, 1995.

Lybecker H, Andersen T: Repetitive hearing loss following dural puncture treated with autologous epidural blood patch, *Acta Anaesthesiol Scand* 39:987–989, 1995.

Neal JM: Update on postdural puncture headache, *Tech Reg Anesth Pain Management* 2:202-210, 1998.

Ready LB, Cuplin S, Haschke RH, Nessly M: Spinal needle determinants of rate of transdural fluid leak, *Anesth Analg* 69:457-460, 1989.

Safa-Tisseront V, Thormann F, Malassine P, et al.: Effectiveness of epidural blood patch in the management of post-dural puncture headache, *Anesthesiology* 95:334-339, 2001.

13

Neural Blockade and Anticoagulation

JOSEPH M. NEAL

INTRODUCTION

Epidural (spinal) hematoma associated with concurrent neuraxial block affects 1 in every 250,000 to 1,000,000 patients, with spinal techniques being somewhat less likely than epidural techniques to cause this complication. However, when neuraxial regional anesthesia is administered in the setting of a pharmacologically or medically altered coagulation status, epidural hematoma may occur in up to 1 in every 1,000 to 10,000 patients. The substantial risks of developing this permanent and devastating complication, which often leads to major neurologic deficits, including paralysis, were underscored when low molecular weight heparin (LMWH) anticoagulants were introduced to the US market in 1993, followed by more than 40 reports over a five-year period of epidural hematoma in the setting of concurrent neuraxial regional anesthesia. When placed into perspective, a previous review of this topic found only 61 reports

between 1906 and 1994. In conjunction with this increased frequency of epidural hematoma, the American Society of Anesthesiologists closed claim database registered a rise in claims associated with neuraxial regional anesthesia. The introduction of ever more powerful thromboprophylactic antiplatelet agents for perioperative and vascular indications continues to challenge the regional anesthetist's vigilance and judgment. Although regional anesthesia procedures have been implicated, it should be remembered that similar concerns apply to neuraxial techniques such as diagnostic lumbar puncture or interventional pain and radiological procedures.

REGIONAL ANESTHETIC BLEEDING COMPLICATIONS

Epidural Hematoma

The anatomy of the epidural space makes this region uniquely susceptible to bleeding complications. Filled with large veins that are frequently punctured by spinal and epidural needles, the narrow dimensions of the epidural space can only accommodate small volumes of expanding hematoma before pressure is exerted on the spinal cord and nerve roots (Fig. 13-1 on p. 152). Furthermore, the hemorrhage is invisible to external examination. When extrinsic pressure exceeds spinal cord perfusion and/or venous pressures, ischemia results and can lead to permanent damage within hours. Epidural hematoma typically develops insidiously; with the first symptoms presenting a median of 3 days after the first LMWH dose is administered. Particularly worrisome, many epidural hematomas manifest around the time of epidural catheter removal. Back pain is a classic sign, but may be present in less than half of patients. More commonly, bowel or bladder dysfunction, sensory changes, and/or motor weakness present after the block

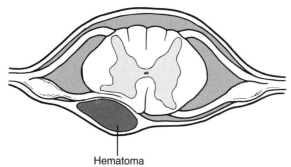

Hematoma

Figure 13-1   Schematic depiction of an epidural hematoma compressing the spinal cord. (Redrawn from Cousins MJ, Veering BT: Epidural neural blockade. In: Cousins MJ, Bridenbaugh PO (eds), *Neural Blockade in Clinical Anesthesia and Management of Pain*, Third Edition, Lippincott-Raven, Philadelphia, 1998, p. 309, Fig. 8-34.)

0.02% in brachial plexus blocks), and except in rare circumstances is not associated with morbidity. Hematoma occurs most frequently after peripheral blocks placed near major vessels, such as axillary, femoral, or supraclavicular blocks. The added risk of performing peripheral nerve block or continuous peripheral catheter placement in anticoagulated patients is unknown. There are no published guidelines, but it is logical to avoid peripheral block in any severely anticoagulated patient (for example, prothrombin time (PT) or activated partial thromboplastin time (aPTT) >2.5 times normal, or platelet count <50,000/mm³). Furthermore, peripheral regional techniques in the anticoagulated patient should be avoided near noncompressible blood vessels (supraclavicular or retrobulbar block) or where an expanding hematoma could compromise respiratory function (interscalene or stellate ganglion block).

dissipates, or recrudesce in the setting of a previously resolving block. If epidural hematoma is suspected, computerized tomography or magnetic resonance imaging confirms the diagnosis (Fig. 13-2). Rapid diagnosis and treatment of epidural hematoma is crucial, as full or partial neurologic recovery is less likely after 8 hours have elapsed between the initial onset of symptoms and decompressive laminectomy (Fig. 13-3 on p. 153) (Box 13-1).

Peripheral Hematoma

The development of bleeding at peripheral nerve block sites is a relatively uncommon event (0.001 to

Clinical Controversy: Peripheral Nerve Blocks in the Anticoagulated Patient

There are no guidelines to identify when it is safe to perform peripheral nerve blockade in the anticoagulated patient

Guidelines pertaining to neuraxial block are likely to be too restrictive for the anticoagulated patient who may benefit from peripheral block

In general, avoid peripheral block if it would not be easy to identify or compress a peripheral hematoma, or if an expanding mass could compromise respiration or vision

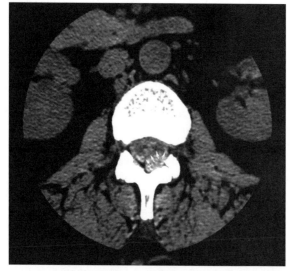
A

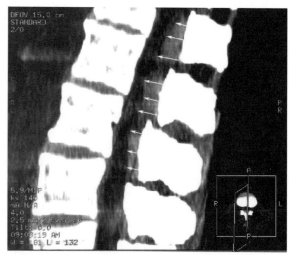
B

Figure 13-2   Lumbar epidural hematoma. A, Axial computed tomography image of a lumbar epidural hematoma. There is a high-density mass in the left posterolateral epidural space compressing the thecal sac (arrows). **B,** Sagittal reconstruction computed tomography image demonstrating the longitudinal extent of the epidural hematoma within the posterior epidural space (arrows).

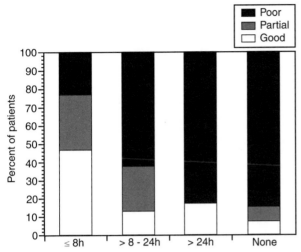

Figure 13-3 **The relationship of symptoms, intervention, and neurological recovery in patients with epidural hematoma.** As the time from symptom development and decompressive laminectomy increases beyond 8 hours, the number of patients with good or partial recovery substantially decreases. (Redrawn from Tryba M: European practice guidelines: thromboembolism prophylaxis and regional anesthesia, *Reg Anesth Pain Med* 23(S2):181, 1998, Figure. 2.)

Box 13-1 **Diagnosis and Treatment of Epidural Hematoma**

Maintain a high index of suspicion when neuraxial block is slow to resolve or recrudesces after partial or full resolution

Back pain is a common sign, but not always present

Sensory changes, progressive motor weakness, and bowel or bladder dysfunction are highly suspicious for neural compression

Diagnosis is confirmed with CT or MRI

Decompressive laminectomy within 8 hours of symptoms improves outcome

---

ANTICOAGULANTS AND CONCURRENT NEURAXIAL ANESTHESIA

The commingling of neuraxial regional anesthetic techniques with anticoagulants requires careful attention to the timing of drug administration and block placement, to the timing of epidural catheter removal, and to postprocedure neurological assessment. While this implies a degree of vigilance over and above that paid to patients with normal coagulation, it should not be taken as a condemnation of neuraxial regional anesthesia in patients who are or may be anticoagulated. Table 13-1 summarizes beneficial tests for evaluating anticoagulated patients prior to technical interventions. The American Society of Regional Anesthesia and Pain Medicine (ASRA) held consensus conferences in 1998 and 2002 to develop evidence and expert opinion-based guidelines for managing anticoagulated patients undergoing concurrent neuraxial regional anesthesia. These guidelines are summarized in Table 13-2 and detailed below.

Low Molecular Weight Heparin

More than any other anticoagulant, LMWH has been linked to perioperative epidural hematoma. Convenient dosing and no requirement for monitoring have made these drugs widely used for thromboprophylaxis and treatment of thrombotic complications. Unfortunately, their pharmacodynamic profile is significantly different from standard heparin, which makes patient management challenging (Box 13-2).

When a single dose of LMWH is given preoperatively, neuraxial block should be delayed for 10–12 (conservatively 24) hours. Post-block administration of LMWH is dependent upon the dosing regimen. Delay administration for 6–8 hours for single daily dosing, or 24 hours for twice daily dosing (preferably after the epidural catheter has been removed). Catheter removal should coincide with

---

Table 13-1 **Coagulation Tests: Appropriateness for Assessing Coagulation Status Prior to Neuraxial Block**

Anticoagulant	Bleeding Time	Platelet Count	Anti Xa	aPTT	INR
LMWH	–	–	Not predictive of bleeding	–	–
Standard heparin	–	If receiving heparin for >4 days	–	Should be near normal	–
Warfarin	–	–	–	–	<1.5 may be acceptable after acute dosage, but chronic warfarin therapy may require INR <1.2
Aspirin and other antiplatelet drugs	–	–	–	–	–

– = Not appropriate; LMWH = low molecular weight heparin; aPTT = activated partial thromboplastin time; INR = international normalized ratio.

Table 13-2   Summary of 2002 ASRA Guidelines for Neuraxial Regional Anesthesia in the Anticoagulated Patient

Anticoagulant	ASRA Guideline	Catheter Removal	Strength of Evidence
LMWH	Preop LMWH/single dose: delay block for 10–12 hours Postop LMWH/single daily dosing: delay LMWH for 6–8 hours Postop LMWH/twice daily dosing: delay LMWH for 24 hours	Single daily dosing: remove catheter 10–12 hours after last LMWH dose; wait ≥2 hours before next dose Twice daily dosing: remove catheter ≥2 hours before first LMWH dose	Pharmacokinetic data. Large series of case reports
Standard heparin	Subcutaneous 5,000 U/first dose: delay heparin injection for 1–2 hours after block placement Intravenous/first dose: delay heparin dose for 1 hour after block placement Intravenous/continuous dose: discontinue heparin infusion for 2–4 hours and check aPTT prior to block placement	Discontinue heparin for 2–4 hours and check a PTT prior to removal	Pharmacokinetic data. Prospective and retrospective case surveys and case reports
Warfarin	New dose: check INR if first dose was given >24 hours previously or if second dose has been given Chronic use: discontinue warfarin for 4–5 days and check INR prior to block (should be near normal)	If warfarin for >36 hours: remove catheter when INR <1.5	Case series and case reports
Aspirin/NSAIDs/COX-2 inhibitors	No issues if patient is not taking other anticoagulants	No issues	Retrospective case surveys
Other antiplatelet agents	Ticlopidine: discontinue for 14 days		
	Clopidogrel: discontinue for 7 days	No recommendation	Pharmacokinetic data
	Eptifibatide/tirofiban: discontinue for 8 hours		
	Abciximab: discontinue for 48 hours		
Thrombolytics/fibrinolytics	Block initiation: avoid within 10 days of drug administration Thrombolytic/fibrinolytic administration: avoid within 10 days of block. If block is received around the time of thrombolytic administration, check neurologic status ≤every 2 hours	No recommendation	Based on surgical recommendations No data
Fondaparinux	Do not combine with neuraxial regional anesthesia	No recommendation	No data
Herbal supplements	No specific concerns	No issues	No data

ASRA = American Society of Regional Anesthesia and Pain Medicine; LMWH = low molecular weight heparin; aPTT = activated partial thromboplastin time; INR = international normalized ratio; NSAIDs = non-steroidal anti-inflammatory drugs; COX-2 = cyclooxygenase-2.

the trough of LMWH activity (10–12 hours after the last dose). Then re-institute LMWH therapy 2 or more hours after catheter removal and documentation of normal neurological examination.

Unfractionated Heparin

Standard thromboprophylactic subcutaneous (sq) heparin (5,000 U every 12 hours) is generally safe with neuraxial anesthesia, providing the initial dose is delayed 1–2 hours after block placement. If sq heparin has been administered for several days, particularly to elderly or debilitated patients, checking an aPTT prior to neuraxial block is advisable, because a small percentage of patients may become therapeutically anticoagulated by these otherwise small doses. Continuous heparin infusions should be discontinued for 2–4 hours and an aPTT checked prior to institution of neuraxial procedures (including catheter

---

Box 13-2   The Pharmacology of LMWH (Enoxaparin)

Half-life is 3–4 hours, but anti-Xa activity remains 50% of baseline at 12 hours and does not normalize until 24 hours

Bleeding time, INR, aPTT, and ACT are not affected by LMWH

Anti-Xa levels are not predictive of bleeding

LMWH is not reversible by protamine

---

removal). Because some patients develop heparin-induced thrombocytopenia, a platelet count may be indicated after receiving continuous heparin for ≥4 days. Patients receiving prolonged perioperative heparin therapy are inappropriate for epidural catheter techniques.

Oral Anticoagulants

Since several doses are required to reach therapeutic levels, neuraxial anesthesia is not contraindicated if a single warfarin dose is given the night before surgery. Indeed, it is unnecessary to check an International Normalized Ratio (INR) if a single dose has been administered <24 hours before the anesthetic procedure. Chronic warfarin use is more problematic. Hold warfarin for 4–5 days prior to surgery and then confirm a normal or nearly normal INR prior to neuraxial anesthesia. For patients receiving warfarin for ≥36 hours, the INR should be <1.5 prior to catheter removal.

Aspirin and Other Antiplatelet Drugs

Aspirin, non-steroidal anti-inflammatory drugs (NSAIDs) of the ibuprophen class, and cyclooxygenase-2 inhibitors present no contraindication to neuraxial anesthesia. Conversely, because of their prolonged and irreversible effects on platelets, other classes of antiplatelet agents are problematic in the setting of neuraxial blockade. Since no firm data exist, recommendations generally follow those made for withholding these drugs prior to surgical procedures. Specifically, ticlopidine is withheld for 14 days and clopidogrel for 7 days. Particular concern is raised because the medical indications for these drugs (such as postcoronary stent placement or postcerebrovascular accident) frequently entail concomitant aspirin or thrombolytic therapy, which further increase the risk of bleeding.

Thrombolytics and Fibrinolytics

Sufficient data are unavailable to guide the timing of neuraxial techniques following thrombolytic or fibrinolytic therapy, or, conversely, the use of these drugs following an invasive neuraxial procedure. Conservatively, up to 10 days should elapse between pharmacologic and technical interventions. Anesthesiologists are most likely to encounter the combined use of thrombolytic agents and neuraxial regional anesthesia in vascular surgery patients. If these drugs have been or may be used in the perioperative period, neuraxial anesthesia is contraindicated. If thrombolytics are unexpectedly used, lower extremity motor and sensory examination should be scheduled at least every 2 hours until the pharmacologic effect dissipates. There is no recommendation regarding the ideal time to remove epidural catheters in these patients, but measurement of a fibrinogen level may be beneficial.

Fondaparinux

Newer anticoagulants (e.g. fondaparinux) are particularly worrisome because of their extended half-lives and "irreversibility." While the actual risks of epidural hematoma are unknown, ASRA guidelines recommend no commingling of these agents with neuraxial anesthesia.

Herbal Supplements

Many herbal supplements have mild anticoagulant effects. However, these drugs in isolation appear to present no increased bleeding risk. Whether they potentiate the risks of other anticoagulants is unknown.

MANAGEMENT CAVEATS

When to be Conservative

Certain clinical scenarios lead to more conservative practice when combining anticoagulant drugs with neuraxial anesthesia. Most typically, conservatism entails prolonging the interval between a neuraxial procedure and LMWH dosing from 12 to 24 hours, or avoiding regional anesthesia altogether. For example, a difficult or bloody epidural approach need not cancel surgery, but should prompt discussion with the surgeon regarding the acceptability of delaying initial LMWH dosing for 24 hours (Box 13-3).

Conservative practice also implies altering epidural dosing regimens or neurological examination protocols when necessary. For instance, a difficult technical procedure or a patient on therapeutic LMWH doses may indicate infusing only epidural opioids or dilute local anesthetic solution, to avoid any diagnostic confusion between neurodeficits induced by local anesthetics rather than an expanding mass. Recent thrombolytic use, re-institution of anticoagulant administration, or postoperative renal failure suggests the need to monitor neurological function every 2 hours for up to 24 hours after neuraxial block or catheter removal. As a matter of

---

Box 13-3 When to be More Conservative With Anticoagulants and Concurrent Neuraxial Anesthesia

When placing the regional block has been difficult, prolonged, or bloody (especially with an epidural needle as compared to a spinal needle)

When the patient is concomitantly taking other anticoagulants

When the patient is taking *therapeutic doses* of anticoagulants, for example, enoxaparin 1 mg/kg or delteparin 200 U/kg

Patients with renal insufficiency

---

routine, normal neurological examination should be documented prior to or after undertaking a neuraxial anesthetic technique (including epidural catheter removal) in the anticoagulated patient.

Combining Anticoagulation Regimens With Neuraxial Regional Anesthesia

Despite legitimate concerns regarding the anticoagulated patient and neuraxial regional anesthesia, it is too simplistic to state that the two modalities should never be combined. Indeed, the previous discussion builds a framework for their safe melding. Preventing thromboembolic complications is an important management goal, but they are not the sole perioperative risk. Regional anesthetic techniques may improve other outcomes (see Chapter 15). The intraoperative use of neuraxial local anesthetics is known to reduce the incidence of thromboembolic and vaso-occlusive complications following hip and peripheral vascular surgery. Regional techniques also improve early rehabilitation by reducing dynamic pain and facilitating ambulation, which in turn further reduces thromboembolic, pulmonary, and gastrointestinal complications. Especially in arthroplastic surgeries, the vigilant and intelligent multimodal combination of neuraxial anesthetics, followed by pharmacologic thromboprophylaxis, and perhaps facilitated by continuous peripheral catheter techniques, increases patient comfort and may improve outcome.

SUGGESTED READING

American Society of Regional Anesthesia and Pain Medicine: Regional anesthesia in the anticoagulated patient – defining the risks, www.asra.com (1–9–2003), 2002.

Horlocker TT: Regional anesthesia in the anticoagulated patient: Defining the risks, *Reg Anesth Pain Med* 28:172–197, 2003.

Neal JM: Controversies in regional anesthesia, *ASA Refresher Courses in Anesthesiology* 28:135–146, 2000.

Neal JM, Rowlingson JC: ASRA consensus conference revisits anticoagulation issue, *Anesthesia Patient Safety Foundation Newsletter* 17:27, 2002.

Vandermeulen EP, Van Aken H, Vermylen J: Anticoagulants and spinal-epidural anesthesia, *Anesth Analg* 79:1165–1177, 1994.

Neurologic Complications

JOSEPH M. NEAL

INTRODUCTION

Patient and practitioner alike fear neurologic injury attributable to regional anesthetic techniques. Fortunately, neurologic complications are extremely rare with most being minor and self-limited; yet there exists the potential for devastating injury. Indeed, in regional anesthesia practice, only the failure to resuscitate local anesthetic-induced cardiac toxicity has greater impact on patient welfare. Although there is no evidence that the incidence of *peripheral nerve* injury secondary to regional techniques is increasing, the American Society of Anesthesiologists Closed Claims Study noted increased claims during the 1990s related to *neuraxial* anesthesia, particularly spinal cord and lumbosacral nerve root injury. The probable reasons for this are twofold. First, a relative reduction in claims for respiratory injury was likely due to improved monitoring. Second, claims for neuraxial injury, particularly those related to chronic pain management, increased coincident with the introduction of powerful anticoagulants. This chapter considers common neurologic complications related to neuraxial and peripheral regional

anesthesia. Emphasis is placed on risk factors, diagnosis, and treatment.

DIFFERENTIAL DIAGNOSIS AND TREATMENT

When a patient experiences postoperative neurologic injury, it is incumbent on the anesthesiologist to consider all possible causes, including pre-existing disease, surgical, and positioning contributions (Box 14-1). Patient factors that increase the risk of perioperative nerve injury include male gender, advanced age, diabetes mellitus, and perhaps pre-existing neurologic disease. Particularly in cases of peripheral nerve injury, surgery may cause direct nerve damage secondary to transection, traction, edema, tourniquets, or constrictive cast application. Certain operations have a notably higher association with post-surgical injury, especially total shoulder replacement and elbow surgeries. Patient positioning may also be implicated in perioperative neural injury. The most common of these is ulnar nerve injury, which is overwhelmingly (85%) associated with general anesthesia. The etiology of ulnar and other perioperative nerve injuries is frequently uncertain, with the exception of spinal cord injury from hematoma or infection.

The urgency to diagnose and treat perioperative nerve injury varies with suspected etiology. Any unexplained motor or sensory deficit, and/or bowel or bladder dysfunction, after a *neuraxial* regional anesthetic technique demands immediate attention, as recovery from expanding epidural (spinal) hematoma or abscess markedly diminishes if spinal cord decompression does not occur within 8 hours. Conversely, isolated neurologic deficits following *peripheral* techniques do not mandate the same urgency. Because the vast majority of peripheral lesions resolve, some authorities recommend delaying electrophysiological

---

Box 14-1 Possible Contributors to Perioperative Nerve Injury

Patient factors
  Male gender
  Advanced age
  Extremes of body habitus
  Pre-existing neurologic disease
  Diabetes mellitus
Surgical factors
  Direct nerve injury – transection, traction
  Secondary nerve injury – tourniquet, cast, edema
Positioning factors
Anesthetic factors
  Vascular injury – ischemic, compressive
  Infectious complications
  Neurotoxicity
  Needle- or catheter-related injury

---

diagnostic workup for 6 to 8 weeks, proceeding only if the deficit is not fully resolved. An equally compelling argument suggests obtaining nerve conduction studies close to the time of injury to rule out treatable causes such as median nerve compression that become unmasked during the perioperative period, or to specifically localize the area of injury. The latter point is particularly cogent when uncertainty exists as to whether the lesion is most compatible with an anesthetic, surgical, or positioning insult. Neurologic consultation is recommended, as most anesthesiologists are unfamiliar with interpreting electrophysiological studies, or with treatment and rehabilitation protocols.

NEURAXIAL NEUROLOGIC COMPLICATIONS

Vascular Complications

Epidural hematoma (see Fig. 13-2 on p. 152) is potentially the most life-altering complication of neuraxial regional techniques. Epidural hematoma concurrent with a neuraxial anesthetic is estimated to occur in one of every 150,000 to 220,000 patients that undergo an epidural or spinal anesthetic, respectively. However, when patients are coagulopathic or taking anticoagulation drugs, the incidence may be as high as 1:1,000 to 10,000. (Details of this topic can be found in Chapter 13.) A high index of suspicion, rapid diagnosis, and early surgical decompression are essential to avoid permanent paralysis. Prolonged recovery from a local anesthetic block or recrudescence of a previously resolving or resolved block suggests an expanding epidural mass. Patients may develop sensory changes, progressive weakness, and/or back pain (Table 14-1). Confirmatory diagnosis with neuraxial imaging (computerized tomography or magnetic resonance imaging) must be obtained in conjunction with immediate neurosurgical consultation. If more than 8 hours pass between symptom onset and decompression, the likelihood of a full or partial recovery decreases dramatically.

Two additional vascular-related mechanisms leading to neuraxial injury have been proposed: reduced spinal cord blood flow (SCBF) and needle injury of the spinal vasculature (Fig. 14-1 and Fig. 14-2 on p. 159 and p. 160). Animal models and extensive human experience have not shown

---

Table 14-1 Presentation of Neurologic Complications Associated With Neuraxial Techniques

	Epidural Hematoma	Epidural Abscess	Transient Neurologic Symptoms	Spinal Vascular Ischemia
History	Anticoagulants; coagulopathy	Inconsistent signs of systemic infection	Lidocaine > other local anesthetics Lithotomy or knee arthroscopy	Atherosclerosis
Onset	Sudden	Over several days, then rapidly progressive	4–8 hours after block resolution	Sudden
Sensory exam	Possible lower extremity deficits	Possible lower extremity deficits	Normal	Usually normal if anterior spinal artery is involved
Motor exam	Progressive weakness	Progressive weakness	Normal	Flaccid paralysis
Symptoms	Back pain variable	Back pain variable; fever	Back or buttock pain with dysesthesia radiating to posterior thighs	Normal
Neuroimaging	Epidural hematoma	Epidural abscess	Normal	Normal or signs of localized neural injury

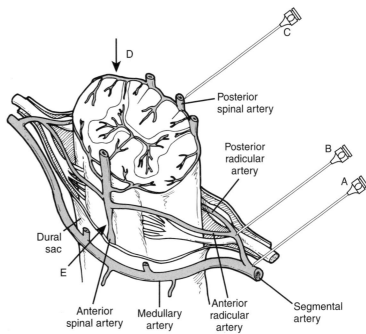

Figure 14-1   Arterial blood supply to the spinal cord, cross-sectional view. Note how the segmental (**A**), radicular (**B**), and possibly the posterior spinal (**C**) arteries are potentially vulnerable to needle injury (as illustrated by needles). Also note on the left side of the figure how vascular anomalies may present: (**D**) fused posterior spinal and posterolateral spinal arteries or (**E**) narrowing of the anterior spinal artery. (Redrawn from Bridenbaugh PO, Greene NM, Brull SJ: Spinal (subarachnoid) neural blockade. In: Cousins MJ, Bridenbaugh PO (eds), *Neural Blockade in Clinical Anesthesia and Pain Management*, Third Edition, Lippincott-Raven, Philadelphia, 1998, p. 211, Fig. 7-10.) (See colour inserts, Plate 6.)

adjuvant epinephrine to significantly alter SCBF. Because SCBF is autoregulated between mean arterial pressure of 50–135 mmHg, hypotension is seldom a factor in spinal cord injury. Direct needle trauma to major radicular arteries (Fig. 14-1) is speculated to contribute to the extremely rare occurrence of anterior spinal artery syndrome, although direct cause-and-effect evidence is lacking (Table 14-1). Indeed, some authorities speculate that ischemic spinal cord injury may require an inciting factor (hypotension, needle trauma) in combination with a spinal vasculature abnormality that impairs collateral circulation.

Infectious Complications

Serious infectious complications can follow neuraxial techniques, presenting either as epidural abscess or meningitis. Epidural abscess (Fig. 14-3 on p. 161) is the most common infectious complication associated with neuraxial techniques, typically presenting several days after placement of an epidural catheter. With permanent (tunneled) epidural catheters, deep track infection or abscess occurs approximately once in every 1,700 catheter days. Localized erythema, tenderness, and mild purulent pericatheter discharge may indicate only superficial infection that will be responsive to oral antibiotics and catheter removal. Especially with tunneled catheters, pain on injection may signal early infection. However, back pain, leukocytosis, or fever may be indicative of deeper infection, necessitating prompt neurologic imaging, parenteral antibiotics, and possible surgical drainage (Table 14-1). The incidence of meningitis following neuraxial techniques is no greater than 1:20,000. The poten-

tial for lumbar puncture to cause meningitis in the setting of bacteremia is controversial, as there are no strong data to suggest a cause-and-effect relationship. Nevertheless, in the absence of overwhelming necessity to choose neuraxial regional anesthesia and/or a continuous catheter technique, doing so in the presence of untreated systemic infection is ill advised. Needle passage through an area of cutaneous infection should be avoided. Once antibiotics have been administered and the patient exhibits an appropriate response (defervescence), neuraxial regional anesthetic techniques are acceptable.

Clinical Caveat: Time Course of an Epidural Abscess

The clinical presentation of early epidural infection can be indolent, with mild backache or fever being the only signs. However, once an epidural abscess begins to expand, sensory and motor changes appear and rapidly progress to paralysis. Prompt consultation with an infectious disease specialist and/or surgical decompression is necessary to prevent permanent neurologic injury.

Transient Neurologic Symptoms

The syndrome of transient neurologic symptoms (TNS; formerly known as transient radicular irritation) is a relatively common malady after spinal anesthesia. Its etiology is unclear, and may not be neurologic in origin. Transient neurologic symptoms refer to back or buttock pain that radiates to the posterior thighs, and occurs after the

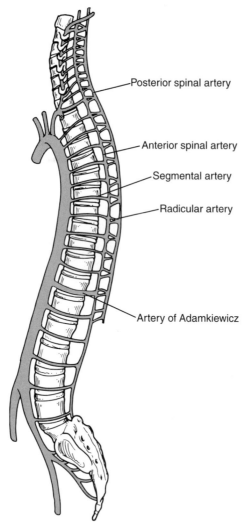

Posterior spinal artery

Anterior spinal artery

Segmental artery

Radicular artery

Artery of Adamkiewicz

Figure 14-2 Arterial blood supply to the spinal cord, longitudinal view. Note the pathway from segmental → radicular → anterior and posterior spinal arteries. (Redrawn from Covino BG, Scott DB: *Handbook of Epidural Anaesthesia and Analgesia*, Grune & Stratton, Orlando, 1985, p. 21, Fig. 1-19.) (See colour inserts, Plate 7.)

resolution of spinal anesthesia. Most TNS resolves within 2 to 3 days, and is frequently more painful than the surgical incision. It is not associated with gross neurologic findings (Table 14-1). Risk factors for TNS include lidocaine, ambulatory surgery, and positions that stretch the sciatic nerve (lithotomy, knee arthroscopy, prone jack-knife). Although most frequently associated with lidocaine, TNS has been reported with all local anesthetics, albeit infrequently with bupivacaine. Following lidocaine spinal anesthesia, TNS is consistently reported in 20 to 35% of patients positioned in lithotomy and ~20% after knee arthroscopy. Baricity, glucose, adjuvants, age, or local anesthetic concentration does not affect TNS. Low-dose lidocaine (20 to 30 mg) with fentanyl may decrease the incidence of TNS, relative to routine clinical doses (>40–100 mg). Thus, TNS is best prevented by avoiding procaine, tetracaine, or "normal dose" lidocaine in patients who will be positioned in lithotomy or for knee

arthroscopy. Spinal anesthesia in these cases can be provided with low-dose bupivacaine 5–6 mg or lidocaine 30–40 mg, each with fentanyl 10–20 μg. When TNS occurs, it is best treated with non-steroidal anti-inflammatory drugs and reassurance.

Neurotoxicity

Direct spinal cord injury from neurotoxic local anesthetics, adjuvants, or preservatives has occurred. Because all local anesthetics, especially lidocaine and tetracaine, are capable of causing concentration- and time-dependent neurotoxicity in isolated animal nerve preparations, this potential to cause clinical injury is cited by some as evidence of a neurotoxic etiology for TNS. Nonetheless, this association remains unproven and is in conflict with certain clinical manifestations of TNS (for instance, TNS is not dependent on local anesthetic concentration). Conversely, supernormal doses of hyperbaric lidocaine and tetracaine have been linked to permanent cauda equina syndrome in some patients who underwent continuous spinal anesthesia using microcatheters. Presumably, maldistribution caused these local anesthetics to remain in close proximity to sacral nerve roots, thereby leading to neurotoxicity.

Commonly used local anesthetic adjuvants (epinephrine) are not inherently neurotoxic, but may potentiate lidocaine toxicity in animal models. Certain preservatives and antioxidants have been identified as neurotoxic. In the 1980s, large doses of 2-chloroprocaine unintentionally deposited within the subarachnoid space caused cauda equina symptoms. This injury was ultimately linked to the formulation's low pH and bisulfite preservative. Not to be confused with the former malady, a separate and distinct syndrome of back pain that presents immediately upon resolution of 2-chloroprocaine epidural anesthesia has also been described. This syndrome is without distinct etiology, but appears to be musculoskeletal in nature. It has been linked to higher volumes of epidural 2-chloroprocaine (≥30 mL) and to the preservative EDTA (ethylenediaminetetraacetate), although cases have been reported in the absence of EDTA. Other commonly used preservatives, antioxidants, and excipients, such as polypropylene glycol or benzyl alcohol, have been variously identified with neurotoxic changes in animal models, but not in humans. This area of neurotoxicity remains poorly studied.

Needle- and Catheter-Related Injury

Direct neuraxial injury secondary to needle or catheter trauma is possible. As previously noted, needles can potentially damage spinal cord feeder vessels, but the significance of this is poorly understood. A more defined issue concerns injury from direct needle contact with, or penetration of, the spinal cord or spinal nerve roots. Paresthesia coincident with the placement of a spinal

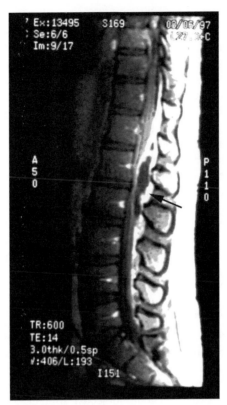

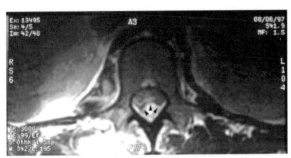

Figure 14-3 **Epidural abscess. A,** Axial MRI demonstrating an epidural abscess with anterior displacement of the dural sac (dark arrows). **B,** Sagittal MRI with gadolinium that demonstrates an epidural abscess (L3 to T9). Arrow shows an area of liquefaction within the abscess. (Reproduced from Rathmell JP, Garahan MP, Alsofrom GF: Epidural abscess following epidural analgesia, *Reg Anesth Pain Med* 25:80, 2000, Figs. 1 and 2.)

needle happens in about 6% of patients, yet the incidence of perioperative spinal cord or nerve root injury is vastly lower than this. Retrospective analyses have either linked paresthesia and/or pain on injection to neuraxial injury, or found no correlation; thus paresthesia *per se* does not specifically predict nerve injury. The use of a continuous catheter during epidural procedures increases both the incidence of paresthesia and the frequency of postoperative nerve injury as compared to single-shot techniques. Of note, neuraxis injury from misdirected needles can also occur in the setting of peripheral approaches, such as interscalene or paravertebral nerve blocks.

PERIPHERAL NEUROLOGIC COMPLICATIONS

The incidence of long-term neuropathy following peripheral nerve block is estimated to be ≤0.4%. Most peripheral nerve injury presents within 48 hours of surgery, but may be delayed for up to 3 weeks. Immediate injury (within 24 hours) is most likely associated with wound hematoma, edema, or nerve laceration. Delayed injury (days to weeks later) represents scar formation or

tissue reaction. Predisposing or exacerbating factors for peripheral nerve injury differ from those noted with neuraxial anesthesia. For instance, neither continuous catheter techniques nor repeat axillary nerve block days to years later increase the frequency of persistent paresthesia. Pre-existing peripheral nerve injury is a more problematic risk factor. Whereas studies are inconclusive regarding the role of systemic nerve disease (diabetes or chemotherapy) as a predictor of perioperative nerve injury, regional techniques in the setting of pre-existing anatomic nerve abnormalities (such as ulnar nerve malposition at the elbow) do not increase the risk of perioperative injury.

Neurotoxicity

Spinal cord and peripheral nerve blood supply (see Fig. 3-4 on p. 27) are markedly different; thus their susceptibility to neurotoxic insult is not only different, but also prevents comparison between systems. Neurotoxicity can be caused by chemical toxicity and/or diminished peripheral neural blood flow (PNBF). Local anesthetics, with or without epinephrine, are neurotoxic in a concentration- and time-dependent fashion in animal isolated peripheral nerve models. In addition, local anesthetics (lidocaine is most commonly studied) decrease PNBF in a concentration-dependent manner, while added epinephrine further reduces PNBF to only 20% of baseline. Vast human experience suggests that commonly used clinical doses of local anesthetic and epinephrine are innocuous, and that normal nerves seemingly withstand significant PNBF reduction without consequence. Indeed, pneumatic tourniquets reduce PNBF to zero for several hours without causing injury. What is unclear, but of theoretical concern, is whether patients with chemotherapy-induced nerve damage or compromised PNBF from diabetes or atherosclerosis are more prone to peripheral neurotoxicity. Human experience again suggests this is not a major concern, but nevertheless one might well consider using lower local anesthetic concentrations and avoiding epinephrine or using a lower concentration (2.5 µg/mL; 1:400,000) in these patient groups.

Needle-Related Injury

The contribution of needle trauma to perioperative peripheral nerve injury remains controversial, particularly regarding the roles of paresthesiae, needle tip design, and the peripheral nerve stimulator (Box 14-2). There is significant debate regarding what the subjective appreciation of a paresthesia signifies: needle touching the nerve, needle entering the nerve, or needle causing indirect pressure on the nerve as it encounters perineural tissues. Paresthesiae *per se* are almost certainly not sentinels of nerve injury, but rather indicate some degree of needle-to-nerve proximity, which the practitioner may interpret as endpoint or warning sign. Large human studies and closed claim analysis are conflicting regarding whether or not nerve injury is consistently associated with concurrent elicitation of a paresthesia. Much clearer is the observation that persistent paresthesia during block placement or pain on injection (indicating intraneural injection) is frequently a factor present in reports of perioperative nerve injury.

Linking needle design to nerve injury is similarly controversial. The commonly held perception that short

beveled (dull) needles cause less nerve injury than long beveled (sharp) needles does not withstand scientific scrutiny. Animal models demonstrate that actual nerve penetration is more difficult to accomplish with a dull needle; but once penetrated, nerves so damaged sustain more intense fascicular disruption and take longer to heal compared with a sharp needle. Similarly, electrophysiological studies normalize much sooner following nerve penetration by a sharp needle. There are no human randomized clinical trials (RCTs) clearly demonstrating a cause-and-effect relationship between paresthesia/needle injury and perioperative nerve injury, or the superiority of one needle design over another.

A final controversy involves the use of peripheral nerve stimulators (PNSs) as an aid for nerve localization during peripheral blockade. Advocates suggest that the PNS is safer and more comfortable for patients; and indeed some studies report a lower incidence of unintentional paresthesia elicitation when a PNS is used. No RCT supports a safety advantage or increased block success rate with the use of a PNS as compared with either paresthesia-seeking or transvascular techniques. Furthermore, a PNS is not protective against nerve injury when used as a localization tool in anesthetized or heavily sedated patients (Fig. 14-4).

Dual insult may be necessary to cause clinically significant nerve injury. Needle-to-nerve proximity *per se*

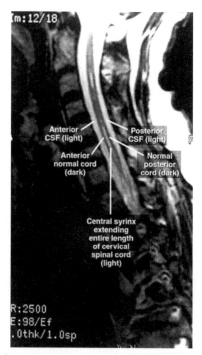

Figure 14-4 Spinal cord syrinx following interscalene block. Magnetic resonance image of a cervical spinal cord central syrinx caused by intramedullary injection of local anesthetic during an interscalene block in an anesthetized patient. (Reproduced from Benumof JL: Permanent loss of cervical spinal cord function associated with interscalene block performed under general anesthesia, *Anesthesiology* 93:1541–1544, 2000.)

Box 14-2 Dispelling the Myths of Preventing Perioperative Nerve Injury

Short beveled (dull) needles are no safer than long beveled (sharp) needles

Paresthesiae *per se* are neither indicative nor predictive of peripheral nerve injury

Peripheral nerve stimulators do not protect against nerve injury

Peripheral nerve stimulators are not protective against intraneural or intraspinal cord injection in anesthetized or heavily sedated patients

may have little clinical significance; in fact, electroneurographers routinely place small electrode needles intraneurally without apparent damage. Similarly, applying local anesthetics, with or without epinephrine, to intact peripheral nerve does not cause injury. However, experimental animal evidence and clinical experience suggests that the combination of nerve–blood barrier disruption (as from an intraneural injection) and a chemical insult (as from a local anesthetic, particularly with epinephrine) may indeed heighten the risk of neural injury. The obvious clinical message is to carefully avoid intraneural injection of local anesthetic solutions, which further implies avoiding peripheral or neuraxial nerve blocks in most sedated or anesthetized patients. The latter point is well documented by case reports of nerve and spinal cord injury following interscalene block in anesthetized patients (Fig. 14-4 on p. 162). Whether this principle holds for other peripheral blocks is uncertain.

Infectious Complications

Perineural infection is distinctly rare after regional anesthetic techniques. Superficial infections after single-shot peripheral nerve block are uncommon, even in otherwise "dirty areas" such as the groin or axilla. Deep tissue infections following either single-shot or continuous peripheral techniques are distinctly rare. Continuous catheter techniques result in no increased infection risk after peripheral block.

SUGGESTED READING

Bergman BD, Hebl JR, Kent J, Horlocker TT: Neurologic complications of 405 consecutive continuous axillary catheters, *Anesth Analg* 96:247–252, 2003.

Cheney RW, Domino KB, Caplan RA, Posner KL: Nerve injury associated with anesthesia. A closed claims analysis, *Anesthesiology* 90:1062–1069, 1999.

Horlocker TT, Wedel DJ: Neurologic complications of spinal and epidural anesthesia, *Reg Anesth Pain Med* 25:83–98, 2000.

Neal JM: Effects of epinephrine in local anesthetics on the central and peripheral nervous systems: neurotoxicity and neural blood flow, *Reg Anesth Pain Med* 28:124–134, 2003.

Neal JM, Hebl JR, Gerancher JC, Hogan QH: Brachial plexus anesthesia: essentials of our current understanding, *Reg Anesth Pain Med* 27:402–428, 2002.

CHAPTER 15

Regional Anesthesia and Outcome

JOSEPH M. NEAL

INTRODUCTION

Regional anesthesia and analgesia have long been postulated to play a significant role in perioperative outcome. The first evidence of this comes from the early 1900s, when the American surgeon George Crile, MD proposed the concept of anociassociation (Fig. 15-1 on p. 165), in which local anesthetic blockade of afferent signals from an injury site was theorized to be an essential component of overall anesthetic management. Since that time researchers have tried to better understand how the pre-, intra-, and postoperative use of local anesthetic blockade impacts morbidity and mortality. Although occasionally taking the argumentative slant of "regional versus general anesthesia," a more reasoned approach embraces the contributions of both modalities, just as Crile did a century ago. This chapter aims to describe the factors influencing perioperative outcome, to understand how various outcomes are impacted by regional techniques, to consider both traditional and non-traditional outcomes, and to include major morbidity as well as the more minor side effects related to ambulatory surgery.

DETERMINANTS OF OUTCOME

A mixture of surgical, patient, and anesthetic factors determine perioperative outcome. Surgical factors primarily determine a patient's risk for perioperative morbidity. Incision site is of paramount importance, with thoracic and upper abdominal incisions causing significantly more physiologic disruption than incisions of the extremities or lower abdomen. Besides causing worse pain, these operations are often associated with tissue manipulation-induced fluid shifts, altered chest wall mechanics, and cardiovascular perturbations from aortic cross clamping. Patient factors also contribute to morbidity, with increased susceptibility to complications seen in the elderly and morbidly obese, and from co-morbidities such as coronary artery disease, diabetes, pulmonary compromise, and renal insufficiency. Anesthesia and analgesia also contribute to morbidity in a variety of ways. Although most intraoperative anesthetic effects such as changes in pulmonary function secondary to inhaled anesthetic agents dissipate shortly after emergence, other factors may significantly impede normal recovery. These include residual neuromuscular blockade or opioid effects, hypothermia, and side effects from epidural analgesia (postural hypotension, motor weakness) and/or opioid analgesia (respiratory depression, sleep disturbance). Thus, perioperative complications are largely determined by surgery type, enhanced in patients with pre-existing disease, and exacerbated by the residual effects of anesthesia and analgesia (Box 15-1).

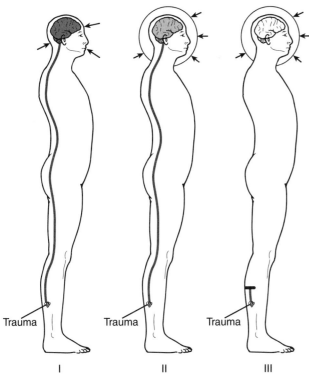

Figure 15-1   George Crile's concept of anociassociation. Optimal anesthesia and analgesia includes blocking afferent messages from the area of trauma with the use of local anesthetic. (Redrawn from Brown DL, Fink R: The history of neural blockade and pain management. In: Cousins MJ, Bridenbaugh PO (eds), *Neural Blockade in Clinical Anesthesia and Pain Management*, Third Edition, Lippincott-Raven, Philadelphia, 1998, p. 23, Fig. 1-25.)

Box 15-1   Determinants of Perioperative Outcome

Surgical factors:
    Incision site – especially thoracic and upper
        abdominal incisions
    Tissue manipulation – third space fluid shifts, edema
    Vascular cross-clamping
Patient factors:
    Pre-existing disease
    Advanced age
    Morbid obesity
Anesthetic factors:
    Temporary effects of inhalational anesthetic agents
    Residual effects of neuromuscular blockade, opioids,
        hypothermia
    Residual effects of analgesia – postural hypotension,
        motor block, respiratory depression

OUTCOME AFTER MAJOR SURGERY

Traditional Outcomes

Mortality

There is little evidence suggesting that regional anesthesia is safer than general anesthesia in terms of overall mortality. Since mortality *per se* is a relatively rare perioperative event, comparative data are mostly gleaned from meta-analysis of major outcome studies or from large quasi-clinical databases, such as Medicare coding records. Although several meta-analyses have identified a small reduction in mortality in patients undergoing regional techniques for specific surgeries such as hip repair, the clinical significance of these findings is debatable.

Analgesia

Regional analgesia techniques clearly offer superior pain control as compared with systemic opioid therapies, even those that are administered via patient-controlled analgesia (PCA). Whether utilizing continuous epidural or peripheral catheters, improved analgesia is most evident in those surgeries associated with significant postoperative pain – major thoracic and upper abdominal procedures, and joint replacement. Yet despite improved analgesia, there is no evidence that pain relief *per se* is a major contributor to improved outcomes in areas most important to health care systems, such as the speed of recovery or the incidence of perioperative complications.

Surgical Stress Response

The perioperative period is a time of intense physiologic stress leading to hypertension, tachycardia, hypercoagulability, decreased immune function, and protein wasting. These physiologic adaptations to stress become maladaptive in the postoperative period, wherein they are associated with ischemia, thromboembolic events, heightened infectious risk, and physical deconditioning. One aim of perioperative management is to attenuate these physiologic perturbations.

The surgical stress response is two pronged. The *peripheral response* entails local release of proinflammatory mediators and systemic messengers such as cytokines and interleukins. These substances cause local inflammation and sensitize the adrenal glands to respond to lower levels of circulating stress messengers. The peripheral arm can be partially blocked through the use of non-steroidal anti-inflammatory drugs and local anesthetic infiltration. The *central response* to stress consists of an afferent–efferent central nervous system loop involving the spinal cord, brain, and hypothalamic-pituitary–adrenal axis (Fig. 15-2 on p. 166). The central response ultimately results in release of adrenal stress hormones (epinephrine, norepinephrine, cortisol, etc.).

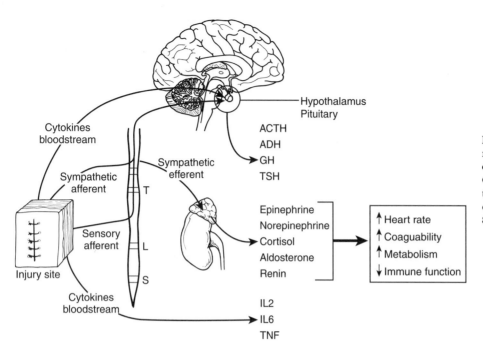

Figure 15-2   The surgical stress response: peripheral and central components. (Redrawn from Liu SS, Carpenter RL, Neal JM: Epidural anesthesia and analgesia. Their role in postoperative outcome, *Anesthesiology* 82:1489, 1995, Fig. 8.)

Importantly, only local anesthetics successfully block this non-nociceptive pathway leading to adrenal gland release, implying that attenuation of the stress response with regional techniques requires the use of neuraxial local anesthetics.

Many outcome studies have associated neuraxial local anesthetic blockade with a decrease in hormonal markers of the stress response. In most of these studies, similar reduction of cardiac, vaso-occlusive, and infectious complications has also been noted in the regional anesthesia group. However, there is no direct evidence for a "cause-and-effect" relationship between regional anesthesia-induced reduction in stress mediators and improved clinical outcome.

Cardiac

Despite creating a favorable myocardial oxygen supply/demand ratio, there is little clinical evidence that links regional anesthesia to improved cardiac outcome. High thoracic segmental local anesthetic blockade (T1–T4) reduces myocardial oxygen demand by promoting bradycardia and reducing inotropy (Fig. 15-3). The same sympathetic blockade improves oxygen delivery

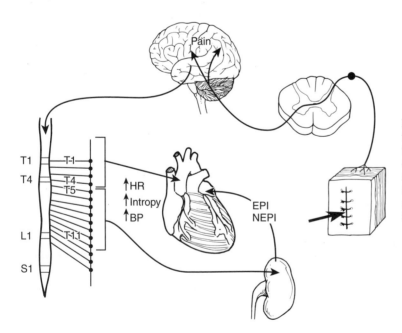

Figure 15-3   Effects of direct and indirect sympathetic stimulation on the heart. Stimulation of T1–T4 thoracic sympathetic nerves worsens indices of myocardial oxygen demand. This can be attenuated with segmental thoracic epidural anesthesia. (Redrawn from Liu SS, Carpenter RL, Neal JM: Epidural anesthesia and analgesia. Their role in postoperative outcome, *Anesthesiology* 82:1475, 1995, Fig. 1.)

by improving blood flow through atherosclerotic coronary arteries. In contrast to lumbar epidural placement that leads to dilation of lower extremity vasculature, a segmental thoracic epidural block preserves lumbar sympathetic tone, thus maintaining normal diastolic coronary perfusion pressure. Yet despite these theoretical advantages, improved cardiac outcome with regional anesthesia has been difficult to prove. One meta-analysis found a small decrease in postoperative myocardial infarction, but most randomized clinical trials fail to link improved cardiac outcome with either the intraoperative or postoperative use of epidural techniques.

Pulmonary

Most studies demonstrate improved analgesia and pulmonary function in patients randomized to the intra- and postoperative use of epidural analgesia with local anesthetic and opioid. Randomized clinical trials and meta-analysis generally support epidural analgesia as a means of reducing the incidence of true adverse pulmonary outcomes, specifically pneumonia and postoperative respiratory failure. However, these results are typically limited to those patient subsets most prone to pulmonary morbidity – the elderly, the morbidly obese, those with thoracic or upper abdominal incisions, and those with pre-existing pulmonary disease. Adjuncts such as incentive spirometry are also critical to improving pulmonary outcome. The effectiveness of epidural analgesia in improving pulmonary outcome likely stems from improved analgesia, limited opioid-induced respiratory depression, and to reversing reflex diaphragmatic inhibition and altered chest wall mechanics (Fig. 15-4).

Gastrointestinal

Individual clinical trials and meta-analysis clearly support the role of thoracic epidural local anesthetics in reducing the frequency and duration of postoperative ileus. Indeed, all studies utilizing thoracic epidural placement for over 24 hours after surgery demonstrate this advantage. Conversely, ileus is more frequent and longer lasting when parenteral opioids are used for pain control. Nevertheless, epidural anesthesia is only part of a regimen for improving gastrointestinal outcome and best results are obtained in a multimodal setting wherein surgeons aggressively feed and ambulate their patients postoperatively. The beneficial effects of epidural analgesia are likely secondary to local anesthetic blockade of sympathetic innervation to the gut, which promotes parasympathetic-induced propulsive activity (Fig. 15-5 on p. 168).

Coagulation

Regional anesthesia reduces thromboembolic and vaso-occlusive complications by up to threefold. Local anesthetics in general, and specifically when used as part of an intraoperative neuraxial technique, promote local blood flow, reduce blood viscosity, enhance fibrinolysis, and attenuate platelet aggregation, albeit at higher than the typical clinical concentrations of local anesthetics. While poorly understood, these effects have been clearly linked to reduced thromboembolic complications following hip fracture repair and to fewer vaso-occlusive events after peripheral vascular surgery, including graft thrombosis, re-operation, and amputation. Particularly with regard to thromboembolic complications, little is known regarding the relative benefit of regional anesthesia as compared with pharmacologic prophylactic regimens, including possible value added by intelligently combining intraoperative regional anesthesia (when clots most commonly form) with postoperative thromboprophylaxis.

Non-traditional Outcomes

Most outcome studies focus on the more traditional morbidities detailed above, but non-traditional outcomes are also important. These outcomes include the effects of anesthetic technique on rehabilitation, patient satisfaction, and cost.

The ultimate goal of perioperative management is rehabilitating patients to their best functional capacity.

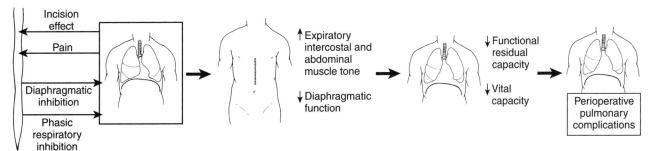

Figure 15-4   The cascade of postoperative pulmonary complications. Pain and incisional effects lead to diaphragmatic inhibition and altered chest wall mechanics, which in turn reduce pulmonary function, and ultimately lead to hypoxemia, pneumonia, and respiratory failure. (Redrawn from Liu SS, Carpenter RL, Neal JM: Epidural anesthesia and analgesia. Their role in postoperative outcome, *Anesthesiology* 82:1482, 1995, Fig. 6.)

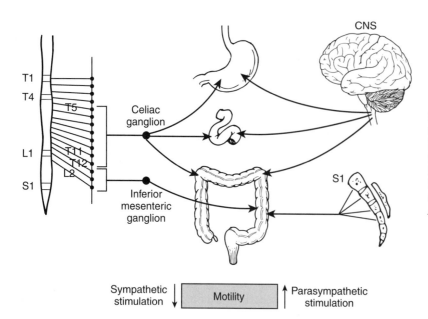

Figure 15-5   Effects of sympathetic stimulation on the gastrointestinal tract. Segmental blockade of T5–L2 sympathetic fibers tips the balance towards parasympathetic stimulation (right side of figure), which promotes gut motility. (Redrawn from Liu SS, Carpenter RL, Neal JM: Epidural anesthesia and analgesia. Their role in postoperative outcome, *Anesthesiology* 82:1487, 1995, Fig. 7.)

Clinical Controversy: Relative Strength of Evidence That Regional Anesthesia/Analgesia Positively Impacts Perioperative Outcome

Weak evidence:
   Mortality
   Cardiac outcome
Equivocal evidence:
   Attenuation of surgical stress response
   Pulmonary outcome, other than a reduced incidence
      of pneumonia
Strong evidence:
   Superior analgesia
   Reduced incidence and duration of ileus
   Reduced thromboembolic and vaso-occlusive events

Specific goals include limiting the physical deconditioning inherent to serious illness, improving the quality of sleep and nutrition, and returning the patient to normal activities. To these ends, there is some evidence to suggest that perioperative regional techniques are beneficial. For instance, clinical trials show that patients who undergo colectomy with epidural anesthesia/analgesia maintain their exercise capacity better than those treated with general anesthesia and parenteral opioid analgesia. Multimodal therapy that includes epidural analgesia has been linked to more rapid return of bowel function, improved nitrogen balance, and better quality of sleep. Total knee replacement patients who received three days of continuous femoral nerve or epidural block completed their physical rehabilitation regimen 20% sooner than those given PCA opioid.

Despite superior analgesia and association with certain measures of outcome improvement, patient satisfaction with regional techniques has been difficult to quantify. Partly due to the vagaries of measurement, improved patient satisfaction with regional analgesia has received little attention in the literature. The actual cost of providing surgical and anesthetic care is also difficult to measure, and consequently it too has received little attention in outcomes literature. The majority of studies that report cost have shown reduced cost of care in those patients randomized to the epidural anesthesia/analgesia arm of their respective clinical trial. Cost analysis must also include those costs associated with providing an epidural analgesia service, and the costs of any related side effects and complications. This issue has only been evaluated by computer modeling, wherein it appears that cost savings are possible when epidural analgesia is provided to ill patients undergoing major surgeries – an observation that curiously parallels our clinical understanding of beneficial outcome.

THE IMPORTANCE OF A MULTIMODAL APPROACH

The influence of anesthetic technique on patient outcome is controversial, confusing, and inconsistent. Scientific understanding of these issues is extremely difficult because modern perioperative outcome is generally outstanding, thus attempting to statistically prove a treatment difference in complication rates that are inherently low requires large numbers of patients. Most randomized clinical outcome trials are inadequately designed and underpowered. Two other methodologies are similarly flawed. Meta-analysis of similarly designed studies can provide adequate patient numbers, but suffers from a lack of rigorous experimental control and dissimilar management protocols. Analysis of quasi-clinical databases, such as Medicare coding records, also provides adequate patient numbers, but is limited by data entry vagaries and lack of standardized research protocols. Overall, existing studies using these various methodologies have been unsuccessful in providing definitive answers regarding the influence of anesthetic choice on perioperative outcome.

By considering the multitude of available information on this topic, and acknowledging its inadequacy, several generalizations can be formulated. First, if anesthetic choice influences outcome following major surgery, it probably does so only in those subsets of patients undergoing major surgery and especially if they have pre-existing disease of the same classification one is trying to prevent. For example, epidural analgesia likely reduces pulmonary complications in patients with preexisting pulmonary risk who are undergoing thoracic or upper abdominal surgery. Conversely, even patients with pre-existing cardiac disease are afforded little if any risk reduction by thoracic epidural anesthesia/analgesia during and following abdominal aortic aneurysm repair.

A second generalization is that a multimodal approach to patient management is crucial to attaining superior outcomes. Multimodal management refers to patient care that involves coordinated, aggressive input from all key players of the perioperative team. From the anesthetic viewpoint, it implies not only the placement of an epidural catheter, but its active management to optimize pain control and ambulation while limiting side effects such as postural hypotension. Further, it means modulating the stress response using various anesthetic approaches, both central and peripheral. Surgeons also play a role, because superior analgesia, improved gut propulsion, and pain-free ambulation are only beneficial if surgical management capitalizes on those gains by promoting early extubation, feeding, ambulation, and stepwise progression towards discharge milestones. Similarly, nurses and physical therapists must make maximal use of analgesia and physiologic advantage to accomplish standardized goals. The importance of multimodal management cannot be overemphasized. Without it, any potential advantage made possible by anesthetic technique is never realized. Indeed, if there is a common theme in outcome studies, it is that the more a team-based multimodal effort is utilized in overall patient management, the more likely outcome improvement is to occur.

OUTCOME AFTER AMBULATORY SURGERY

The likelihood of major cardiac, respiratory, or gastrointestinal morbidity occurring after ambulatory surgery is quite small. Nevertheless, important side effects can

---

Clinical Caveat: Importance of Multimodal Management

Interpretation of perioperative outcome literature suggests that multimodal management of the patient is essential if physiologic gains from regional anesthesia/analgesia are to result in less morbidity. Without a multidisciplinary commitment to using superior analgesia, improved ambulation, or reduced ileus as a means of moving patients along a standardized pathway towards the achievement of discharge milestones, none of these goals will be reached. Such milestones include early extubation, ambulation, feeding, and hospital discharge, along with physical rehabilitation, resumption of exercise, and return to work.

---

impact the outpatient setting, where pain control, prevention of postoperative nausea and vomiting (PONV), and time to discharge are the principal indicators of patient satisfaction.

Analgesia

Patients and caregivers expect adequate pain control after ambulatory procedures. Indeed, failure to control pain is a primary reason for unplanned hospital admission. The use of local anesthetic block is a valuable adjunct for managing these patients, particularly to the extent that it reduces side effects inherent to opioid analgesia, such as PONV, sedation, and respiratory depression. Local anesthetic block does not necessarily imply individual peripheral nerve or plexus block. Local anesthesia via subcutaneous infiltration, intra-articular instillation, or surgeon-placed field block can frequently accomplish the same goal.

Postoperative Nausea and Vomiting

Besides uncontrolled pain, PONV is a frequently cited reason for unplanned admission and patient dissatisfaction. Regional anesthesia's role in reducing PONV is somewhat dependent on adjunctive management of sedation and analgesia. With the exception of intraoperative nausea and vomiting associated with neuraxial anesthesia, regional techniques *per se* are not strongly linked to PONV, and therefore it is intuitive that PONV occurs less frequently when regional anesthetics are used. However, proof for this contention is inconsistent because of the difficulty in separating the influence of perioperative sedation and analgesic routines from the regional anesthetic. Concurrent intraoperative sedation with benzodiazepines, opioids, or barbiturates increases the risk of PONV, as does the postoperative use of opioids after the regional block has dissipated. Thus, while regional anesthesia techniques in isolation can clearly reduce the incidence of PONV, the adjunctive use of emetogenic drugs tends to counteract this advantage.

Discharge Time

Comparative studies consistently demonstrate that discharge times are shortest when monitored anesthesia care is combined with local anesthetic infiltration by the surgeon. The use of neuraxial or peripheral nerve blocks can favorably or unfavorably impact discharge time from several aspects. The intelligent selection of local anesthetic is key to controlling readiness for discharge following neuraxial blocks. Since "dose is duration," spinal anesthetics that employ higher dose lidocaine (50–75 mg) result in slower discharge times than those using lower dose lidocaine (30–40 mg) with adjuvant fentanyl. Similarly, bupivacaine spinal anesthesia (unless used in low 3–6 mg doses with fentanyl) prolongs time to discharge, as does the selection of epidural lidocaine as compared with 2-chloroprocaine. Long-acting neuraxial anesthesia also impacts discharge time if voiding is required before patient discharge. Recent evidence suggests that voiding requirements may not be mandatory except in patients at risk for postoperative urinary retention – those with prostatic hypertrophy and/or undergoing perirectal or inguinal hernia surgeries. Peripheral nerve blocks typically facilitate rapid discharge. It is unnecessary to require resolution of peripheral block prior to discharge, provided the anesthetized limb is adequately protected from trauma or stretch injury.

SUGGESTED READING

Kehlet H: Multimodal approach to control postoperative pathophysiology and rehabilitation, *Br J Anaesth* 78:606–617, 1997.

Liu SS, Carpenter RL, Neal JM: Epidural anesthesia and analgesia. Their role in postoperative outcome, *Anesthesiology* 82:1474–1506, 1995.

Neal JM, McDonald SB: Regional anesthesia and analgesia: outcome and cost effectiveness. In: Neal JM, Mulroy MF, Liu SS (eds), *Problems in Anesthesia*, Lippincott, Williams & Wilkins, Philadelphia, 2000, pp. 188–198.

Norris EJ, Beattie C, Perler BA, et al.: Double-masked randomized trial comparing alternate combinations of intraoperative anesthesia and postoperative analgesia in abdominal aortic surgery, *Anesthesiology* 95:1054–1067, 2001.

Rigg JR, Jamrozik K, Myles PS, et al.: MASTER Anaesthesia Trial Study Group. Epidural anaesthesia and analgesia and outcome of major surgery: a randomized trial, *Lancet* 359:1276–1282, 2002.

Rodgers A, Walker N, Schug S, et al.: Reduction of postoperative mortality and morbidity with epidural or spinal anaesthesia: results from overview of randomised trials, *BMJ* 321:1–12, 2000.

Wu CL, Fleisher LA: Outcomes research in regional anesthesia and analgesia, *Anesth Analg* 91:1232–1242, 2000.

SPECIALITY CONSIDERATIONS

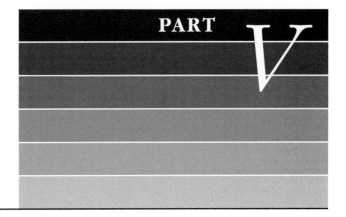

CHAPTER 6

Obstetric Anesthesia

CHRISTOPHER M. VISCOMI

INTRODUCTION

Anesthetic care of the pregnant mother and her developing fetus presents the anesthesiologist with unique challenges along with the opportunity for a gratifying physician–patient relationship. Many anesthesiologists are wary of obstetric anesthesia in the contemporary litigious environment. Indeed, in the USA, cesarean delivery results in malpractice claims against anesthesiologists more often than any other surgical procedure. Anesthesia is the sixth leading cause of obstetric death in the USA. Among anesthesia-related maternal deaths, general anesthesia for cesarean delivery is grossly over-represented: the maternal anesthetic mortality rate with general anesthesia is nearly 17 times that of regional anesthesia (Box 16-1).

Given the excellent safety record of general anesthesia for most surgical procedures, why is general anesthesia seemingly so dangerous for cesarean delivery? Morbid obesity, emergency surgery, and pre-eclampsia are the three primary risk factors for maternal anesthetic death. These factors are related to request for general anesthesia, a higher incidence of difficulties with regional anesthesia, and relative contraindications to regional anesthesia (thrombocytopenia with pre-eclampsia). Thus, those patients who require general anesthesia for cesarean delivery are likely just the group one would suspect to be at highest risk for complications. In addition, due to the mucosal edema of the airway during pregnancy, endotracheal intubation of the parturient is notoriously difficult. Failed endotracheal intubations occur ten times more frequently in the pregnant patient compared to the non-pregnant surgical population. Normal physiologic changes that occur during pregnancy lead to high oxygen consumption and relaxation of lower esophageal sphincter tone (resulting in esophageal reflux). In combination, these factors both place the parturient at risk for hypoxia and aspiration on induction of general anesthesia.

To avoid the dangers of general anesthesia for cesarean delivery, the anesthesiologist must be knowledgeable and skillful in the use of regional anesthesia for routine and high-risk obstetric anesthesia. Regional anesthesia is likely to yield a safe, comfortable childbirth experience and an appreciative patient.

LABOR PAIN PATHWAYS

First Stage of Labor

Labor pain can be thought of as two distinct sequential pain experiences (Fig. 16-1). First-stage pain primarily relates to regular uterine contractions with stretching and dilation of the cervix. The first stage of labor can be divided into latent and active phases. The latent phase begins with the onset of regular uterine contractions and ends when cervical dilation accelerates (after 4–5 cm of cervical dilation); the active phase begins at this point and ends when cervical dilation is complete. Pain fibers from the uterus coalesce near the cervix in the right and left cervical plexi. A "paracervical block" can be used to anesthetize the cervical plexus directly.

Visceral afferent fibers travel from the paracervical region to join the hypogastric plexus, a loose collection of nerve fibers that transmit both afferent (visceral nociceptive) and efferent (sympathetic motor) impulses to structures within the pelvis. From the hypogastric plexus, pain transmission is carried toward the spinal cord in the lumbar paravertebral sympathetic chain. Nociceptive impulses enter the spinal cord via the dorsal nerve roots of T_{10}-L_1 before ascending toward higher centers via the spinothalamic tracts.

Second Stage of Labor

Near the end of the first stage of labor, the fetal head begins to descend causing perineal distention and activation of somatic nociceptive pathways. These somatic pain impulses are transmitted primarily via the pudendal nerves, which originate from the second through fourth sacral nerves. The somatic pain that arises during the latter part of the first stage and the second stage of labor occurs in addition to ongoing visceral pain of uterine contractions. Bilateral pudendal nerve blocks are occasionally employed during the second stage of

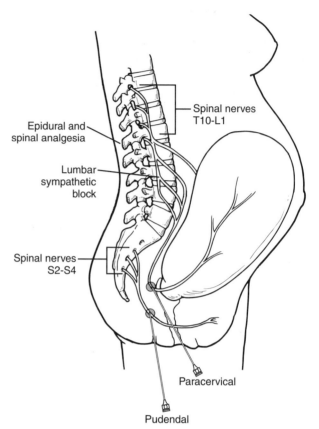

Figure 16-1   Major nociceptive pathways carrying pain signals during labor and delivery. Pain during the first stage of labor enters the central nervous system via the T10–L1 nerve roots; these visceral afferent signals from the uterus travel via the hypogastric plexus and can be blocked using paracervical block. Closer to the neuraxis, lumbar sympathetic block can be used to block pain during the first stage. Pain during the second stage of labor travels to the S2–S4 spinal nerve roots via the pudendal nerve and can be relieved via blockade of the pudendal nerve at the ischial spine. Neuraxial blocks (spinal and epidural analgesia) can successfully block pain throughout both stages of labor.

labor; they will relieve the pain of vaginal distention, but will have no effect on the pain of uterine contraction (Box 16-2).

Box 16-2   The Stages of Labor

	STAGE 1	STAGE 2
Definition	From onset of labor through complete dilation of the cervix	From complete dilation of the cervix through delivery
Pain type	Visceral	Visceral and somatic
Nerve roots carrying nociceptive signals	T_{10}-L_1	S_2-S_4

Psychologic Approaches to Analgesia during Labor and Delivery

Patient education, a supportive environment, and training with non-pharmacologic analgesic techniques all appear to have positive impact on labor pain, particularly during the latent phase (early first stage). Nulliparous patients who have undergone prenatal education report about 15% less pain compared to patients who have not had such training. Severe pain during early labor is predictive of a long labor and a high probability of operative vaginal delivery (vacuum extraction or forceps) or cesarean delivery.

Parenteral Pharmacologic Therapy

Opioids form the mainstay of maternal systemic analgesia. Nearly all opioids have been used to provide analgesia during labor, including morphine, meperidine, fentanyl, and remifentanil. Because of a shorter redistribution half-life, these last two agents (fentanyl and remifentanil) are typically administered via an intravenous patient-controlled analgesia (PCA) device.

Morphine has limited application in contemporary obstetric practice because of higher rates of maternal and neonatal respiratory depression compared to meperidine or fentanyl. Meperidine is probably the most commonly used opioid in labor. Normeperidine, the principal metabolite of meperidine, has significant analgesic and respiratory depressant effects. Normeperidine levels peak in the fetus one to three hours after maternal intramuscular injection, leading some to advocate against maternal administration if delivery is anticipated within one to three hours. However, large studies examining the administration of meperidine during labor via an intravenous PCA device showed no association with delayed respiratory depression in neonates.

Partial agonist and mixed agonist–antagonist opioids such as butorphanol and nalbuphine are employed at some centers. These agents have an inherent "ceiling effect" on both analgesia and respiratory depression. At low doses, they act primarily as agonists at the κ-opioid receptor, providing analgesia and causing some depressant effects on respiration. At higher doses, they competitively antagonize the binding of other opioids at the μ-opioid receptor, reversing analgesia and respiratory depression. These agents do provide modest analgesia and they may infer some safety against the respiratory depressant effects of pure opioid agonists. However, significant respiratory depression can still occur in opioid naïve patients with the agonist–antagonist agents. These agents will precipitate opioid withdrawal symptoms when they are given to patients who are regularly taking opioids (via prescription for chronic pain or in those abusing opioids like heroin).

Paracervical Block

Clinical uses. This block is performed almost exclusively by the obstetrician to control first-stage labor pain, but it is rarely performed in contemporary obstetric practice because of its associated high rate of fetal bradycardia. Perhaps the most common use of this block is for cervical dilation and uterine curettage (d&c). In combination with light sedation, a paracervical block provides good analgesia for d&c in patients that are not optimal candidates for spinal or general anesthesia.

Anatomy. Visceral pain fibers from the uterus and cervix coalesce in the lateral fornix of the upper vaginal canal. This collection of nerves is termed the cervical plexus or Frankenhauser's ganglion (Box 16-3).

Technique. A 14 cm 22 gauge needle is used, and care must be taken to limit needle penetration to the submucosa (Fig. 16-2 on p. 176). One instrument (the Iowa trumpet) is used for paracervical and pudendal blocks, and limits the advance of the block needle beyond the "trumpet." Local anesthetic (5–10 mL) is injected at three and nine o'clock. Duration of analgesia varies from 45 to 90 minutes.

Complications. Because of proximity to the uterine artery, paracervical injection may lead to high levels of local anesthetics in the fetus. Indeed, up to 70% of fetuses will have arrhythmias (principally *bradycardia*) within ten minutes of injection. Fetal deaths from bupivacaine cardiotoxicity have also been reported. In addition, injections have occasionally been made directly into the fetal scalp. Because anesthesia lasts only 45–90 minutes,

---

Box 16-3 Paracervical Block

Cervical plexus (Frankenhauser's ganglion) lies just beneath the mucosa in the lateral fornix of the vagina, where the vaginal mucosa meets the cervical mucosa

With the cervix viewed from the introitus with the position nearest the anterior abdominal wall defined as the twelve o'clock position, local anesthetic is injected submucosally at the three and nine o'clock positions in the lateral fornix

There is a high rate of fetal bradycardia associated with paracervical block, likely due to high local anesthetic concentrations reaching the fetus

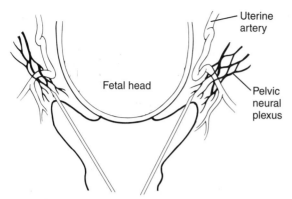

Figure 16-2   Neurovascular anatomy associated with paracervical block. (Redrawn from Bloom SL, Horswill CW, Curet LB: Effects of paracervical blocks on the fetus during labor: a prospective study with the use of direct fetal monitoring, *Am J Obstet Gynecol* 114: 218, 1972.)

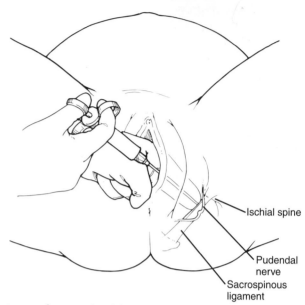

Figure 16-3   Pudendal nerve block, transvaginal approach. (Redrawn from Cousins MJ, Bridenbaugh PO (eds): *Neural Blockade*, Third Edition, Lippincott-Raven, Philadelphia, 1998, p. 573.)

frequent re-injection may be necessary. Finally, uterine artery hematoma, cervical abscess, and ureteral trauma have all been reported with paracervical block.

Pudendal Nerve Block

Clinical uses. Pudendal nerve blocks are useful in the second stage of labor to control the pain of perineal distention. This block technique is also useful for urgent forceps delivery, although the presence of the fetal head in the vagina can make needle placement difficult or impossible. The block is also useful for providing analgesia for repair of more extensive episiotomy incisions or lacerations. As with paracervical block, the pudendal block is almost always placed by the obstetrician.

Anatomy. The pudendal nerves arise from the second through fourth sacral nerve roots and exit the pelvis via the greater sciatic foramen just superior to the ischial spine. They supply sensation to the distal portion of the vagina and the perineum. The pudendal artery and vein lie in close proximity to the nerve. The posterior femoral cutaneous nerve and the sciatic nerve lie somewhat posterior and lateral to the pudendal nerve at the level of the ischial spine.

Technique. The most common approach is transvaginal (Fig. 16-3). With the patient in the lithotomy position, the ischial spine is palpated on one side, and the 22 gauge block needle is advanced posterior to the ischial spine, with a slight posterior and lateral orientation of the needle. Advancing the needle 1–1.5 cm should place the needle tip through the sacrospinous ligament. After negative aspiration, 10 mL of a fast-acting local anesthetic (1% lidocaine or 2% chloroprocaine) is deposited on each side.

Complications. The pudendal artery and vein lie in close proximity to the nerve, thus intravascular injection can easily occur. The sciatic nerve lies just posterior and

---

Box 16-4   Pudendal Nerve Block

Pudendal nerve block provides good pain control during the second stage of labor, during forceps delivery, and for episiotomy repair

Complications include direct injection into the fetal scalp, maternal intravascular injection, and sciatic nerve block and/or injury

---

lateral to the ischial spine. One to five percent of patients note transient pain in the sciatic nerve distribution after pudendal nerve blocks (Box 16-4).

Lumbar Sympathetic Nerve Block

Pain during the first stage of labor is transmitted via sympathetic afferent fibers that enter the central nervous system after traversing the lumbar paravertebral sympathetic chain. Before epidural analgesia was popularized, bilateral lumbar sympathetic blocks were occasionally utilized for the first stage of labor pain. Needle placement without x-ray guidance (available in most pain clinics, but rarely used in obstetrics) can be difficult and is uncomfortable. The brief duration of analgesia (45–60 minutes) and the widespread availability of spinal and epidural analgesia have all but eliminated the use of selective lumbar sympathetic blockade during labor. The anatomy and technique of lumbar sympathetic blockade are discussed in more detail in Chapter 11.

NEURAXIAL TECHNIQUES FOR LABOR

Neuraxial techniques (spinal and epidural analgesia and anesthesia) are the mainstays of contemporary obstetric anesthetic practice.

Spinal Analgesia

Spinal analgesia can provide effective pain relief during labor. It is a particularly useful technique when delivery is expected within two hours. Spinal analgesia is also a means of providing pain relief in smaller hospitals where trained anesthesia personnel are not available to staff a full labor epidural service.

The advantages of spinal analgesia include rapid onset of analgesia, potential for minimal motor block, little or no risk of systemic local anesthetic toxicity, minimal drug transfer to the fetus, and modest anesthesiologist staffing demands. The major constraint of spinal analgesia during labor is related to its limited duration, which can be problematic when the remaining duration of labor is unknown. When labor outlasts the duration of the spinal analgesic, the block must be repeated or the patient will deliver in pain. Efforts to overcome this fundamental limitation involve using either larger doses of the spinal drugs or agents with longer duration. Both approaches carry risks: larger doses often lead to more side effects, and the use of drugs with longer duration often results in effects that far outlast labor and delivery (Box 16-5).

The most common agents used for spinal analgesia during labor are longer-acting local anesthetics (most commonly bupivacaine), lipophilic opioids (most commonly fentanyl or sufentanil), and adjuvant drugs, such as epinephrine. Drugs are almost always used in combination to gain rapid onset, sufficient duration, and additive or synergistic analgesic effects. Synergy between spinally administered local anesthetic and opioid is most potent for visceral pain (first stage of labor) and less so for somatic pain (second stage labor). Clinically, these drug combinations provide good to fair analgesia during the first stage of labor, and fair to poor analgesia during the second stage of labor.

Bupivacaine is the most common local anesthetic used for spinal labor analgesia. Small doses (1.5-3 mg) of an isobaric solution are generally used. Higher bupivacaine doses cause significant motor block and increase the risk of hypotension. Opioids are also frequently used, either alone or in combination with bupivacaine. Fentanyl (10-25 μg) or sufentanil (2-5 μg) provide a rapid analgesic effect with approximately 90 minute duration. Higher doses of sufentanil (10 μg) were once routinely used, but were associated with a higher incidence of fetal bradycardia and occasional maternal respiratory depression. When delivery is not expected for more than two hours, morphine may be used. Intrathecal morphine has been associated with delayed respiratory depression as much as 18 hours after injection. Urinary retention, pruritus, and nausea/vomiting are all significantly more common with this drug than with either fentanyl or sufentanil. Some practitioners administer continuous infusions of low-dose naloxone or oral naltrexone after delivery to diminish the side effect profile of intrathecal morphine. Including epinephrine in the intrathecal injectate increases analgesic duration (by as much as 45 minutes with some drug combinations). However, the incidence of nausea and motor block increase with the addition of epinephrine.

Box 16-5 Spinal Analgesia for Labor

ADVANTAGES

Technically simple
Rapid onset of analgesia
Low likelihood of systemic local anesthetic toxicity
Minimal fetal drug transfer
Minimal motor block
Modest staffing demands

DISADVANTAGES

Must be repeated if labor continues beyond the duration of analgesia
Side effects are common with long-acting drug combinations
Long-acting drug combinations may outlast labor
Analgesia is often insufficient during the second stage of labor

---

Clinical Pearl: Spinal Analgesic Drug Combinations

DELIVERY EXPECTED IN 1–2 HOURS

Isobaric bupivacaine 2.5 mg
Sufentanil 2.5 μg
Epinephrine 50 μg

DELIVERY EXPECTED IN >2 HOURS

Isobaric bupivacaine 2.5 mg
Sufentanil 2.5 μg
Morphine 0.1 mg
Epinephrine 50 μg
Oral naltrexone 25 mg after delivery

Epidural and Combined Spinal–Epidural Analgesia

Epidural and combined spinal–epidural (CSE) techniques are the most common and effective techniques for providing analgesia during labor and anesthesia for cesarean delivery. Modern techniques allow rapid initiation of analgesia, minimal motor block, patient autonomy using patient-controlled epidural analgesia (PCEA), flexibility for varying clinical situations that evolve, and unlimited duration of effect.

Epidural analgesia and anesthesia using local anesthetics have been in widespread use for many decades. Early practitioners who used this technique for labor analgesia tended to use high concentrations of local anesthetic alone. While this afforded excellent labor pain relief, it was often at the expense of significant motor blockade and frequent hypotension. Initiating analgesia with minimal motor block is an essential element in contemporary obstetric analgesia. This can be accomplished by one of two means: using high-volume, low-concentration epidural medications or by using CSE analgesia. Both techniques involve the analgesic synergy of a local anesthetic (typically, bupivacaine or ropivacaine) in combination with a lipophilic opioid (typically, fentanyl or sufentanil) (Box 16-6).

The most common risks associated with epidural analgesia during labor result from the consequences of sympathetic blockade or the unrecognized misplacement of the epidural catheter in a vein or the intrathecal space. Hypotension after initiation of epidural or CSE techniques occurs in approximately 10% of cases and typically is most pronounced at 15–20 minutes after initiation of neural blockade. Because uterine blood flow is directly proportional to uterine arterial pressure (i.e. there is no autoregulation), maternal hypotension can lead to inadequate fetal–placental perfusion. After initiation of labor analgesia, patients should be placed in a full or partial lateral position. This prevents aortocaval compression by the gravid uterus, which may dramatically impede venous return. Hypovolemia should be corrected by using intravenous hydration prior to placing the block. An intravenous bolus of crystalloid solution (e.g. 500 mL of Lactated Ringer's solution) modestly reduces the incidence of significant hypotension following initiation of either spinal or epidural analgesia. If the maternal blood pressure falls in excess of 20% of the pre-block level or any new fetal heart rate abnormalities appear, small doses of an intravenous vasopressor should be used to correct the hypotension. The most common agent used is ephedrine (5–10 mg intravenously); small doses of phenylephrine (50 μg) have been shown to cause significant uterine arterial constriction in experimental animals, but use of this agent has been repeatedly demonstrated to be safe in humans.

Clinical Caveat: Hypotension after Placement of a Labor Epidural

The incidence of hypotension may be reduced with adequate hydration prior to initiating epidural analgesia and an intravenous bolus of crystalloid immediately before block placement (e.g. 500 mL of Lactated Ringer's solution)

After block placement, the mother should be placed in the lateral decubitus position to reduce aortocaval compression

Maternal blood pressure decrease of more than 20% should be treated promptly with an intravenous vasopressor (e.g. ephedrine 5–10 mg)

Any decline in maternal blood pressure that is accompanied by a new fetal heart rate abnormality should be treated promptly with supplemental oxygen, intravenous crystalloid, and a vasopressor

---

Placement of the epidural catheter into an epidural vein occurs in approximately 5% of obstetric patients. This frequency is much higher than in the nonobstetric population due to epidural vein engorgement caused by compression of the vena cava by the gravid uterus. If intravenous placement goes unrecognized, systemic local anesthetic toxicity, manifest as seizures or cardiac toxicity, may result. Intravenous placement typically occurs with initial epidural catheter placement, but may occur hours later, likely due to catheter movement as the patient changes position. Epidural vein cannulation can be reduced by two practices. First, loss-of-resistance technique using a saline-filled syringe rather than an air-filled syringe has a lower rate of venous cannulation. Second, use of epidural catheters with soft, pliable tips rather than those that are stiff or have a metal stylette lowers the rate of venous cannulation. If venous cannulation does occur, blood will often spontaneously appear in the epidural catheter. Gentle aspiration of the catheter may also reveal blood. The reliability of aspiration of the catheter revealing venous cannulation is highly dependent on catheter design. Older single-orifice catheters were unreliable: only 50% of intravenous catheters could be identified via catheter aspiration. Conversely, modern multiorifice catheters will allow visible blood aspiration in 90–99% of intravenous cannulations. It is important to keep in mind that an

---

Box 16-6 Advantages of Epidural Analgesia for Labor

Rapid initiation of analgesia
Minimal motor block
Unlimited duration
Adaptable to various clinical scenarios

epidural catheter may well be intravenous even when there is no blood seen during aspiration through the catheter.

To detect intravenous or intrathecal catheter placement, many clinicians utilize a "test dose" via the epidural catheter. The goal of a test dose is to administer a drug that will reliably identify intravascular or intrathecal cannulation without undue risk to mother or fetus. A common test dose used to rule out intravenous placement is 3 mL of 1:200,000 epinephrine (15 μg). A rapid increase in maternal heart rate (>20 beats per minute) within 30 seconds identifies epidural vein injection. Because maternal heart rate also increases during active contractions, some recommend timing test dose injection with the end of the previous contraction. Even with this approach, interpretation of epinephrine test doses in the parturient can be challenging. Furthermore, the hemodynamic changes that accompany a true intravenous bolus of 15 μg of epinephrine may be problematic in patients with pregnancy-induced hypertension. Therefore, epinephrine-containing test doses are relatively contraindicated in the pre-eclamptic population. The prudent clinician always "fractionates" local anesthetic boluses given via the epidural catheter. This term means dividing the intended dose into 3-4 smaller doses administered over 5-10 minutes. Any previously functioning epidural catheter that suddenly becomes ineffective should be suspected of having migrated into an epidural vein.

Epidural catheters can also be unknowingly placed in the intrathecal space. If local anesthetic doses used to produce epidural analgesia are given intrathecally, total spinal anesthesia manifesting as hypotension and respiratory arrest may follow. The local anesthetic dose required for typical spinal anesthesia is approximately 15% of the dose required for epidural anesthesia, and therefore, if a typical epidural dose is unintentionally administered spinally, a rapid spinal block involving the phrenic nerve, all sympathetic nerve fibers, and the brainstem will occur. This is clinically termed "total spinal anesthesia." Prevention of total spinal anesthesia is similar to the previous discussion of intravascular epidural catheters. Spontaneous flow of cerebrospinal fluid (CSF) can sometimes be observed from either the epidural needle or catheter. Epidural catheters should always be "aspirated" prior to any dose administered. The appearance of clear to blood-tinged fluid suggests intrathecal placement of the epidural catheter. Many clinicians utilize a "test dose" to identify spinal placement. This test dose contains an amount of local anesthetic that would provide a recognizable and safe spinal anesthetic if injected intrathecally. Because of the large differences in dose requirements, this dose of local anesthetic should be insufficient to cause a significant epidural block. Lidocaine 45 mg is frequently chosen for this purpose. Typically, 3 mL of 1.5% lidocaine with 1:200,000 epinephrine is administered as a combined intravascular and intrathecal test dose. A rapid rise in maternal heart rate suggests an intravascular catheter, while a significant sensory block developing over 2-5 minutes suggests an intrathecal

catheter. Epidural blocks that seem unusually high or "dense" suggest unintentional spinal placement.

Clinical Caveat: Avoiding Systemic Local Anesthetic Toxicity and Total Spinal Anesthesia

Loss-of-resistance using a saline-filled syringe and use of a soft, unstyletted epidural catheter are associated with lower rates of intravascular cannulation

Multiorifice epidural catheters are more reliable in identifying intravascular cannulation with catheter aspiration compared to single-orifice catheters

Carefully observe and aspirate both the epidural needle and the epidural catheter for spontaneous return of blood or CSF

Give an appropriate test dose. Three milliliters of 1.5% lidocaine with 1:200,000 epinephrine is commonly chosen. Use a pulse oximeter to objectively evaluate heart rate changes. Observe and question patient for 4-5 minutes about a sudden sensory change in the lower extremities and pelvis

Fractionate local anesthetic dose into 3-5 mL increments given every 4-5 minutes. After each increment, observe for any signs of intravascular or intrathecal placement

Always be suspicious. A sudden, poorly functioning labor epidural may have migrated intravenously. An unusually "dense" sensory or motor block may indicate an unintentional intrathecal catheter placement or migration

Suggested Labor Epidural Dose Regimens

Modern obstetric analgesia aims for substantial decrease (but not elimination) of labor pain/pressure and avoidance of maternal motor block. Maternal motor block is suspected (but not proven) of increasing the likelihood of malrotation of the fetal head (presentations other than occiput anterior) and impaired maternal pushing ability.

After initial epidural bolus dosing, patients can be started on either a continuous epidural infusion (CEI) or patient-controlled epidural analgesia (PCEA) pump. The goal of both devices is to provide sufficient, but not excessive, analgesia. PCEA is rapidly gaining popularity in obstetric analgesia. PCEA allows substantial patient control, which enhances satisfaction. Patients typically consume less total drug with PCEA compared to CEI, require fewer anesthetic personnel interventions, have no increased side effects, and have very high satisfaction. PCEA is particularly useful near the end of the first stage of labor, when descent of the fetal head activates pain transmission via the pudendal nerve (S_{2-4}). This requires extension of the epidural to block the sacral nerve roots (Box 16-7). One common regimen for epidural dosing during labor is shown in Box 16-8.

Box 16-7   Advantages of Patient-controlled Epidural Analgesia (PCEA) in Labor

Patient autonomy
Less total drug consumed
Anesthetic staffing savings
No increased side effects
Excellent patient satisfaction

Box 16-8   Recommended Labor Epidural Dosing

Aspirate catheter
Test dose: 3 mL 1.5% lidocaine with 1:200,000 epinephrine
If test dose is negative, give 15 mL of 0.125% bupivacaine plus 100 μg of fentanyl (17 mL total) in divided doses over 10 minutes
Start infusion of 0.0625% bupivacaine with 2 μg/mL fentanyl at 15 mL/hour
OR
Begin PCEA: 10 mL/hour continuous infusion
  8 mL bolus
  10 minute lockout
  34 mL/hour maximum
  Using 0.0625% bupivacaine with 2 μg/mL fentanyl

Combined Spinal–Epidural Analgesia (CSE)

Perhaps the greatest technical advance that has improved obstetric anesthesia during the last 20 years is the increased use of CSE analgesia. Prior to the late 1980s, spinal analgesia and anesthesia was reserved for cesarean delivery and rarely used as a part of labor analgesia, principally due to the high chance of postdural puncture headache in the parturient. With the development of pencil-point spinal needles (Whitacre, Sprotte, Gertie Marx), headache rate for 25–27 gauge needles has fallen below 2%. With the effectiveness of intrathecal opioid and local anesthetic combinations for providing analgesia and the lower rate of postdural puncture headache, spinal analgesia has become more useful in obstetrics.

Although some clinicians utilize "single-shot" spinal analgesia for labor, there are numerous limitations of this technique (see the discussion earlier in this chapter). However, it is possible to combine the advantages of spinal analgesia (fast onset of analgesia, profound potency of opioids delivered intrathecally) with the duration and flexibility of an epidural catheter. In addition to the faster onset and greater potency of spinal analgesia, there are a number of

additional benefits of CSE. Total neuraxial drug consumption in labor is decreased. This is principally due to minimal need for epidural medications in the first two hours after the spinal injection. Furthermore, there is an increased effectiveness of epidural medications after use of the CSE technique, presumably from facilitated epidural drug entry into the CSF via the dural opening produced during spinal placement. Another advantage of CSE is a decreased unintentional dural puncture ("wet-tap") rate with the epidural needle. Two separate studies have shown this effect at teaching centers, where dural puncture rates are typically 1–4%. The explanation for this is not entirely obvious. In this author's opinion, the likely explanation lies in the ability for the inexperienced anesthesia provider who is faced with an ambiguous loss-of-resistance to use spinal needle placement to confirm proper needle location (see Case Study box).

Case Study: How Do I Identify the Epidural Space When the Loss-of-Resistance is Less Than Convincing?

At 4:15 am, a very fatigued anesthesiology resident is attempting to place a labor epidural in a moderately obese parturient in active labor. At a depth of 5 cm, a partial loss-of-resistance to injection of saline is noted. With this "confusing" loss-of-resistance, the young doctor considers several options:

1. Continue advancing the epidural needle, knowing that an unintentional dural puncture (wet-tap) could result
2. Thread an epidural catheter at this depth. The resident has little confidence that the epidural needle is properly sited, and fears the next hour could be spent confirming errant placement, followed by replacement of the epidural catheter
3. Place a 5 inch 25 gauge Whitacre spinal needle through the epidural needle. This technique essentially uses the spinal needle like a "blind man's cane," defining the tissues deep to the tip of the epidural needle. The passage of the long spinal needle will likely provide one of three outcomes:
   CSF will be obtained, confirming that the loss-of-resistance was indeed entry into the epidural space
   The spinal needle passes easily, but no CSF is obtained. This tells the operator that the epidural needle can be cautiously advanced another 0.5–1 cm without undue fear of dural puncture
   The spinal needle encounters bone. A common "false" loss-of-resistance (loss-of-resistance that is not indicative of entry into the epidural space) is periostium

This "option 3" appears to minimize risk of dural puncture and will also diminish the likelihood of placing a nonfunctional catheter.

CSE techniques have also been associated with several other favorable outcomes. Perhaps due to minimal local anesthetic motor block, CSE labor analgesia is associated with faster cervical dilation compared to conventional epidural labor analgesia. CSE techniques have a lower rate of epidural catheter replacement during labor compared to conventional epidural catheter placement. This outcome is probably consequent to confirmation of epidural needle location by obtaining CSF via the long spinal needle. Finally, failure of an epidural to provide adequate anesthesia for cesarean delivery is more likely after conventional epidural catheter placement as compared to CSE.

Some disadvantages of CSE labor analgesia are apparent. The expense of the spinal needle adds a few dollars to the equipment costs. This may be offset by reduced drug consumption and fewer replaced epidural catheters later in labor. It is more difficult to identify subarachnoid placement of an epidural catheter when CSE analgesia is employed. One of the main reasons to "test dose" is to identify intrathecal placement of the epidural catheter. This test dose is usually accomplished by giving a small local anesthetic dose (e.g. 45 mg of lidocaine) via the epidural catheter and observing for rapid development of spinal analgesia/anesthesia (see the discussion earlier in this chapter). Critics of CSE believe that because the initial CSE dose is administered prior to placing the epidural catheter, and results in rapid spinal analgesia, it is difficult to rule out unintentional intrathecal placement of the epidural catheter. No clinical studies exist which confirm or refute this criticism. A final criticism of CSE analgesia is that ineffective epidural catheters are not discovered until the initial intrathecal block has dissipated. This is typically about 90 minutes after initiation of CSE labor analgesia. This is a clinical trade off: fewer epidural block failures with CSE, but those that do occur are not immediately apparent.

Combined Spinal–Epidural Labor Analgesia: Pharmacologic Options

In comparison to 15 years ago, the recommended doses for labor epidural analgesia have significantly decreased. Similarly, the intrathecal injectate was initially 10–20 μg of sufentanil, often combined with 2.5–5.0 mg of bupivacaine. Although analgesia was rapid, side effects were pronounced. Occasional maternal respiratory arrests occurred, likely secondary to rapid cephalad migration of sufentanil in the CSF. Pruritus was nearly universal. Motor block was much more common with bupivacaine doses >2.5 mg.

Over time, it has become evident that much lower intrathecal doses provide excellent analgesia with fewer side effects. Intrathecal injection is intended to provide rapid analgesia without motor block, whereas use of the epidural catheter provides extended duration of analgesia.

With this in mind, low-dose local anesthetic–lipophilic opioid combinations accomplish the goals of CSE. Bupivacaine 1.5–2.5 mg is frequently combined with fentanyl 6–10 μg or sufentanil 2.5 μg. Some practitioners utilize 0.0625% bupivacaine with fentanyl 2 μg/mL for epidural infusions. For the intrathecal injection, one simply uses 3 mL of this solution (1.9 mg of bupivacaine, 6 μg of fentanyl).

An important technical element is orientation of the aperture of the pencil-point spinal needle cephalad: significantly better analgesia is obtained as compared to caudal orientation. This is likely because opioid receptors are in the spinal cord, not the cauda equina.

CONTRAINDICATIONS TO REGIONAL ANESTHESIA DURING LABOR AND DELIVERY

Coagulopathy

Presence of a significant coagulopathy merits concern due to the risk of epidural hematoma, and resultant neurologic injury. The most common coagulation disturbance of pregnancy is thrombocytopenia, occurring in 1–2% of parturients. The most common etiology is pre-eclampsia, particularly in the subset of patients with pre-eclampsia known as the HELLP syndrome (*H*emolysis, *E*levated *L*iver enzymes, *L*ow *P*latelets). In prior years, many anesthesiologists refused to provide regional anesthesia if the platelet count was lower than $100,000 \times 10^9$/L. This arbitrary limit has been largely abandoned. Pregnancy is a hypercoagulable state, with elevated levels of most coagulation factors. Even with moderate levels of thrombocytopenia, very few pregnant women have a clinical coagulopathy. When confronted with a woman with thrombocytopenia, the prudent anesthesiologist performs a coagulation-directed history and physical examination. Recent onset of easy bruising or bleeding gums with tooth brushing suggests platelet dysfunction. Venopuncture and intravenous sites should be examined for evidence of impaired coagulation. Visual inspection of the nail beds, palate, and sclera in search of petechiae should be carried out. In only a small percentage of women with platelet counts >50,000 is there any historical or physical evidence of coagulopathy.

Examination of the airway is also extremely important. The pre-eclamptic patient often has significant airway edema, and difficult intubation is likely. When considering the risks of regional anesthesia, the prudent consultant also considers the risks of general anesthesia if regional anesthesia is not provided. Because of both the paucity of reports of epidural hematomas in parturients, and the clear risks of general anesthesia, many anesthesiologists will consider placing epidural catheters in pre-eclamptic women with moderate thrombocytopenia (platelet counts between $50,000–100,000 \times 10^9$/L). Fig. 16-4 provides an

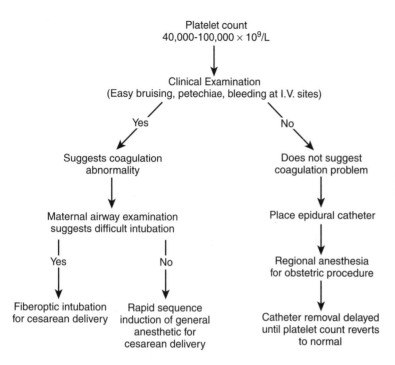

Figure 16-4   Approach to the parturient with thrombocytopenia.

algorithm for anesthetic management of the parturient with thrombocytopenia.

Infection

The use of neuraxial regional anesthesia in the presence of either systemic sepsis or cellulitis at the lumbar puncture site is ill advised because the circumstances pose an unknown risk of seeding the neuraxis with microorganisms. The hemodynamic instability associated with septic shock combined with the sympathetic blockade of regional anesthesia could also prove catastrophic.

Much more common than either systemic sepsis or localized cellulitis during labor is chorioamnionitis. Chorioamnionitis is typically a polymicrobial infection of the amniotic fluid and placental components, often seen during prolonged pre-delivery rupture of the membranes. The diagnosis of chorioamnionitis is made clinically, with a maternal fever combined with a tender uterus suggesting the diagnosis. Chorioamnionitis that is not associated with systemic sepsis (hypotension, oliguria, altered mental status, and rigors) does not contraindicate epidural or spinal anesthesia. Several large studies have utilized epidural analgesia in patients with suspected chorioamnionitis being treated with systemic antibiotics; there have been no reported cases of epidural abscess or meningitis in association with this approach.

Bleeding and Hypovolemia

Uncorrected hypovolemia is another contraindication to regional anesthesia. During parturition, hemorrhage is the most common cause of significant hypovolemia. Maternal hemorrhage is a leading cause of maternal mortality, most commonly due to placenta previa (placental position directly overlying the cervix leading to placental detachment and bleeding early in labor) and abruptio placenta (partial or complete premature separation of the placenta from the uterine wall). With attempted vaginal birth after previous cesarean delivery (VBAC), uterine rupture can also lead to life-threatening hemorrhage. The blood loss with placenta previa is usually obvious. However, bleeding with abruptio placenta and uterine rupture is not always evident via vaginal bleeding. Instead, hypotension and tachycardia combined with severe abdominal pain suggest the diagnosis. Placental abruption is accompanied by disseminated intravascular coagulopathy (DIC) in 10% of cases. In the postpartum period, uterine atony and uterine inversion may be associated with significant bleeding, which may contraindicate regional anesthesia. In all cases, maternal volume resuscitation and correction of coagulopathy must precede consideration of regional anesthesia.

Fetal Distress

Severe fetal distress suggests the need for general anesthesia for emergent cesarean delivery. Most commonly, prolonged fetal bradycardia leads to this request. The anesthesiologist must remember that the primary concern is the health of the mother. Therefore, when the airway examination strongly suggests that endotracheal intubation will be difficult, a regional anesthetic may still be appropriate.

REGIONAL ANESTHESIA FOR ELECTIVE CESAREAN DELIVERY

Whenever possible, regional anesthesia should be utilized for abdominal delivery. Outcome studies suggest that regional anesthesia is safer for the mother, with approximately a 94% decrease in anesthetic-related maternal mortality compared to general anesthesia. Maternal awareness during the birth and more immediate mother–newborn bonding are well appreciated. Pain control during the postoperative period is facilitated by regional anesthesia. The addition of short-acting lipophilic opioids to epidural or spinal anesthesia provides 2–6 hours of postoperative analgesia. Alternatively, adding morphine (3–4 mg in the epidural, or 0.1–0.2 mg in the spinal) provides 10–15 hours of analgesia. Neonatal outcome is also improved. Apgar scores are better after regional anesthesia compared to general anesthesia. Fewer babies need active resuscitation after maternal regional anesthesia versus general anesthesia.

This choice between epidural and spinal anesthesia for cesarean delivery has been greatly simplified by the development of pencil-point spinal needles, which have dural puncture headache rates <2%. For elective cesarean delivery, spinal anesthesia is usually most appropriate. In comparison to epidural anesthesia, spinal anesthesia has a higher success rate, is easier to perform, has a more rapid onset, has minimal potential for systemic toxicity, and typically results in a more comfortable intraoperative patient.

Clinical Caveat: Advantages of Regional Anesthesia for Cesarean Delivery

Lower maternal mortality versus general anesthesia
Better hemodynamic control
Awake and alert mother
Early bonding with neonate
Higher neonatal Apgar scores
Less need for active neonatal resuscitation
Better postoperative pain control

Epidural anesthesia may be preferable in a few patients presenting for elective cesarean delivery. Patients with significant systemic disease, particularly diabetes, pre-eclampsia, and chronic hypertension, may benefit from the slower onset and more controlled hemodynamics of epidural analgesia. Furthermore, epidural anesthesia has been shown to reduce the catecholamine levels that are associated with pregnancy-induced hypertension. Motor block is typically less profound with epidural anesthesia, which may benefit patients with severe pulmonary disease (e.g. cystic fibrosis). When a lengthy surgical duration is anticipated, epidural anesthesia may be preferable, as redosing can provide anesthesia of unlimited duration. Although spinal morphine can provide 12–24 hours of postoperative analgesia, postoperative epidural infusion can also provide analgesia for more involved surgical procedures (Box 16-9).

The main role of epidural anesthesia for cesarean delivery is the laboring parturient that requires semi-urgent abdominal delivery. If a woman has been receiving epidural labor analgesia, it is quite reasonable to provide epidural anesthesia. This practice saves the patient a second anesthetic procedure. Also, many anesthesiologists will incrementally dose the epidural in the labor room (with appropriate monitoring) while the operating room is prepared. This allows the patient to arrive in the operating room already anesthetized, thereby promoting greater operating room efficiency.

Clinical Caveat: Spinal versus Epidural Anesthesia for Elective Cesarean Delivery

SPINAL ANESTHESIA ADVANTAGES

Technically easier
Fewer block failures
Rapid onset
Minimal risk of systemic toxicity
More comfortable patient

EPIDURAL ANESTHESIA ADVANTAGES

Titratable
Less hypotension
Indefinite duration
Prolonged postoperative analgesia

Clinical Caveat: Contraindications to Regional Anesthesia for Cesarean Delivery

Infection: systemic sepsis or cellulitis at lumbar
    puncture site
Uncorrected hypovolemia
Significant maternal coagulopathy
Severe fetal distress

ANESTHESIA AND ANALGESIA FOR MISCELLANEOUS OBSTETRIC PROCEDURES

Cervical Cerclage

A nonfunctioning ("incompetent") cervix is a leading cause of early second-trimester miscarriage. Therapy is usually placement of a purse-string suture (cerclage) in the cervix at about 12 weeks gestation, followed by removal at approximately 37 weeks gestation. Both placement and removal of cervical cerclage are typically performed with low-dose spinal anesthesia. Hyperbaric lidocaine 20 mg plus fentanyl 20 μg is typically effective and of appropriate duration.

External Cephalic Version

Approximately 3–5% of fetuses will be in the breech or transverse lie position in the last six weeks of pregnancy. Because these fetal presentations typically result in cesarean delivery, attempts to reposition the fetus manually are often attempted. These attempts, termed "external cephalic version," typically involve gentle transabdominal pressure simultaneously applied to fetal head and buttocks (Fig. 16-5). The obstetrician attempts to "roll" the fetus into a position amenable to vaginal delivery. Several recent reports suggest improved external version success rates with regional analgesia. External versions are usually performed at approximately 36 weeks gestation. At earlier gestational ages, the fetus will often return to the original lie sometime after the version. With attempts at version much beyond 36 weeks, success rates are low. Again, low doses of spinal analgesia are sufficient. Isobaric lidocaine 10–20 mg plus fentanyl 20 μg usually provides excellent procedural analgesia.

Postpartum Tubal Ligation

Postpartum tubal ligation is easily accomplished in the days following delivery, before the uterus recedes into the pelvis. Regional anesthesia is optimal for this procedure because of the same physiologic changes of pregnancy that make general anesthesia worrisome for cesarean delivery as well as concerns over maternal transfer of drugs to the breast-feeding infant.

If the patient has an epidural catheter in place, it may be used for the tubal ligation. However, the success of using the epidural is affected by the interval from delivery until tubal ligation. Intervals longer than six hours lead to lower success rates. Thus, if the delivery to tubal ligation interval is greater than six hours or the epidural did not function well during labor, spinal anesthesia is the more effective technique (Box 16-10).

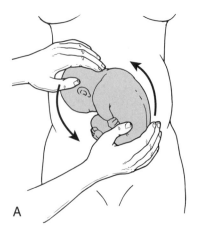
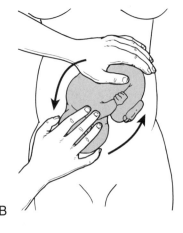

A   B

Figure 16-5   External cephalic version. External cephalic version is accomplished by gently "squeezing" the fetus out of one area of the uterus and into another. Here, the "forward roll," often the most popular, is illustrated. (Redrawn from Gabbe SG, Niebyl JR, Simpson JL: *Obstetrics: Normal and Problem Pregnancies*, Third Edition, Churchill Livingstone, New York, 1996, p. 489.)

Box 16-10   Regional Anesthesia for Postpartum Tubal Ligation

SPINAL ANESTHESIA

Hyperbaric 5% lidocaine 1 mL
Fentanyl 20 μg

EPIDURAL ANESTHESIA

2% lidocaine 20 mL
Epinephrine 1:400,000
Fentanyl 100 μg

CONCLUSIONS

Obstetric analgesia and anesthesia is a uniquely challenging and rewarding field. The anesthesiologist must consider numerous facets of physiology, pharmacology, drug transfer, and coexisting disease, all within an emotionally charged environment. Despite these multiple challenges, one can dramatically improve patient safety and comfort with expertise in regional anesthesia.

SUGGESTED READING

Benumof JL, Saidman LJ: *Anesthesia and Perioperative Complications*, Mosby, St. Louis, 1999.

Brown DL: *Atlas of Regional Anesthesia*, Second Edition, WB Saunders, Philadelphia, 1999.

Chestnut DH: *Obstetric Anesthesia: Principles and Practice*, Second Edition, Mosby, St. Louis, 2001.

Gabbe SG, Niebyl JR, Simpson JL: *Obstetrics: Normal and Problem Pregnancies*, Third Edition, Churchill Livingstone, New York, 1996.

Hahn MB, McQuillan PM, Sheplock GJ: *Regional Anesthesia: An Atlas of Anatomy and Techniques*, Mosby, St. Louis, 1996.

Stoelting RK, Miller RD: *Basics of Anesthesia*, Fourth Edition, Churchill Livingstone, Philadelphia, 2000.

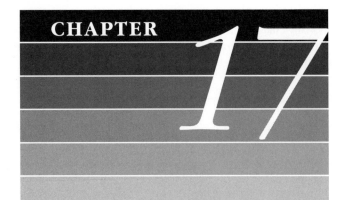

CHAPTER 17

Regional Anesthesia in Pediatrics

CHRISTOPHER M. VISCOMI

INTRODUCTION

The use of regional anesthesia in infants and children has grown in popularity in recent years. Most techniques are used in conjunction with general anesthesia to provide a pain-free awakening and rapid recovery. Much of the increase in popularity of using peripheral nerve blocks stems from the ability to provide superior analgesia and facilitate the rapid discharge of same-day surgery patients. Our familiarity with the appropriate conduct of spinal and epidural analgesia in infants and children is gaining momentum. Postoperative apnea is less frequent in high-risk patients such as neonates and ex-premature infants who undergo spinal anesthesia. Other pulmonary complications (atelectasis, oxygen desaturation, and pneumonia), particularly in premature infants and children with cystic fibrosis, can also be reduced with the use of continuous

epidural analgesia for postoperative pain management (Box 17-1). Safe and effective use of regional anesthesia in infants and children relies on a sound understanding of the developmental pharmacology of local anesthetics and the developmental anatomy of the region to be blocked.

DEVELOPMENTAL PHARMACOLOGY OF LOCAL ANESTHETICS

Local anesthetics in clinical use fall into one of two major groups: the amides and the esters (see detailed discussion in Chapter 2). The amides undergo degradation in the liver, while the esters are hydrolyzed by plasma cholinesterase. These metabolic pathways account for many of the differences in pharmacokinetics of local anesthetics that occur in children, particularly neonates, as compared to adults.

Amide local anesthetics in common clinical use include lidocaine, bupivacaine, and ropivacaine. In small children and infants, the potential for toxicity plays a major role in the selection of agent and the dose employed. Compared with adults, the neonatal liver has a limited capacity for drug metabolism. While single doses of either bupivacaine or lidocaine result in similar peak plasma concentrations as those seen in adults, there is a larger volume of distribution of these agents in infants and children, resulting in a prolonged elimination half-life. This is of little consequence following single administration, but results in significant risk of drug accumulation during repeated injections or infusions of amide local anesthetics.

The pharmacokinetics of ester local anesthetics are also affected by age. The level of plasma cholinestersase and activity of this enzyme are reduced in neonates, not attaining adult levels until 3 to 6 months of age. This may prolong metabolism of chloroprocaine, but its rapid metabolism is only slightly altered. Some investigators have thus suggested chloroprocaine as a particularly safe

186

Box 17-1 Advantages of Regional Anesthesia in Infants and Children

Peripheral nerve blocks can provide for pain-free recovery and early hospital discharge following many surgeries

Spinal anesthesia in infants is associated with a lower incidence of postoperative apnea compared with general anesthesia

Postoperative epidural analgesia can reduce pulmonary complications in high-risk patients (e.g. those with obesity or cystic fibrosis)

agent for use in neonates. Another enzymatic system with reduced activity in neonates is methemoglobin reductase. This enzyme is responsible for maintaining hemoglobin in a reduced state capable of carrying oxygen. Hepatic metabolism of prilocaine to o-toluidine can induce the production of methemoglobin, rendering red cells incapable of transporting oxygen. Although prilocaine is no longer in general use in the USA, it is a component of the topical agent EMLA (eutectic mixture of local anesthetics) commonly used to provide topical anesthesia for intravenous placement in children. To avoid toxicity, EMLA must be applied only to normal intact skin in appropriate doses (<10 kg: maximum of 100 cm^2 surface area (SA); 10–20 kg: maximum of 600 cm^2 SA; >20 kg: maximum of 2,000 cm^2 SA).

The potential for systemic toxicity of local anesthetics is increased in infants and children, largely due to lower level of plasma proteins. Concentrations of both albumin and α_1-acid glycoprotein which are primarily responsible for binding local anesthetics are significantly reduced in neonates and do not reach adult levels until 3–6 months of age. This results in as much as 30% higher free (unbound) local anesthetic concentrations in infants under 6 months of age. Neonates may be even more susceptible to the toxic effects of local anesthetics. In experimental neonatal animals, lidocaine plasma levels that produce respiratory and cardiovascular depression are about half those that produce similar toxicity in adults. Likewise, young dogs have a decreased threshold to both cardiac toxicity and seizures induced by bupivacaine. No data on relative toxicity of local anesthetics in adults as compared with infants and children are available in humans. Nonetheless, based largely on animal data, experts recommend a 30% reduction in local anesthetic doses in infants under 6 months of age. This is particularly important when continuous infusions are used for postoperative analgesia and equates to a maximum hourly rate for bupivacaine of 0.25 mg/kg. Avoiding local anesthetic toxicity by paying close atten-

tion to the total dose administered, considering the effect of injection site on blood levels, and the treatment of local anesthetic toxicity are similar to considerations for adults and have been discussed in detail in Chapter 2.

Clinical Caveat. Local Anesthetic Toxicity in Infants and Children

Based largely on evidence from experimental animals, children below the age of 6 months or approximately 60 weeks post-conceptual age appear to be more susceptible to the systemic toxic effects of local anesthetics.

Systemic factors contributing to increased local anesthetic toxicity in children include:

Toxicity (respiratory depression, seizures, or cardiovascular depression) may occur at lower plasma concentrations in neonates

Reduced protein binding (lower levels of albumin and α_1-acid glycoprotein than in the adult) results in higher free (unbound) concentrations of local anesthetic

Recommendations for avoiding local anesthetic toxicity in children:

Do not exceed maximum dose recommendations

Reduce maximum dose recommendations for adults by 30%

When using continuous infusions of bupivacaine, do not exceed 0.25 mg/kg/hour

NEURAXIAL BLOCKADE IN INFANTS AND CHILDREN

Anatomy

Several anatomic differences between adults and children are directly relevant to the performance of spinal and epidural anesthesia. The conus medullaris (the inferior extent of the spinal cord where it ends in the cauda equina) lies adjacent to the L3 vertebral body in the newborn and gradually achieves the adult position of L1–2 by 1 year of age (Fig. 17-1 on p. 188). Thus, spinal anesthesia is typically carried out through the L4–5 or L5–S1 interspaces in children under the age of one. The sacrum is less angulated in infants as compared to adults (Fig. 17-1 on p. 188) which makes the approach to the epidural space from the caudal canal more direct. This difference in angulation may account for the ease with which an epidural catheter can be threaded cephalad to the thoracic region in children up to 5 years of age. In

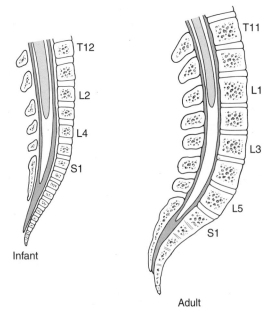

Figure 17-1 Anatomic differences between adults and children that affect the performance of spinal and epidural anesthesia. An infant's sacrum (left) is flatter and narrower than an adult's (right). The tip of the spinal cord (conus medullaris) ends at L3 in the neonate and does not achieve the normal adult position of L1-2 until approximately 1 year of age. (Redrawn from Cote CJ: *A Practice of Anesthesia for Infants and Children*, Third Edition, WB Saunders, Philadelphia, 2001, p. 642.)

older children and adults, catheters tend to coil within the sacral or low lumbar epidural space. The distance from the skin to the subarachnoid space is very short in neonates (approximately 1.4 cm) and progressively increases with age (Fig. 17-2). Cerebrospinal fluid (CSF) volume relative to total body weight is much greater in neonates than the adult (12–14 mL/kg in full-term newborn versus 2 mL/kg in adults). This may account for the relatively large doses of local anesthetic (on a mg/kg

basis) that are required for spinal anesthesia in infants (Box 17-2).

Spinal Anesthesia in Infants and Children

Clinical Uses

Spinal anesthesia has been performed in infants and children for more than 100 years. With the widespread availability and improved safety of general anesthesia, the technique lost favor. In recent years, investigators have documented a significant incidence of postoperative apnea following general anesthesia, particularly in premature infants. This has led to a resurgence in the popularity of this technique as large series of infants receiving spinal anesthesia have demonstrated the ease and success of the technique along with fewer or no episodes of postanesthetic apnea.

Spinal anesthesia is used most commonly for orthopedic procedures on the lower extremities, and lower abdominal and perineal surgery. The most common surgical procedures performed under spinal anesthesia in infants are inguinal hernia and hypospadias repair. The technique has also proven successful for reduction of smaller gastroschisis defects, umbilical hernia repair, and myelomeningocele repair (in which the local anesthetic is injected directly into the sac and supplemented with direct application by the surgeon).

Block Technique

After routine monitors are placed, the patient is placed in the sitting position. An assistant holds the infant in place by grasping both shoulders and creating an accentuated posterior curve in the lower spine (similar to the slumped position for spinal anesthesia in adults) (Fig. 17-3 on p. 189). Care must be taken to support the head and neck in infants as forward flexion will cause upper airway obstruction. The sitting position will aid in identifying correct needle placement by

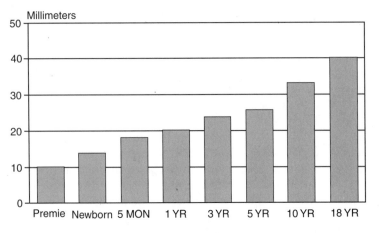

Figure 17-2 Changes in the distance from the skin to the subarachnoid space with age. (Redrawn from Cote CJ: *A Practice of Anesthesia for Infants and Children*, Third Edition, WB Saunders, Philadelphia, 2001, p. 643.)

Box 17-2   Anatomic Differences Between Children and Adults That Affect Spinal and Epidural Anesthesia

The tip of the spinal cord lies more caudad in neonates (L3) than in adults (L1-2) - spinal anesthesia should be carried out via the L4-5 or L5-S1 interspace

The sacrum is less angulated in neonates than in adults - entry into the epidural space via the sacral hiatus and caudal canal is less angulated and catheters can be threaded to the thoracic epidural space with ease in children up to 5 years of age

The distance from the skin to the subarachnoid space gradually increases with age - the spinal needle will enter the subarachnoid space at an average depth of 1 cm in the premature infant, 2 cm in the 1 year old, 3 cm in the 10 year old, and not attain the adult average of 4 cm until 18 years of age

The volume of CSF relative to total body weight is large in infants (14 mL/kg) versus adults (2 mL/kg) - thus the relative doses of spinal anesthetic required (mg/kg) are much larger in infants than in adults

increasing the hydrostatic pressure within the subarachnoid space. The skin and subcutaneous tissues are anesthetized with 1% lidocaine over the midline within the L4-5 or L5-S1 interspace. A 22 gauge 1.5 inch styletted spinal needle is then advanced. The depth of the subarachnoid space averages just 1 cm from the skin in premature infants and 1.4 cm in term newborns (Fig. 17-2 on p. 188). The stylette is removed and position confirmed by free return of CSF. For accurate dosing, the local anesthetic dose is drawn up in a tuberculin syringe. Care is taken to administer the dose slowly in order to avoid turbulence that can result in cephalad mixing of the local anesthetic and a high anesthetic level. The needle is removed and the patient is immediately placed in the supine position. After administration of the spinal anesthetic, the patient's legs should not be elevated. Lifting the legs produces an extreme head-down tilt and will cause hyperbaric local anesthetic to spread cephalad and can result in total spinal anesthesia.

The proportional dose (mg/kg) of local anesthetic required for subarachnoid block in infants and children is much higher than that required for adults. As discussed previously, this is likely related to the relatively large volume of CSF relative to total body weight that is found in infants relative to adults. The duration of spinal anesthesia is about one-third to one-half of that using

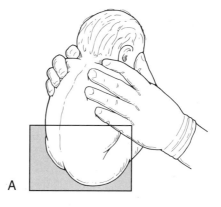
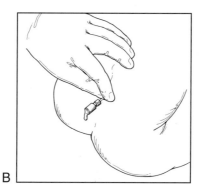
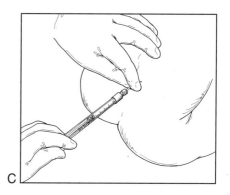

Figure 17-3   Lumbar puncture in the neonate or infant is easily performed in the sitting position. A, An assistant holds the child firmly by the shoulders accentuating the lumbar curvature and supporting the infant's head with both thumbs. **B,** After infiltrating the skin with 1% lidocaine, lumbar puncture is performed with a 22 gauge 1.5 inch styletted needle at the L4-5 or L5-S1 interspace. Position of the needle is confirmed by free flow of CSF. **C,** The spinal dose of local anesthetic is injected with a tuberculin syringe. Care must be taken not to inject rapidly or a high level of blockade might result.

Box 17-3 Local Anesthetics for Spinal Anesthesia in Neonates and Infants

ANESTHETIC DRUG	DOSE (MG/KG)
1.0% tetracaine in 5% dextrose	0.6–1.0 (infants)
	0.3–0.4 (children 12 weeks–2 years)
	0.2–0.3 (children older than 2 years)
0.5% bupivacaine (isobaric)	0.80 (neonates)
	0.3–0.5 (children ages 2 months–12 years)
0.75% bupivacaine in 8.25% dextrose	0.6
5.0% lidocaine in 7.5% dextrose	1–3

the same drug in an adult. The drugs used most commonly for spinal anesthesia in infants are tetracaine, bupivacaine, and lidocaine. Reported doses of tetracaine range from 0.22 to 1.0 mg/kg with most experts recommending the higher dose to attain an adequate level. The most common agent in clinical use is hyperbaric tetracaine with epinephrine. The solution is prepared by first drawing epinephrine (1:1,000) into the syringe and expelling the contents leaving a residual epinephrine "wash" within the syringe. Equal volumes of 1% tetracaine and 10% dextrose are then drawn into the syringe. Doses of other agents used in infants are shown in Box 17-3.

There is little information about dosing for spinal anesthesia in children because spinal anesthesia is used much less commonly beyond the neonatal period. When regional anesthesia is used in older children, it is most often combined with a light general anesthetic. Spinal doses of 0.3 to 0.5 mg/kg of 0.5% isobaric bupivacaine have been recommended for children 2 months to 12 years. Doses of 0.3 to 0.4 mg/kg of hyperbaric tetracaine have been used for spinal anesthesia in children 12 weeks to 2 years and 0.2 to 0.3 mg/kg in those older than 2 years. There are limited available data regarding dosing for spinal anesthesia in children. However, it is clear that the dose requirements decrease with increasing age.

Complications

Complications following spinal anesthesia in infants include total spinal anesthesia, postdural puncture headache, and neurologic sequelae. Total spinal anesthesia can be produced by rapid drug administration or by lifting the infant's legs soon after spinal placement. This can occur when a surgical assistant lifts the patient to apply a grounding pad for electrocautery to the child's back. Total spinal anesthesia is manifest as apnea and loss of responsiveness without a decline in blood pressure in infants. As compared with adults, decline in blood pressure during spinal anesthesia in infants is uncommon. Postdural puncture headache is unusual in children, even with the use of larger needles. In pediatric oncology patients who required lumbar puncture with 20 gauge needles, headache was rare in children under the age of 13 years. However, the peak incidence of postdural puncture headache is during the teenage years. The incidence in infants, who are preverbal, is unknown. Neurologic sequelae following spinal anesthesia are rare; there have been no cases detected in over 1,200 consecutive spinal anesthetics in infants at the University of Vermont.

Case Study: Infant Spinal Anesthesia for Bilateral Inguinal Hernia Repair

A 3-month-old, 6 kg infant presents for elective bilateral inguinal hernia repair. The child was born prematurely at 34 weeks gestational age, and was observed uneventfully in the newborn nursery for 48 hours after birth. The surgeon and the child's parents favor spinal anesthesia. Spinal anesthesia is carried out in the sitting position using a 22 gauge, 1.5 inch Quincke spinal needle and 4 mg of hyperbaric tetracaine with epinephrine is given. The patient is placed immediately supine, the blood pressure cuff is placed on one leg and an intravenous line placed in the other leg. The child rests comfortably with a pacifier throughout surgery. There is no observed change in oxygen saturation, heart rate, or blood pressure during the 90 minute surgery. No further anesthetic medications are necessary. The child is taken to the postanesthesia care unit, where spontaneous movement returns to the legs by 120 minutes after the spinal anesthetic injection.

Epidural Anesthesia

Clinical Uses

Epidural anesthesia administered by the caudal, lumbar, or thoracic route can be used for the same types of surgery as is spinal anesthesia. However, epidural anesthesia is used most commonly in infants and children for postoperative pain management.

Block Technique

The most common technique for epidural placement in infants is using a caudal approach. The sacrum in infants is flat and less angulated than in adults, thus a smaller degree of angulation is needed to pass a needle or epidural catheter into the epidural space via the caudal approach. The technique for epidural placement directly at the lumbar and thoracic levels in older children is similar to that for adults, with the caveat that the depth of the epidural space from the skin's surface does not reach that found in the adult until age 18 years.

For caudal epidural placement, the patient is placed in the lateral decubitus or prone position. The cornua of the sacral hiatus can be palpated as two bony ridges, 0.5 to 1 cm apart near the superior extent of the gluteal crease (Fig. 17-4). A 22 gauge, styletted needle or intravenous catheter 1.5 inches in length is used. The needle is inserted in the sacrococcygeal ligament at an angle of approximately 45° from the plane of the sacrum in a cephalad direction (Fig. 17-4). A slight "pop" is felt as the needle advances through the sacrococcygeal ligament, and then the angle of the needle is reduced to bring the needle's direction closer to the axis of the caudal canal. The needle is advanced an additional 1–2 cm into the caudal canal, and the stylette is removed. The caudal canal contains a network of veins and it is important to administer a test dose to rule out intravascular injection, even during single-shot caudal block. After confirming that no blood or CSF can be withdrawn on aspiration, a test dose of local anesthetic containing 1:200,000 epinephrine is administered. During injection, the area over the sacrum is palpated to detect subcutaneous injection outside of the caudal canal in the subcutaneous tissues. The amount of drug needed to produce blockade to a given dermatomal level is more dependent on volume than concentration and varies widely from patient to patient (see Clinical Caveat box).

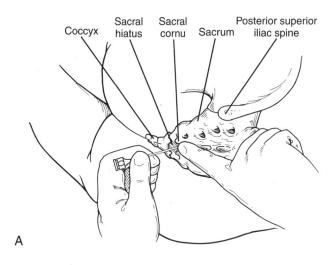

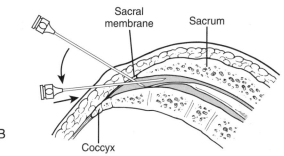

Figure 17-4   Caudal block. **A,** The patient is positioned in the lateral decubitus position and the sacral cornua are palpated. A needle is advanced at an angle of 45° from the plane of the sacrum through the sacrococcygeal ligament until a distinct "pop" is felt. **B,** The angle is then decreased to lie more parallel to the plane of the sacrum and the needle is advanced into the caudal canal. (Redrawn from Cote CJ: *A Practice of Anesthesia for Infants and Children*, Third Edition, WB Saunders, Philadelphia, 2001, p. 649.)

Clinical Caveat: Calculating the Dose of Local Anesthetic Needed for a Single-Shot Caudal Block

Volume (mL) = 0.05 mL/kg/dermatome to be blocked

Thus, in a 10 kg child in whom one wishes to produce a T10 dermatomal level, one would use a volume of (0.05 mL/kg/dermatome) × (10 kg) × (12 dermatomes) = 6 mL

Another simple method is to administer 1 mL/kg (up to 20 mL) of 0.125% bupivacaine with 1:200,000 epinephrine to provide a T4–T6 level

---

Catheter insertion for a continuous technique is performed using a similar technique. A 16 to 18 gauge intravenous catheter is inserted into the caudal canal. Using care to maintain sterility, the length of epidural catheter needed to reach the desired level is measured by holding the catheter over the patient's back between the sacral hiatus and the final position before inserting the catheter. The epidural catheter is inserted through the intravenous catheter and advanced to the predetermined position. The catheter should advance easily once inside the caudal canal. The intravenous catheter is removed and the catheter is aspirated to assure no blood or CSF can be withdrawn. A test dose of local anesthetic containing 1:200,000 epinephrine is administered before giving epidural doses of local anesthetic.

Clinical Caveat: Can Epidural Test Doses Reliably Detect Intravascular Needle or Catheter Placement in Children?

In awake adult patients, injection of a "test dose" of solution containing 15 μg of epinephrine (3 mL of 1:200,000 solution) will result in an increase in heart rate within 1 minute of administration. When the same solution is administered during general anesthesia, the efficacy of the test dose in detecting intravascular injection is reduced. Only 75–85% of children receiving 15 μg of epinephrine during general anesthesia with halothane or sevoflurane had an increased heart rate. A rise in heart rate of 10 beats per minute or more is a reliable indication of intravascular injection.

Pretreatment with atropine before test dose administration increased the reliability of the test dose to better than 90%. An increase in systolic blood pressure by more than 10% occurred in all patients along with changes in T wave amplitude. Thus, experts recommend:

Pretreat with atropine before the test dose is administered

Test dose with epinephrine 5 μg/kg

Elevation of heart rate (>10 beats/minute) or systolic blood pressure (>10%) within 1 minute following the test dose indicates intravascular injection

Change in the amplitude of the T wave also reliably indicates intravascular injection

Even following administration of a negative test dose, epidural dosing should proceed with slow injection in increments with attention toward detecting intravascular injection with each dose

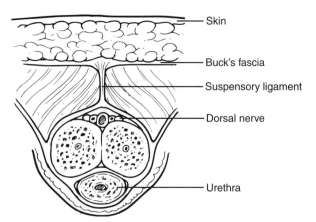

Figure 17-5   Anatomy of the dorsal penile nerve. Cross-section at the base of the penile shaft demonstrating the bilateral dorsal penile nerves adjacent to the midline vascular structures and just deep to the suspensory ligament and Buck's fascia. (Redrawn from Cousins MJ, Bridenbaugh PO: *Neural Blockade*, Third Edition, Lippincott-Raven, 1998, p. 631.)

Block Technique

There are two commonly used techniques for penile block: (1) a ring technique, and (2) block of the dorsal penile nerve (Fig. 17-6). To perform the ring technique, a 27 gauge needle is used to inject a subcutaneous ring of local anesthetic circumferentially around the base of the penile shaft. Block of the dorsal penile nerve is performed with a 27 gauge needle

PENILE NERVE BLOCK

Anatomy

The distal two-thirds of the penis is innervated by the dorsal penile nerves which are bilateral and adjacent to the midline (Fig. 17-5). The dorsal penile nerves are distal branches of the pudendal nerves, which arise from the sacral plexus (S2, 3, 4). At the base of the penis, these nerves divide into multiple filaments that encircle the shaft before reaching the glans. The base and proximal part of the penis are innervated by the genitofemoral and ilioinguinal nerves.

Clinical Uses

Penile nerve block is used for analgesia following procedures on the distal two-thirds of the penis including circumcision, hypospadias repair, and urethral dilation. Pain following procedures on the proximal penis is better managed with caudal block.

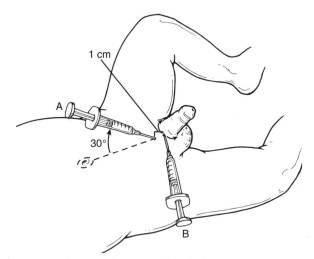

Figure 17-6   Penile nerve block. A, Dorsal penile nerve block: a 27 gauge needle is inserted over the pubic symphysis at an angle of 30° from the abdominal wall and advanced just beyond the inferior margin of the symphysis. The needle penetrates the suspensory ligament and is advanced 1 cm further where 1–4 mL of local anesthetic is deposited. **B,** Ring block: using a 27 gauge needle, local anesthetic is placed subcutaneously around the circumference of the base of the penile shaft. (Redrawn from Cote CJ: *A Practice of Anesthesia for Infants and Children*, Third Edition, WB Saunders, Philadelphia, 2001, p. 659.)

inserted over the symphysis pubis in the midline with a 30° angulation from the skin's surface directed in a caudad direction until it contacts the inferior margin of the symphysis. The needle is walked inferior to the pubic symphysis, where it passes posteriorly through the suspensory ligament of the penis (about 1 cm further in depth). After careful aspiration 1–4 mL of local anesthetic is injected.

Complications

The major complication associated with penile block is compromise of blood flow. Vasoconstrictors such as epinephrine should never be used for this block. Intravascular injection of the small volume of local anesthetic used for this block is unlikely to result in significant systemic toxicity.

ILIOINGUINAL/ILIOHYPOGASTRIC NERVE BLOCK

Ilioinguinal/iliohypogastric nerve block is another technique commonly used to provide analgesia after hernia repair. The anatomy and technique for this block have been discussed in detail in Chapter 7.

CONCLUSIONS

Regional anesthesia and analgesia are valuable techniques for providing intraoperative anesthesia and postoperative analgesia in infants and children. Most regional techniques that are useful in adults can be adapted for use in children. Several references with in-depth discussion of regional anesthesia techniques less commonly employed in children are provided below. Spinal anesthesia is proving to be a remarkably safe and simple method for providing surgical anesthesia in infants. Most other regional techniques are combined with general anesthesia in children. Many of these techniques are simple and effective. With a firm understanding of the anatomic and physiologic differences between adults and children, these regional techniques offer a valuable tool for practicing anesthesiologists.

SUGGESTED READING

Geiduschek JM: Pediatrics. In: *Regional Anesthesia and Analgesia*, WB Saunders, Philadelphia, 1996, pp. 558–575.

Krane EJ, Dalens BJ, Murat I, et al.: The safety of epidurals placed during general anesthesia, *Reg Anesth Pain Med* 23:433–438, 1998.

McGown RG: Caudal analgesia in children: five hundred cases for procedures below the diaphragm, *Anaesthesia* 37:806–818, 1982.

Polaner DM, Suresh S, Coté CJ: Pediatric regional anesthesia. In: Coté CJ, Todres ID, Ryan JF, Goudsouzian NG (eds), *A Practice of Anesthesia for Infants and Children*, Third Edition, WB Saunders, Philadelphia, 2001, pp. 636–674.

Sartorelli KH, Abajian JC, Kreutz JM, et al.: Improved outcome utilizing spinal anesthesia in high-risk infants, *J Pediatr Surg* 27:1022–1025, 1992.

Stafford MA, Wilder RT, Berde CB: The risk of infection from epidural analgesia in children: a review of 1620 cases, *Anesth Analg* 80:234–238, 1995.

Viscomi CM, Abajian JC, Wald SL, et al.: Spinal anesthesia for repair of meningomyelocele in neonates: a case series, *Anesth Analg* 81:492–495, 1995.

CHAPTER *18*

Acute Pain

JAMES P. RATHMELL

INTRODUCTION

Regional anesthetic techniques have gained popularity in recent years, not only for surgical anesthesia, but also for analgesia in the immediate postoperative or posttraumatic period. These methods provide excellent pain control while minimizing the systemic side effects attributable to parenteral opioids. In some high-risk patients, continuous regional analgesic techniques can reduce perioperative morbidity and mortality (see detailed discussion in Chapter 15). Continuous regional anesthetic techniques have come into more widespread use for a number of reasons, particularly advances in training and technology. Physicians in anesthesiology training programs universally gain some exposure to these techniques. A significant training period in pain medicine is a core portion of anesthesiology training and familiarity with regional techniques is required in all residency

programs. The advent of microprocessor-controlled infusions pumps, first for intravenous patient-controlled analgesia and then their ready extension to provide continuous epidural analgesia, have made this approach feasible in nearly every hospital within the USA. Assembling the infrastructure to support an acute pain service is more difficult, and is common in larger institutions, particularly those conducting high-risk procedures where regional anesthesia is likely to be of particular benefit. In this chapter, we review the organization of a formal acute pain service, common analgesic techniques for controlling perioperative pain (from oral opioids through continuous regional techniques), and then examine specific strategies for treating pain poorly controlled in those receiving regional anesthesia and assuring their safety during the conduct of these techniques.

ANESTHESIOLOGY-BASED ACUTE PAIN SERVICES

During the past decade, there has been increasing public attention toward the widespread under treatment of pain. There have been a number of national educational efforts aimed at improving practitioners' skills in properly assessing and treating pain. Several national organizations, including the Joint Council for Accreditation of Health care Organizations (JCAHO) and the Veterans' Administration system have adopted mandates to develop systematic means of assessing and treating pain in the patients they care for. At the same time, the subspecialty of pain medicine has been developing. Indeed, many of the pioneers who have promoted this new subspecialty have been the leaders of major education and public awareness campaigns about pain. In the USA, the American Board of Anesthesiology created a formal subspecialty designation in Pain Medicine in 1993, and now a decade of trained subspecialists are in practice. In most large institutions, formal acute pain services for hospitalized patients have been established. Typically, an anesthesiologist has been the lead practitioner for these services.

In the late 1970s and early 1980s, epidural administration of opioids and patient-controlled analgesia (PCA) were introduced into clinical practice. Clinicians in many parts of the world quickly recognized the value of these methods for improving postoperative pain control and made them available to patients. Since the introduction of these techniques, it has become apparent that establishing an effective acute pain service has more to do with organization than it does with expertise in any one technique.

The exact structure and services offered by the acute pain service will vary from institution to institution (Box 18-1, Box 18-2). In larger institutions, an anesthesiologist is designated as the leader and will visit all patients who are receiving epidural analgesia daily and remain available 24 hours a day. In many smaller institutions, a nurse or other practitioner is designated to manage the service and consults with a physician as needed. Both models have been well described and can be used effectively to improve perioperative and other acute pain management in hospitalized patients (Box 18-3). The basic tools of the acute pain trade include oral and systemic analgesics, including PCA, intrathecal opioid administration, and epidural analgesia.

Box 18-1   Essential Elements of an Acute Pain Service

At least one practitioner with knowledge and expertise in assessing and treating acute pain. Many institutions have an anesthesiologist in the lead. This practitioner may visit all patients on the service daily or assist a dedicated nurse or other practitioner when problems arise. This leader should be closely involved in setting guidelines for pain management within the institution.
Ready availability of expertise and a recognized system for getting help when it is needed. Most services will designate an "on-call" provider who is available 24 hours a day to answer questions and assist with poorly controlled pain.

Box 18-2   Typical Services Offered by an Acute Pain Service

Assistance with patient-controlled analgesia
Management of postoperative epidural analgesia and follow-up after administration of intrathecal opioids
Consultation for uncontrolled pain in hospitalized patients

Box 18-3   Principles Common to Acute Pain Services

Belief in the importance of postoperative pain relief and the improvement in function that accompanies it
Recognition of the large degree of interpatient variability
Belief in the need to provide comprehensive education
Belief that regular pain assessment and documentation are essential
Belief in the importance of collaborative efforts
Recognition of the value of institutional protocols
Recognition that side effects are common and may interfere with optimal pain control
Recognition of the need to track the quality and safety of postoperative analgesia

---

ACETAMINOPHEN AND THE NON-STEROIDAL ANTI-INFLAMMATORY DRUGS (NSAIDS)

Acetaminophen

Acetaminophen is a *para*-aminophenol derivative with analgesic and antipyretic properties similar to the NSAIDs. Acetaminophen does not produce any significant peripheral inhibition of prostaglandin production. Acetaminophen causes no significant gastrointestinal toxicity or platelet dysfunction and there are few side effects within the normal dose range. Acetaminophen is entirely metabolized by the liver and minor metabolites are responsible for the hepatotoxicity associated with overdose. The most common oral analgesics used to treat moderate to severe pain incorporate acetaminophen in combination with one of the opioids.

NSAIDs

NSAIDs are an important class of drugs that can effectively treat mild to moderate pain, particularly pain associated with inflammatory conditions. They are widely used and, in the form of salicylic acid, the NSAIDs have been a recognized part of pain treatment for hundreds of years. Drugs classified as NSAIDs have diverse chemical structures, but all share the ability to inhibit the enzyme cyclooxygenase and thereby inhibit the formation of prostaglandins from arachidonic acid.

NSAIDs produce analgesia by inhibiting the formation of prostaglandins. When cell membranes are damaged, arachidonic acid is produced by the action of phospholipases on membrane phospholipids. Arachidonic acid is, in turn, further converted by the enzymes cyclooxygenase and lipoxygenase. Cyclooxygenase is present in most tissues and converts arachidonic acid to prostaglandins and other inflammatory mediators. The lipoxygenase system leads to leukotriene synthesis, another group of inflammatory mediators, some of which are involved in pain transmission. The NSAIDs block cyclooxygenase and reduce prostaglandin production. Prostaglandins play a key role in sensitization of both the peripheral and central nervous system and the apparent mechanism for analgesia produced by the NSAIDs is the prevention of sensitization by diminishing prostaglandin production.

Mammalian cells contain at least two different cyclooxygenase isoenzymes (Fig. 18-1). Type I cyclooxygenase (COX-1) is a constitutively expressed enzyme that is present in varying amounts in most cells, including vascular endothelium, platelets, and renal tubules. COX-1 levels remain fairly constant within cells. Type II cyclooxygenase (COX-2) is almost undetectable in most tissues under normal conditions, but increases 10- to 80-fold during inflammation. Significant levels of COX-2 are present under normal physiologic conditions within the brain and renal cortex. COX-1 serves a key role in cellular homeostasis and is the primary form of the enzyme present in platelets, the kidney, stomach, and vascular smooth muscle. In recent years, extensive investigative efforts have led to the isolation of numerous NSAIDs with high selectivity for COX-2 inhibition. The goal in developing the COX-2-selective NSAIDs was to reduce the formation of prostaglandins associated with pain and hyperalgesia while leaving unaffected those needed to preserve normal function of the gastrointestinal mucosa and kidney, and to preserve normal platelet function. The NSAIDs can be classified according to their inhibition of COX and their selectivity for the COX-2 isoenzyme (Box 18-4).

Although there appears to be no tolerance or physical dependence associated with the NSAIDs, they are associated with significant toxicity. Most clinically significant toxicities involve the gastrointestinal (GI), renal, hematologic and hepatic systems. Dyspepsia is the most

common side effect, and nonselective NSAIDs lead to asymptomatic ulcers in 20–25% of users within one week of administration. Complicated ulcers, including perforated ulcers, upper GI bleeding, and obstruction occur in a significant number of long-term NSAID users. The ulcerogenic potential of NSAIDs lies in the inhibition of COX-1 and prostaglandin synthesis that affect secretion of GI mucus and bicarbonate, as well as epithelial cell turnover and repair. Several factors increase the risk of NSAID gastropathy and development of gastroduodenal ulcers (Box 18-5).

Renal impairment occurs in some patients taking NSAIDs and results in reduction in renal perfusion due to inhibition of prostaglandin synthesis. In patients with contraction of their intravascular volume, renal perfusion is maintained through the vasodilatory effects of prostaglandins. Common conditions associated with intravascular volume contraction include congestive heart failure, acute blood loss, and hepatic cirrhosis; those with chronic hypertension and diabetes may also be at higher risk (Box 18-6). Renal toxicity may manifest as acute interstitial nephritis or nephrotic syndrome. Acute renal failure occurs in as many as 5% of patients using NSAIDs; renal impairment typically resolves with discontinuation of NSAID therapy, rarely progressing to end-stage renal disease.

Hematologic toxicity associated with NSAIDs primarily takes the form of inhibition of normal platelet function. The prostaglandins produced by cyclooxygenase

---

Box 18-4 Classification of NSAIDs Based on COX Inhibition and Selectivity ○

Aspirin: Irreversible inhibition of both COX-1 and COX-2
Ibuprofen, naproxen: Reversible, competitive inhibition of both COX-1 and COX-2
Indomethacin: Slower, time-dependent, but reversible inhibition of both COX-1 and COX-2
Rofecoxib, celecoxib, valdecoxib: Slow, time-dependent, and highly selective COX-2 inhibition

---

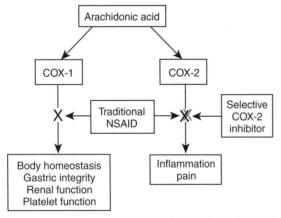

Figure 18-1   The arachidonic acid cascade and the effects of cyclooxygenase-1 and -2 inhibition.

Box 18-5 Factors That Increase the Risk of NSAID-Induced Gastropathy

Age over 60 years
Prior history of peptic ulcer disease
Steroid use
Alcohol use
Use of multiple NSAIDs
The first 3 months of use

are in turn converted to thromboxane A_2 (TXA_2) by platelets and prostaglandin I_2 (PGI_2) by the vascular endothelium. TXA_2 activates platelets and produces vasoconstriction while PGI_2 inhibits platelets and produces vasodilation. Platelet activity is thus a balance between the effects of TXA_2 and PGI_2 activity. By inhibiting TXA_2, NSAIDs block platelet activation. Aspirin irreversibly acetylates cyclooxygenase, and thus the platelet inhibition resulting from aspirin use persists for the 7 to 10 days required for new platelet formation. Non-aspirin NSAIDs induce reversible platelet inhibition that resolves when most of the drug has been eliminated. Blood loss during surgery may be somewhat greater in patients using NSAIDs; however, studies in various surgical populations have produced conflicting results. There does not appear to be any increased risk of hematoma formation when performing peripheral or neuraxial blocks in patients using NSAIDs (see Chapter 13 for further discussion).

Hepatic toxicity may also result from NSAID use. Minor elevations in hepatic enzyme levels appear in 1–3% of patients. The mechanism appears to be immunologic or metabolic mediated direct hepatocellular injury, with dose-related toxicity occurring with both acetaminophen and aspirin. Periodic assessment of liver function is recommended in those on long-term NSAID therapy.

Large clinical trials have demonstrated the safety of the new class of COX-2-selective NSAIDs. Gastrointestinal complications are reduced to the level of that seen with placebo and there is no inhibition of platelet activity with the COX-2-selective agents. Renal and hepatic toxicity are similar to that seen with the nonselective NSAIDs.

Clinical Controversy: Are COX-2-Selective NSAIDs Safer Than Non-selective NSAIDs?

Gastrointestinal toxicity: COX-2-selective agents dramatically reduce the incidence or gastrointestinal complications (perforated ulcers, gastrointestinal bleeding, and perforation). Dyspepsia is common with both non-selective and COX-2-selective agents

Platelet inhibition: COX-2-selective NSAIDs do not interfere with platelet function. Aspirin produces irreversible platelet inhibition, while other NSAIDs inhibit platelet function while significant blood levels of the drug remain

Renal toxicity: Both COX-1 and COX-2 enzymes are present in the kidney and regulate renal blood flow. Renal impairment can occur with both non-selective and COX-2-selective NSAIDs

Hepatic toxicity: Mild hepatocellular injury may occur with all NSAIDs.

Box 18-6 Factors That Increase the Risk of NSAID-Induced Renal Toxicity

Hypovolemia
Acute blood loss
Chronic diuretic use
Low cardiac output (congestive heart failure)
Hepatic cirrhosis
Pre-existing renal insufficiency

NSAIDs are used most widely to treat the pain and inflammation associated with rheumatic and degenerative arthritides. They also serve as a useful adjunct to opioids for providing control of acute pain. Addition of an NSAID can often reduce opioid requirements and related side effects in the postoperative period. Numerous agents are available for oral administration and several are available without prescription. Thus, they are among the most common first-line analgesics.

Ketorolac is currently the only parenteral NSAID approved for clinical use in the USA. It is a potent analgesic and antipyretic and several studies have demonstrated its usefulness in treating moderate postoperative pain. Ketorolac is a non-selective NSAID, and despite parenteral administration is associated with GI toxicity similar to other NSAIDs. Paracoxib, an intravenous prodrug to the oral COX-2-selective NSAID valdecoxib, is available in Europe and pending the outcome of additional clinical studies will likely become available in the USA. The chemical classification, names, and half-lives of common NSAIDs are shown in Table 18-1. Familiarity with the dosing and administration of several oral NSAIDs as well as ketorolac is an important tool for those treating acute pain. Addition of an NSAID to an opioid regimen during the perioperative period can often improve analgesia and reduce opioid-related side effects. While it is important to avoid NSAIDs in those at significant risk for toxicity, many patients having surgery can benefit from their addition.

SYSTEMIC OPIOIDS

The opiates are among the most universally effective agents available for treating pain. Morphine, the prototypical opiate, is derived from the milk of the scored seed pod of the oriental poppy, *Papaver somniferum*. Several other compounds can be derived directly through chemical modification of morphine (Fig. 18-2 on p. 198). Those drugs derived directly from morphine are termed the *opiates*. Other synthetic compounds have been produced that act via opiate receptors – all compounds that act via opiate receptors are termed the *opioids*. Because

Table 18-1 Classification of Non-steroidal Anti-inflammatory Drugs by Chemical Structure

Class	Drug		
	Generic Name	Brand Name(s)	$T_{1/2\beta}$ (Hour)
Non-selective NSAIDs			
Propionic acids	Naproxen	Alleve, Anaprox, Naprosyn	12–15
	Ibuprofen	Motrin	2–2.5
	Ketorolac	Toradol	5.5
Indoleacetic acids	Indomethacin	Indocin	6
	Sulindac	Clinoril	1.5
Phenylacetic acids	Diclofenac	Cataflam, Voltaren	1–2
Salicylic acids	Salsalate	Disalcid, Monogesic, Salflex	3.8
	Choline magnesium trisalicylate	Trilasate	7
Naphthylalkenone	Nabumetone	Relafen	26
Oxicam	Piroxicam	Feldene	48.5
Pyrroleacetic acid	Tolmetin	Tolectin	1
COX-2-selective NSAIDs			
Furanone	Rofecoxib	Vioxx	17
Benzenesulfonamide (pyrazole)	Celecoxib	Celebrex	11
Benzenesulfonamide (isoxazole)	Valdecoxib	Bextra	8–11

the opioids are universally effective for relieving pain, they form the cornerstone of effective pain management. However, the opioids are associated with significant side effects and their long-term use is clouded by tolerance and the possibility of addiction.

Opioids produce analgesia by binding to a group of specific receptors within the central nervous system. These receptors are a part of the normal nociceptive system that modulates pain perception within the body. There are groups of naturally occurring compounds within the body that bind to and activate the opioid receptors, called the endogenous opioids. The endogenous opioids are all simple peptides containing the amino acid sequence *tyrosine–glycine–glycine–phenylalanine* and are formed through cleavage of larger precursor molecules. Three distinct groups of endogenous opioids have been identified: the enkephalins, the endorphins, and the dynorphins. They are derived from different precursors and bind to distinct receptor subsets (Table 18-2). The endogenous opioids bind primarily to the μ-receptors, leading to analgesia and the side effects typical of all opioids: respiratory depression, cardiovascular, and GI effects. (For a more detailed discussion of the anatomic localization and function of opioid receptors in modulation of nociceptive input, see Chapter 1.)

Side effects associated with opioid analgesics include respiratory depression, cardiovascular effects, sedation, pupillary constriction, nausea and vomiting, and constipation. All μ-agonists produce dose-dependent reduction in responsiveness of the brain stem respiratory centers to increases in arterial carbon dioxide tension (P_aCO_2). There is a group of agonist–antagonist opioids that act as agonists

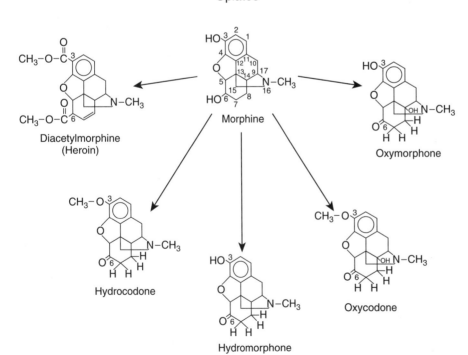

Opiates

Diacetylmorphine (Heroin)

Morphine

Oxymorphone

Hydrocodone

Hydromorphone

Oxycodone

Figure 18-2   The opiates: morphine and its derivatives.

Table 18-2 Classification Schema for Opioid Receptor Types and Their Proposed Actions

Receptor type	Endogenous Ligand	Action
μ	β-endorphin	Analgesia (spinal and supraspinal)
		Respiratory depression
		Cardiovascular effects
		Gastrointestinal effects
δ	Enkephalin	Spinal analgesia
κ	Dynorphin	Spinal analgesia
		Sedation

at lower doses, but exhibit a "ceiling effect" such that no further effect on respiration or additional analgesia is produced beyond a certain dose. Clinically, opioid-induced respiratory depression manifests as reduction in breathing rate and, at high doses, apnea. Opioids are mood-altering drugs, producing a feeling of warmth and well-being, drowsiness, and euphoria. μ-Receptor agonists all produce pupillary constriction. The opioids cause nausea and vomiting by direct stimulation of the chemoreceptor trigger zone within the area postrema in the medulla. Opioids also reduce the propulsive peristaltic contractions of the small and large intestines, leading to constipation.

Cardiovascular effects take the form of a dose-dependent bradycardia caused by central stimulation of the vagal nucleus within the medulla. Except for meperidine, opioids do not suppress myocardial contractility at clinically useful doses. Morphine, and to a lesser extent meperidine and codeine, have a direct effect on vascular smooth muscle and an indirect effect through histamine release, producing arteriolar vasodilation and venodilation (Box 18-7).

With continued use of substantial amounts of opioids, larger doses of the drug are required over time to produce the same physiologic effects. This phenomenon is called tolerance and is characteristic of the entire class of opioids. Physical dependence is characterized by the precipitation of a distinct withdrawal (abstinence) syndrome when the opioid is discontinued. Manifestations of opioid withdrawal include diaphoresis, hypertension, tachycardia, abdominal cramping, nausea, and vomiting. Physical dependence occurs in any individual given a large enough dose of opioid for a long enough period of time and it is not synonymous with addiction. Addiction is popularly conceived as a compulsion or overpowering drive to obtain a drug in order to experience its psychologic effects (see Clinical Controversy box for the formal definition of addiction). Opioid addiction is rarely induced iatrogenically, and fears of addiction should not be used as an excuse to limit opioid dosing during attempts to control pain acutely.

Clinical Controversy. Acute Pain Management in the Patient with Opioid Tolerance or a History of Opioid Addiction

Addiction is defined by the World Health Organization as:

A state, psychic and sometimes also physical, resulting from the interactions between a living organism and a drug, characterized by behavioral and other responses that always include a compulsion to take the drug on a continuous or periodic basis in order to experience its psychic effects, and sometimes to avoid the discomfort of its absence. Tolerance may or may not be present.

This formal definition is similar to the popular conception of addiction as a compulsion or overpowering drive to obtain a drug in order to experience its psychologic effects. Addiction is *not* synonymous with physical dependence. While all individuals who are taking opioids for an extended period of time will exhibit withdrawal symptoms when the drug is abruptly discontinued, few will exhibit the compulsive behavior and psychologic dependence characteristic of addiction. Opioid addiction rarely occurs iatrogenically. Two groups of patients present particular challenges to the clinician in the perioperative period: those who have been taking large doses of opioids for chronic pain and those with current or previous addiction. Simple rules of thumb for managing the opioid-tolerant patient or those with a history of addiction include the following:

Consider regional anesthetic techniques (spinal opioids, epidural infusions) to improve analgesia and minimize systemic opioid effects. Keep in mind that higher than usual doses of neuraxial opioid may be required in those with significant tolerance.

Use adjunctive analgesics whenever possible to reduce total opioid requirements (e.g. NSAIDs).

Administer opioid analgesics liberally to control pain in the immediate postoperative period. *Do not* attempt to limit the opioid dose or wean opioid analgesics in the immediate postoperative period. Those with significant tolerance will invariably require higher than average doses to control acute pain.

Use the preoperative opioid doses as a baseline requirement and administer additional doses beyond this to control acute pain. This baseline requirement can be administered as a continuous intravenous infusion as part of patient-controlled analgesia or by continuing the preoperative long-acting opioid in addition to use of PCA.

Consider consultation with a substance abuse specialist during hospitalization for those with ongoing opioid abuse or a history of addiction.

Closely coordinate (communicate) the plan for pain management with the patient's primary care provider before hospital discharge. While acute escalation in the opioid requirement is often necessary in the perioperative period, a plan for weaning the opioids to their previous levels should be established *before* the patient is discharged from the hospital.

Box 18-7   Side Effects Associated with Opioid Analgesics

Respiratory depression – dose-dependent reduction in responsiveness of the brain stem respiratory centers to increases in arterial carbon dioxide tension (P_aCO_2); manifests as reduction in breathing rate and at high doses, apnea

Sedation – mediated through the limbic system

Pupillary constriction – excitatory action on the autonomic segment of the Edinger–Westphal nucleus of the occulomotor nerve

Nausea and vomiting – direct stimulation of the chemoreceptor trigger zone within the area postrema in the medulla

Constipation – reduction in the propulsive peristaltic contractions of the small and large intestines

Bradycardia – central stimulation of the vagal nucleus within the medulla

Oral Opioids

Oral opioids are common agents used for control of mild to moderate pain in those who are able to continue oral intake. Many agents are available as combination preparations containing an opioid along with acetaminophen. The duration of analgesic action for the orally administered opioids is similar and in the range of 3–4 hours. Commonly used oral opioids are listed in Table 18-3. In those with opioid tolerance or greater than average opioid requirements, oral opioid alone (without acetaminophen) should be used to avoid hepatic toxicity.

Intravenous Opioids

Control of moderate to severe pain or treatment of those who are unable to tolerate oral intake often requires use of intravenous opioids. The pharmacokinetic profiles of opioid analgesics administered intramuscularly are similar but somewhat more erratic due to variations in muscle blood flow compared to that seen with intravenous administration (Fig. 18-3); however, there is significant discomfort with intramuscular (IM) administration. Common agents used for control of moderate to severe pain and their approximate equianalgesic doses are shown in Table 18-4. There is no maximum dose for any of the pure opioid agonists (either orally or parenterally), and the dose can be increased until acceptable analgesia is produced or intolerable side effects ensue. Patients who require large doses of opioids should be closely monitored during initial dose titration as marked respiratory depression and apnea may occur unexpectedly.

Table 18-3   Common Oral Opioid and Opioid–Acetaminophen Combinations Used to Treat Mild to Moderate Pain

Drug	Equianalgesic Oral Dose (mg)	How Supplied
Acetaminophen	–	325, 500, 625 mg tabs; 500 mg/15 mL elixir
Codeine	60	15, 30, 60 mg tabs; 15 mg/5 mL elixir
Acetaminophen with codeine	–	300–15, 300–30, 300–60 mg tabs; 120–12/5 mL elixir
Hydrocodone	20	(Available only in combination with acetaminophen)
Acetaminophen with hydrocodone	–	500–2.5, 500–5, 500–7.5, 660–10 mg tabs; 500–7.5/15 mL elixir
Oxycodone	10	5 mg tabs; 5 mg/5 mL elixir
Acetaminophen with oxycodone	–	325–5, 500–5 mg tabs; 325–5/5 mL elixir
Morphine	10	15, 30 mg tabs; 10, 20 mg/5 mL elixir
Hydromorphone	2	2, 4, 8 mg tabs; 5 mg/ 5 mL elixir

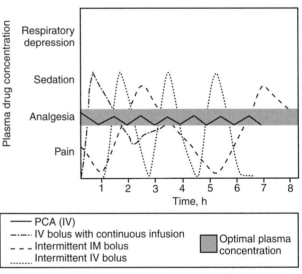

— PCA (IV)
–·–·– IV bolus with continuous infusion
– – – Intermittent IM bolus
········· Intermittent IV bolus
☐ Optimal plasma concentration

Figure 18-3   Relationship between the plasma drug concentration and pharmacologic effect of opioid analgesics. PCA, patient-controlled analgesia; IV, intravenous; IM, intramuscular. (Redrawn from Tuman KJ, et al.: *Hosp Formulary* 23:580, 1988.)

Patient-Controlled Analgesia

Patient-controlled analgesia (PCA) utilizes patient self-administration of opioid analgesia via a patient-activated infusion device. This method for delivering analgesics

Table 18-4	Common Opioids Used Orally or Parenterally to Treat Moderate to Severe Pain	
Drug	**Equianalgesic Parenteral Dose**	**Equianalgesic Oral Dose**
Fentanyl	100 µg	–
Hydromorphone	1.5 mg	7.5 mg
Morphine	10 mg	30–60 mg
Meperidine	75 mg	300 mg

has evolved with the introduction of computer-controlled, programmable infusion pumps. The PCA paradigm holds that the timely administration of small intermittent doses of analgesics will allow maintenance of optimal plasma drug concentration while minimizing side effects and periods of poor analgesia associated with intermittent intravenous (IV) or IM administration (Fig. 18-3 on p. 200). Typical PCA devices can be programmed to deliver a specified dose of opioid and then "lock out" further administration for a specified interval; most devices can also be programmed to administer a continuous basal infusion suitable for meeting the background requirements of those with opioid tolerance. Guidelines for PCA administration of common opioid analgesics are shown in Table 18-5. PCA provides superior analgesia in many settings where hospitalized patients experience acute pain. Patients are very accepting of this technology and are typically quite satisfied with the close degree of control of pain that PCA allows. The addition of a basal infusion to the PCA dosing regimen should be reserved for those patients with opioid tolerance – routinely including a basal infusion does not improve analgesia, but simply increases the total opioid dose used and the frequency of opioid-related side effects (Box 18-8).

Table 18-5	Guidelines for Opioid Administration via IV PCA	
Drug (Concentration)	**Typical Demand Dose (Range)**	**Typical Lockout Interval (Range)**
Morphine (1 mg/mL)	1.0 mg (0.5–3.0 mg)	10 minutes (5–12 minutes)
Meperidine (10 mg/mL)	10 mg (5–30 mg)	10 minutes (5–12 minutes)
Fentanyl (10 µg/mL)	10 µg (10–20 µg)	10 minutes (5–10 minutes)
Hydromorphone (0.2 mg/mL)	0.2 mg (0.1–0.5 mg)	10 minutes (5–10 minutes)

Box 18-8	Patient-Controlled Analgesia

Advantages:
 Allows each patient to control their own pain relief
 Provides for rapid administration of analgesic immediately on patient request
 Has a high degree of patient acceptance and satisfaction
 Reduces total opioid dose and related side effects
Disadvantages:
 Requires the patient's ability to understand and follow directions
 Requires availability of specific PCA infusion pumps
 Subject to programming errors that can cause over- or underdosing

NEURAXIAL ANALGESIA

The pharmacology and clinical use of intrathecal and epidural opioids and local anesthetics has been covered extensively in earlier chapters (see Chapters 9, 10, and 15). In this section, we focus on the practical aspects for using neuraxial techniques to provide postoperative analgesia.

Intrathecal Opioids

Administration of intrathecal opioids can provide prolonged analgesia after a single injection. When a surgical procedure is to be carried out using spinal anesthesia, the addition of an opioid to the local anesthetic serves as a practical and effective means for improving postoperative analgesia. The technique is limited by the frequency of side effects at higher doses, and the inability to provide complete analgesia for more extensive and painful procedures.

There are two general classes of opioids used for spinal analgesia: those that are hydrophilic (e.g. morphine) and those that are lipophilic (e.g. fentanyl, sufentanil). The hydrophilic opioids are slower in onset (peak analgesic effect occurs between 20 and 60 minutes), but persist at significant levels within the CSF for prolonged periods of time. The prototypic hydrophilic agent is morphine. While it produces prolonged analgesia, it has also been associated with a small incidence of delayed respiratory depression occurring as late as 18–20 hours after administration. This is believed to be due to the persistence of significant levels of the drug within CSF for up to 24 hours and the rostral spread of drug within the CSF (see Fig. 9-13 on p. 107). Morphine 0.1–0.3 mg can provide analgesia for 8–24 hours; however, patients should remain hospitalized and observed periodically to detect and promptly treat delayed respiratory depression with this agent. Respiratory depression produced by neuraxial opioids usually begins with a decrease in respiratory rate, and an increase in tidal volume. The increase in tidal volume is not sufficient to offset the decrease in respiratory rate, thus P_aCO_2 rises. Hypoxemia is a late manifestation of opioid toxicity, thus pulse oximetry is a poor means for detecting impending respiratory arrest.

The lipophilic opioids have a rapid onset (peak analgesic effect within 5 to 10 minutes) and short duration of analgesic action (2 to 4 hours). Delayed respiratory depression has not been observed with the lipophilic opioids. Fentanyl 10–25 µg or sufentanil 2.5–10 µg is often combined with small doses of local anesthetic to provide surgical anesthesia and postoperative analgesia for outpatient surgery.

Epidural Opioids

Opioid analgesics also provide effective analgesia when administered into the epidural space. They can be administered as single-bolus injections, but it is far more common to place a catheter and administer combinations of opioid and low-dose local anesthetic to provide for continuous analgesia following surgery. Intermittent injections are technically simpler and may be used when there is no equipment or administrative infrastructure available to support continuous epidural infusion. It is imperative to understand the dermatomal extent of analgesia that can be expected from each agent and to place the injection at or near the midpoint of the dermatomal location of the surgical incision (see Fig. 9-13 on p. 107). Hydrophilic agents such as morphine can be placed in the lumbar region and still provide analgesia for incisions that extend to the thoracic region, while fentanyl will not spread to the same extent. However, if the epidural injection or infusion is administered outside of the dermatomal distribution of the incision, addition of local anesthetic will not provide additional analgesia. Local anesthetics provide analgesia only within the dermatomes adjacent to the site of injection. Typical doses for epidural administration of opioids are shown in Table 18-6.

Continuous Epidural Infusion and Patient-Controlled Epidural Analgesia

Continuous epidural infusions of opioids or opioid–local anesthetic combinations result in fewer fluctuations in concentration of the analgesic drug and allow for patient-controlled supplementation via patient-controlled epidural analgesia (PCEA) using programmable infusion pumps identical to those used for IV PCA. Appropriate catheter location and choice of agents is essential for optimizing analgesia (see Clinical Caveat box). Common

Clinical Caveat: Optimizing the Placement of Injection and Choice of Agent for Neuraxial Analgesia

Hydrophilic opioids such as morphine tend to spread extensively within the CSF and produce a wide band of analgesia, while lipophilic opioids like fentanyl provide only a limited band of analgesia adjacent to the level of injection (see Fig. 9-13 on p. 107). Factors to consider when choosing the location of the injection and the best agent include:

Location of injection:

Intrathecal – always carried out below L2 to avoid the conus medullaris

Epidural – optimal location is always to place the single-shot injection or the catheter in the middle of the dermatomal band corresponding to the surgical incision. In some cases, practitioners still do not have expertise or comfort with placing a catheter at the thoracic level, thus choosing an agent that spreads from the lumbar region may be the best available technique (e.g. lumbar epidural placement of morphine for post-thoracotomy pain).

Choice of agent:

Intrathecal – tailor the agent to the procedure being performed. Morphine will provide more prolonged analgesia, but carries a small risk of respiratory depression and should be reserved for hospitalized patients. Fentanyl and sufentanil provide shorter duration of analgesia and are suitable for outpatient procedures.

Epidural opioid–morphine and other hydrophilic opioids (meperidine, hydromorphone) can be used to provide a wide dermatomal spread. Thus, when there is an extensive incision (e.g. esophagogastrectomy) or a lumbar injection is placed for thoracic surgery, one of these hydrophilic agents should be used. When the single-shot epidural injection or catheter tip is located within the dermatomes corresponding to the surgical incision, either the hydrophilic or the lipophilic opioids can be used. The hydrophilic agents will have a longer duration of action following single-shot administration.

Epidural local anesthetic–opioid combinations – epidural local anesthetic will provide a sensory block and analgesia only in the dermatomes adjacent to the site of injection. Thus, when the epidural injection is placed at a site distant from the dermatome corresponding to the surgical incision, there is no additional benefit in adding local anesthetic to the opioid. For instance, infusing local anesthetic in addition to a hydrophilic opioid through a lumbar epidural catheter for pain control following thoracotomy will likely only produce motor block in the lower extremities and some degree of hypotension without improving the analgesia provided by using the epidural opioid alone.

| Table 18-6   Epidural Administration of Opioids or Opioid–Bupivacaine Combinations |

	Intermittent injection		
Drug	Dose	Onset (minutes)	Duration (hours)
Morphine	0.5–5 mg	20–60	8–24
Meperidine	25–100 mg	5–10	6–8
Hydromorphone	0.2–1 mg	10–15	10–12
Fentanyl	50–100 μg	4–10	4–6
Sufentanil	10–60 μg	7–10	2–4

	Continuous infusion		Patient-controlled epidural analgesia (PCEA)	
	Starting Rate (mL/hour)	Range (mL/hour)	Bolus Dose (mL)	Lockout Interval (minutes)
Morphine 0.002–0.005% + bupivacaine 0.0625–0.125%	6–8	4–12	1	10
Hydromorphone 0.0005–0.001% + bupivacaine 0.0625–0.125%	6–8	4–12	1	20
Fentanyl 0.0002–0.0005% + bupivacaine 0.0625–0.125%	6–8	4–12	1	20

epidural opioid and opioid–bupivacaine combinations are listed in Table 18-6. As discussed above, intravenous PCA relies on the patient-administered intermittent bolus doses to provide analgesia, and continuous infusions are seldom needed. In contrast, when using PCEA, the continuous infusion provides the majority of the analgesia, and small intermittent patient-administered doses are used to supplement analgesia.

Sedation, pruritus, nausea and vomiting, and urinary retention are common in patients receiving epidural or intrathecal opioids. Standing orders should be in place for addressing these common, minor side effects (Box 18-9).

Despite the excellent analgesia afforded by continuous epidural infusions and use of PCEA, patients experience inadequate pain relief from time to time, and a systematic approach to responding must be in place. A member of the acute pain service should be immediately available to assess the patient and determine the cause for inadequate analgesia. A common algorithm for responding to inadequate analgesia in patients receiving epidural analgesia is shown in Box 18-10. The patient is first assessed by direct observation and it is ascertained that the epidural catheter has not been dislodged. A bolus dose of the opioid–local anesthetic solution equivalent to the amount being given over 30–60 minutes is then given. If analgesia remains inadequate 20–30 minutes after this bolus dose, a test dose of 2% lidocaine (5–10 mL given incrementally)

is given to test for epidural location of the catheter. The patient must be monitored continuously for at least 20 minutes after bolus dosing using concentrated local anesthetic solution and a means of treating the hypotension that may ensue must be readily at hand. If the patient develops no identifiable sensory block within 20 minutes, the epidural should be replaced or discontinued and

---

Box 18-9   Standing Orders for Management of Common Side Effects Associated with Neuraxial Opioid Administration

Nausea: Ondansetron 1–4 mg IV or dolansetron 12.5 mg IV (nalbuphine 1–3 mg IV or butorphanol 0.25–0.5 mg IV every 4 hours as needed may also be effective)
Pruritus: Diphenhydramine 25–50 mg IV every 4 hours as needed, nalbuphine 1–3 mg IV or butorphanol 0.25–0.5 mg IV every 4 hours as needed
Urinary retention: Keep indwelling urinary catheter in place until discontinuation of epidural analgesia
Sedation or respiratory depression: Notify acute pain service *immediately*, for respiratory rate less than 6/minute, place supplemental oxygen 4 L/minute via nasal cannula and administer naloxone 0.4 mg IV

Box 18-10   Management of Inadequate Analgesia in Patients Receiving Continuous Epidural Analgesia

Assess the patient directly at the bedside to determine the cause for inadequate analgesia. If unable to respond in a timely fashion, consider alternative means for providing analgesia (e.g. order a one-time intravenous dose of opioid by telephone; consider discontinuing epidural infusion and beginning IV PCA). Remember that it is better to provide some analgesia, even if it is less effective than epidural analgesia, when one cannot get to the bedside quickly.

Examine the patient for signs of a unilateral block or a dislodged or disconnected epidural catheter.

Administer a bolus dose of the opioid or opioid–local anesthetic in use for continuous infusion. Choose the dose based on the severity of pain and use between 1/2 and 1 hour's worth of the medication (e.g. 4–8 mL bolus of fentanyl 0.0004%/bupivacaine 0.0625% in a patient receiving 8 mL/hour).

If there is no improvement in pain relief within 20–30 minutes, consider test-dosing the epidural catheter with 5–10 mL of 2% lidocaine. *Do not* administer a test dose unless the patient can be attended continuously and monitored with blood pressure checks at least every 5 minutes for 20 minutes after the bolus is given. Means for treating hypotension must be readily available (intravenous access, ready availability of a vasopressor such as ephedrine or phenylephrine).

If no sensory or motor block appears within 20 minutes, replace or discontinue epidural and begin an alternative means for providing analgesia (e.g. IV PCA).

If a unilateral sensory block develops, withdraw the epidural catheter slightly and re-administer an epidural bolus of the medication in use for continuous infusion.

If a bilateral sensory or motor block develops, re-administer an epidural bolus of the medication in use for continuous infusion and increase the epidural infusion rate. Be alert for causes of inadequate analgesia (e.g. a lumbar epidural catheter in use for pain following thoracotomy). Consider changing the opioid in use if the catheter location is suboptimal or there is an extensive incision.

---

replaced with an alternative means for providing analgesia (usually IV PCA). If the patient develops a unilateral block, the catheter should be withdrawn slightly and re-dosed. If the patient develops a bilateral sensory block, an additional epidural bolus should be given and the infusion rate increased.

Although the goal of epidural analgesia is to provide excellent pain relief and minimize side effects, there are several serious complications associated with its use. Subarachnoid catheter migration can lead to increasing levels of sensory block and total spinal anesthesia. The need for respiratory monitoring to detect respiratory depression is a subject of great controversy. Some institutions limit the use of epidural infusions to the intensive care and postanesthesia care units. There is ample evidence that patients can safely receive epidural opioids while on the regular hospital ward, provided that an anesthesiology-based acute pain service is responsible for all adjustments of analgesic and sedative medications.

Indwelling epidural catheters can become infected directly at the skin entry site or through hematogenous seeding of the catheter tip within the epidural space. Superficial site infection is common and rarely needs treatment beyond the removal of the catheter. Extension of a superficial infection or direct seeding of the catheter tip to produce an epidural abscess is rare. Epidural hematoma formation is also uncommon, but may follow epidural placement or removal in a patient receiving systemic anticoagulants. Both epidural abscess and hematoma present with worsening back pain and neurologic deficit (urinary retention, sensory and/or motor loss in the lower extremities). The recognition and management of these complications are discussed in detail in Chapter 14.

Clinical Caveat: Checklist for Daily Management of Patients Receiving Epidural Analgesia

Examine the bedside nursing record for adjustments and supplemental analgesics as well as medications for side effects required since the last assessment. Check vital signs for evidence of persistent fever or hypotension

Assess for adequate analgesia and side effects by directly questioning the patient. Be alert for sedation, pruritus, nausea/vomiting, and urinary retention

Examine the patient to detect signs of unilateral block or excessive sensory or motor block

Examine the epidural catheter site for signs of infection and the presence of an intact occlusive dressing

Interrogate the infusion pump to assess the patient's use of supplemental doses; ensure that it is properly programmed. Examine the infusion bag directly to be certain the medication ordered is what the patient is receiving

Document any interaction in detail in the patient's chart and order any changes needed. Include when one anticipates changing or discontinuing therapy

CONTINUOUS PERIPHERAL NERVE BLOCKS

Recent improvements in catheter and needle systems have increased the success rate for placing indwelling catheters adjacent to specific nerves to provide continuous regional analgesia. Catheters that incorporate an electrode into the distal tip allow for nerve stimulation through the catheter as it is being threaded into place. This assures that the catheter tip remains in close proximity to the nerve as it is being positioned. A detailed knowledge of the technique for placing single-shot blocks is essential before attempting to place peripheral catheters. Continuous peripheral nerve block techniques are gaining in popularity, but are not yet in widespread use. Studies have demonstrated the effectiveness of these continuous techniques for providing analgesia following a number of surgeries. Several combinations have proven particularly successful. Continuous femoral nerve block following total knee arthroplasty provides good analgesia and reduces the need for supplemental analgesics. Because the posterior aspect of the knee joint is innervated by contributions from the obturator and sciatic nerves, femoral nerve block usually must be supplemented with intravenous analgesics. Brachial plexus block using continuous infusion has also proven effective for surgery on the shoulder and upper extremity. Continuous peripheral nerve blocks are carried out by infusing local anesthetic alone (0.125–0.25% bupivacaine) at a rate of 8–12 mL/hour. Supplemental IV analgesics can be administered as needed.

CONCLUSIONS

The success of an acute pain management service relies on the administrative structure and the availability of personnel to respond when analgesia is inadequate more than it relies on any one technique. Regional anesthetic techniques, particularly continuous epidural analgesia, can provide excellent analgesia following surgery and they are safe and effective when carried out under the organization of a formal pain service.

SUGGESTED READING

Lichtenstein DR, Wolfe MM: Cox-2-selective NSAIDs: New and improved? *JAMA* 284:1297–1299, 2000.

Lubenow TR: Analgesic techniques. In: Brown DL (ed), *Regional Anesthesia and Analgesia*, WB Saunders, Philadelphia, 1996, pp. 644–657.

Rawal N, Nerggren L: Organization of acute pain services: a low-cost model, *Pain* 57:117–123, 1994.

Ready LB, Oden R, Chadwick HS, et al.: Development of an anesthesiology-based postoperative pain management service, *Anesthesiology* 68:100–106, 1988.

Ready LB, Rawal N: Anesthesiology-based acute pain services: a contemporary view. In: Brown DL (ed), *Regional Anesthesia and Analgesia*, WB Saunders, Philadelphia, 1996, pp. 632–643.

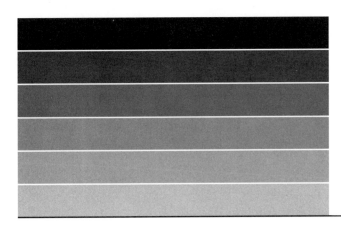

Index

Note: Page numbers in *italics* refer to figures and tables/boxed material.

A

Abdominal pain, 134
Aβ fibers, 6, 7
Abscess, epidural *see* epidural abscess
Acetaminophen, 195
Action potential
  components, 4, *5*
  ionic mechanisms, 4, 14
  local anesthetic effects, 4, *5*, 14
  sensory neurons, 3
Adamkiewicz's artery, 137
Addiction, opioids, 199, *199*
Additives, 25–31
  actions, 25
  alkalinization, 29–30, *30*
  allergic response, 15
  antioxidants, 30
  discharge time and, 170
  dosing, *27*
  epinephrine *see* epinephrine
  excipients, 30
  neuraxial effects, 25–27, 28, 29
  peripheral effects, 27–28, *28*
  preservatives, 18, *18*, 21, 30, 160
  spinal anesthesia, 124–125
  toxicity, *18*, 21, 30, 160
  see also specific additives
Aδ fibers, 6, 7, 115
Adrenergic receptors, *130*
  epinephrine effects, 25, *26*
  nociception, 9–10
Afferent fibers, 3, 6, 7, 115
Airway anesthesia, 54–58
  anatomical issues, 54–55, *55*
  clinical uses, 54
  glossopharyngeal block, 55–57, *56*, *57*
  laryngeal block, 57, *57*
  nasal septum/cavity block, 55, *56*
  transtracheal, 57, *58*
  see also specific nerves/techniques
Alcohol, neurolysis, 135

Alkalinization, 29–30, *30*
Allergy
  additives *vs.* anesthetics, 15
  dental anesthesia, *49*
Allodynia, 8, *8*
  neuropathic, *131*
A–adrenergic receptors
  clonidine agonism, 28
  epinephrine agonism, 25, *26*
  vasoconstriction, *130*
Alveolar nerve
  inferior, 45–46, 51
  posterior superior, 49
American Board of Anesthesiology, acute pain
  services, 194
American Society of Anesthesiologists (ASA)
  Closed Claims Database, 126, 151
  standards for monitoring, *36*
American Society of Regional Anesthesia and
  Pain Medicine (ASRA), anticoagulation
  guidelines, 153, *154–155*
Amide anesthetics, 19–20, 186
  metabolism, 186
  properties, *14*, *16*
  stereoisomerism, 14
  structure, 13–14, *14*
  toxicity, 186
  see also specific agents
Analgesia, 194–205
  acute pain services, 194–195, *195*
  epinephrine effects, 25
  neuraxial techniques, 201–204
    caudal blocks, 111, 112, 191, *191*
    epidural opioids, 202–204, *203*
    inadequate, 203–204, *204*
    optimization, *202*
    patient-controlled, 202–204
    pediatric epidural analgesia,
      111, 190
    postdural puncture headache, 148
    side-effect management, *203*
    spinal opioids, 201–202

Analgesia *(Continued)*
  NSAIDs *see* non-steroidal anti-inflammatory
    drugs (NSAIDs)
  obstetric *see* obstetric anesthesia/analgesia
  opioids *see* opioids/opiates
  outcome measure, 165, 169
  patient-controlled *see* patient-controlled
    analgesia (PCA)
  peripheral techniques
    continuous blocks, 205
    ilioinguinal/iliohypogastric blocks,
      81, *82*, 193
    intercostal nerve block, 75
    lumbar plexus blocks, 96
    sympathetic blocks, *130*
    thoracic paravertebral nerve block, 80
  systemic, 175, 197–201
  see also specific drugs/techniques
Anal surgery, jackknife position, 121, *122*
Ankle nerve block, 91–92, *92*
  anatomical considerations, 91, *91*, *92*
  complications, 92
  patient selection, 91
Anociassociation concept, 164, *165*
Anticoagulation, 151–156
  antiplatelet agents, 155
  bleeding complications, 151–153
  coagulation tests, *154*
  fibrinolytics, 155
  fondaparinux, 155
  herbal supplements, 155
  low molecular weight heparin, 153, *155*, 156
  neuraxial anesthesia and, 151, 153–155
    ASRA guidelines, 153, *154–155*
    management caveats, 155–156, *156*
  oral anticoagulants, 155
  peripheral anesthesia and, 152, *152*
  thrombolytics, 155
  unfractionated heparin, 153
Antiplatelet agents, 155
Arachidonic acid cascade, 195–196, *196*
Arachnoid meninges, 115, *117*